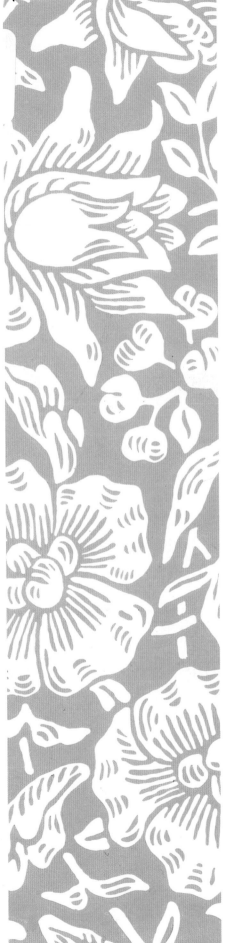

D0565369

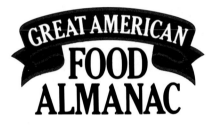

GREAT AMERICAN
FOOD
ALMANAC

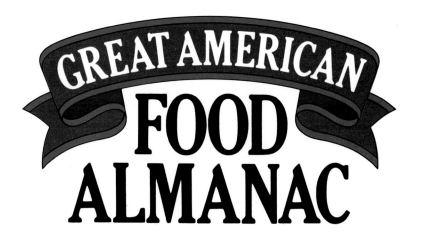

GREAT AMERICAN
FOOD
ALMANAC

by Irena Chalmers
with Milton Glaser
and Friends

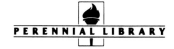

PERENNIAL LIBRARY

HARPER & ROW, PUBLISHERS, New York

Cambridge, Philadelphia, San Francisco, Washington,
London, Mexico City, São Paulo, Singapore, Sydney

Editorial Staff

Carlotta Kerwin
MANAGING EDITOR

Pamela Mitchell
ASSISTANT TO THE EDITOR

Richard Atcheson
Janet Black
Franklin Brill
Shannon Brownlee
Laura Stanton Bross
Catherine Gonick
Helen Scott-Harman
Mindy Heiferling
Lyn Stallworth
Robert Ostermann

Harkavy Information Service

Design Staff

Monica Banks
ASSISTANT ART DIRECTOR

Ann Titus
PRODUCTION MANAGER

George Leavitt
Juan Suarez-Botas
Carol Layton
Ruth Hiller
Lauren Nadler
Marc Rosenthal

Picture Research

Laurie Platt Winfrey
Lyssa Papazian
Carousel Research Inc.

Copyright © 1986 by Irena Chalmers

All rights reserved. Printed in the United States of America. No part of this book may be used or re-produced in any manner whatsoever without written permission except in the case of brief quotations embodied in critical articles and reviews. For information address Harper & Row, Publishers, Inc., 10 East 53rd Street, New York, N.Y. 10022. Published simultaneously in Canada by Fitzhenry & Whiteside Limited, Toronto.

FIRST EDITION

Library of Congress Cataloging-in-Publication Data

Chalmers, Irena.
    The great American food almanac.

    1. Food. 2. Diet—United States. 3. Cookery, American. I. Title.
TX360.C49 1986   641.3′0973   86–45085
ISBN 0-06-181151-3   86 87 88 4 3 2 1
ISBN 0-06-096067-1 (pbk.)   86 87 88 4 3 2 1

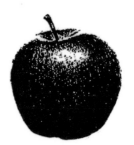

For
Hilary and Philip
—and for
Robert
For
George and Joe

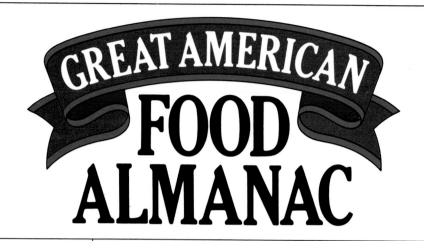

GREAT AMERICAN FOOD ALMANAC

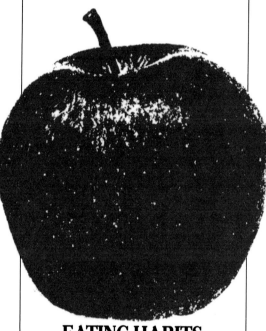

WHAT'S BEEN HAPPENING
9
The Ways We Eat
The Old and the New
Diet and Indulgence
Innovation and
Technology
Less Amounting to
More
More Resulting in
Less
The Implications of
Time and the Meaning
of Longer Life Being
Measured in
Microwavable
Microseconds

PEOPLE
15
These are A Few Among
The Many Who
Influence the Way We
Eat Today
The Food Stars—Who
They Are
and How They Seduce
Us
The Writers Who
Inform Us
The Researchers Who
Think for Us
The Entrepreneurs Large
and Small Who Provide
for Us

EATING HABITS
25
What America Eats
Junk Food
Diet and Nutrition
Fad Foods

FOOD MARKETS
53
Supermarkets
Health Food Stores
Specialty Food Stores
Green Markets
Mom-and-Pop Stores
Farmers' Markets
City Markets
Food by Mail

BIG BUSINESS OF FOOD
77
Conglomerates
Fast-Food Chains
Packaging and
Labeling
Irradiation
Advertising
Food Industry Associations

EATING OUT
105
Hotel Dining
The New Restaurants
Firehouse Food
Picnics and
Barbecues
Catered Affairs
Spa Food

EATING IN
133
Family Food
What's New in the Kitchen
Take-Out Food
Hunger in America

COOKING SCHOOLS
149
Professional
Amateur

AGRIBUSINESS
155
Genetic Engineering
Hydroponics
Exotic Fruits
and Vegetables
Biosphere

AQUABUSINESS
173
Aquaculture
Today's Catch
Food Festivals

FOOD SERVICE
183
Executive Dining Rooms
Train Food
Airline Food
School and
College Food
Hospital Food

THE PRINTED WORD
199
Cookbooks
Writing Them,
Buying Them, Selling Them
Bestsellers

FOOD ON VIDEO
209
Teletext and
Videotex
Videotapes
Software

COTTAGE INDUSTRIES
217
Specialty Food Packagers
Growers and Distributors

PREDICTIONS
230

SCATTERED THROUGHOUT:

RUMINATIONS
Anecdotes
Stories
Likes and Dislikes

AND FOR GRAZING:
Lists
Cartoons
Quizzes
Quotes
Trivia
Trends

. . . AND RECIPES

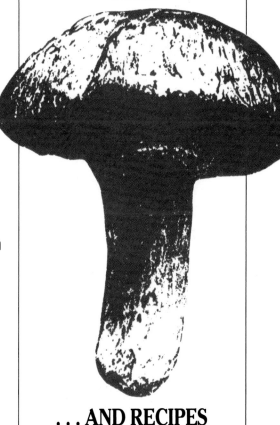

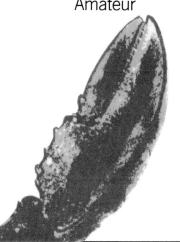

WHAT'S BEEN HAPPENING

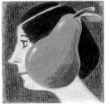

We are in the midst of an extraordinary revolution today, this minute—a social revolution that is making astonishing, radical changes in how we live now and how we will live in the future. We will be as altered as the French after the fall of Louis XVI, as the Russians after the abdication of the Czar. The difference is that this revolution is benign. At the moment, we are hardly feeling a thing. But that is also what they said about the guillotine.

Fully two-thirds of the people in the nation eat today just as they ate ten years ago, so that, on the surface, very little appears to have changed. However, those individuals who constitute that other third are increasingly vocal in their demands for new products eaten in different ways, while *still* wanting to retain the old—a concept that has the supermarket shelves spilling over with new-old diversities, freshly packaged for our delectation.

A dichotomy exists at all levels of the human food chain. There is a kind of nutritional schizophrenia abroad in our land, in which we indulge in a diet of denial from Monday through Friday—clothed and posturing resplendently in self-righteousness—and then on the weekend we wallow in hedonistic, glorious excess.

We are buying more diet books than ever, and we are in the curious position of realizing that never before have so many advertising dollars been spent to promote products that exemplify Mies van der Rohe's contention that "less is more." As a result, the American public has become accustomed, for the first time, to spending more for less. Now we buy because the package promises to deliver less salt, less sugar, less alcohol, less caffeine, fewer calories, fewer chemicals . . . and absolutely no additives or preservatives whatever. There is even a rumor that V-8 Juice is cutting back to offer us V-5½!

From this evidence, you might suppose that we would end up with a lot of good, pure fresh food. But this is not precisely the case.

Every true statement has another truth at the opposite swing of the pendulum. Note that, in 1985, we as a nation consumed exactly half the amount of sugar we spooned up a decade ago. Yet statistics show that we swallowed 113 pounds of sweeteners last year. Each.

We are Puritans at heart and want to eat in exactly the same way they did. Certainly, we eat the trendy new foods, but in times of stress we yearn longingly for the foods of our childhood. Mashed potatoes and gravy are making a big comeback. But, of course, the commodity our forefathers had in such plenty that we lack altogether is time. We either want fast food—cooked and eaten in a few minutes—or we want it prepared in advance, so that it is ready for us at the end of the day. It could be argued that a long, slow-simmered stew is just another variation on fast food because all it needs is to be reheated when we are hungry.

This knowledge of our past eating patterns and presently unfulfilled longings accounts for the predictable success of Lean Cuisine and its many imitators in this country, where we want *everything* immediately and with success guaranteed or our money back. The kitchen helpers who take the guesswork out of our food preparation now work at Stouffer's and robots are taking over many of the chores.

We *are* a curious lot. We deny ourselves a doughnut, ostensibly for health reasons and because we want to be slim and healthy and young and admired—and then we cheerfully devour a DoveBar and laugh at our "wickedness." DoveBars are all right to eat because they are fashionable and all our friends are "into" them too. Our apparent concern for nutrition is at war with the plain fact that 30 percent of us are overweight. Yet we waddle on.

We are positively bombarded with information about nutrition. But I wonder whether we've actually progressed very far from those golden days when the Pilgrims ate fresh turkey cooked over an open fire (though not mesquite) and drank homemade cider. Today our turkey is frozen, prebasted and microwave-ready, with a pop-up thermometer to let us know when it is dinner time. And with this prefabricated turkey we drink a can of Diet Pepsi.

Of course, there *has* been a change. It was not so long ago, after all, in the days before we knew better, that huge, succulent steaks were held in high esteem as one of the great triumphs of the U.S.A. We also slathered butter on our bread, sour cream on our baked potatoes and drank milk with every meal.

Yes, things have certainly changed. Now we are revering all those boring, cheap ethnic foods that those who had achieved some measure of success left firmly behind them as they climbed the ladder to the American Dream. Now we will only eat red meat if it is cooked into something Mexican, or if it comes in the form of hamburger and turns brown in color so that somehow it doesn't count as meat and therefore must be good for us.

Even our milk is fat-free, skimmed or "Skinny," and the calcium we used to be urged to drink it for seems to have become one of the most sought-after minerals. But it is now being popped in tablet form into the mouths of everyone from pregnant mothers to senior citizens. Soon we will be hearing that too much calcium causes some other dread disease. Whatever happened to our passion for zinc, I wonder?

I wonder, too, about fish. We are all enraptured with eating fish these days, yet no one has ever given a fish an anesthetic, checked its cardiovascular system, monitored its blood pressure and said it is OK to have six times a week. When the scientists come to analyze fish as minutely as they have our domesticated animals, will they be finding that too much fish is bad for us too?

Today's new foods and eating patterns have not developed in a vacuum. There was a certain inevitability about it all. Social scientists have determined that it took hundreds of thousands of years for man to travel from a spoken language to a written one. It took another 5,000 years beyond that for the printing press to be invented. Then, a mere 500 years later, up popped the visual image in the form of television. It is barely ten years since the introduction of the videocassette recorder, which today can be found in 35 percent of American homes.

I mention this passage of time imploding upon itself in terms of technological development, because this rapid change applies to every field of endeavor. This is *itself* the force that feeds the revolution of which I speak.

As we sit in front of the video screen, we eat very differently from the time when we were more physically active. The day of the family meal—certainly in the big cities around the nation—has virtually gone, and it is now mainly at Thanksgiving, at Christmas and at other special, festive occasions that we gather around a shared table. Increasingly, we bring home small quantities of ready-prepared food from the take-out store, or we buy partially or totally processed foods at the supermarket. One-third to one-half of all meals in America are eaten away from home, and 40 cents of every American food dollar is spent on eating out.

Those of us who live in urban communities are starting to act much like the Chinese in Hong Kong. As real estate and mortgage financing costs continue to rise, we are obliged to live in smaller and smaller spaces and to pay more for that space. To escape our tiny apartments, we use restaurants and cafés as our second homes.

Kitchens are getting smaller and smaller too, and as we peer into the future, we can see that the day is not far off when the kitchen will disappear altogether. The compact microwave oven, which serves to reheat food, will perch on top of the television as part of the home entertainment center. As food becomes shelf-stable, we will have less use for the refrigerator and none at all for the freezer. We will need only a small adjunct box to flash-cool our food, and a poker-like device to chill our cocktails. Ice cubes will be used merely to clink in the glass.

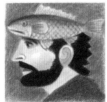

Today, there are 50 million women in America who work for a living. These women have little or no time or energy to prepare an evening meal. They look today for convenience, and cost is no longer the deciding factor in their food purchases. Traditional family buying patterns have changed radically. In at least 30 percent of homes, the male mate now shares the burden of shopping.

There are 20 million single households in the country today and a new category has emerged on the census records: single people living together for non-sexual purposes. It is estimated that, by the end of the century, fully 35 percent of American households will be single households. All indications are that fewer children will be born in the next decade. One consequence, of course, is that all businesses will find it more difficult to hire junior-level help. There will be more switching to self-service. Companies that now make baby food will be looking for, and no doubt finding, other products and markets.

And what will these other markets be? One will most certainly be the elderly. Their ranks are swelling hugely, and already it is forecast that, by the next decade, over *100,000* Americans will live beyond the age of 100. There are already 56,000 American centenarians and by the year 2080 there will be 1.9 million. One day, it will not be unusual for people to live to 125 and beyond, as more attention is paid to their diet.

Changes in the composition of the work force will further rattle the expectations of the food industry. The professional, well-educated class will grow larger, and the ranks of those inheriting wealth will also swell, as only one or two children acquire the assets from *two* working parents. At the other end of the scale, laborers and blue-collar workers who lack the continuing education necessary to enter the social technocracy will drop further back in their earning potential.

Each year we see a rise in the number of food stamps that are being redeemed, and though there are always rumors of people abusing the program to buy lobsters and Twinkies, most folk on food stamps probably shop no less wisely than the rest of us. One thing we do know is that social groups who experience economic hardship and the consequent psychological disadvantages, display a strong need for sugar and and all other sweet things.

What we choose to buy may be less a personal choice than we think. We are, as a nation, all of us, in all walks of life, receiving the same messages from advertisers. Thus we may, for example, be persuaded that it really is all right for us to eat breakfast away from home—even though such a thought may, at first, seem quite un-American.

Just give a moment's thought to this:

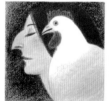 eredith, the giant publisher of *Better Homes & Gardens*, has just bought *The Ladies' Home Journal*. Now, *Better Homes & Gardens* has a circulation of eight million. Are you counting? *Woman's Day* and *Family Circle* each have circulations of roughly seven million. Add in *Gourmet, Food & Wine, Cook's, The Pleasures of Cooking, Bon Appétit* and the new *Good Food* magazines—and realize that just seven or eight food editors, most of whom are personal friends, most of whom live in New York, attend many of the same functions, dine out at the same restaurants and belong to the same clubs, are speaking to—and influencing—some 30 *million* people! And let me tell you—if they say that American Food is *in*, you had better believe it. Until the moment when they say it's *out. . . .*

Actually, I don't think they will ever say it is *out*.

I mention this fact about just a handful of people influencing a nation not to deplore it or celebrate it, but simply to make the point that it *is* so, and is all part of the interlocking of groups and elements that shapes our lives. I find nothing sinister in it, and much that is fascinating. The consumers, too, play their role. Just as advertisers and public relations firms and writers exert an influence on consumers, in turn, consumers exert considerable influence on the large food companies. But the interactions are so subtle that it is often difficult to know who is influencing whom, which are the chickens, and which, finally, are the eggs.

Speaking of chickens, it is true that we are eating more poultry, but this is not wholly because we have decided on our own that poultry is a healthier source of protein. For this we have to thank Frank Perdue.

We are influenced by the economic realities of raising chickens, just as much as by the power of advertising. So Frank Perdue does hold our hearts in his hand, and has power over our minds, too. He is one of the innovative technocrats who have pioneered the raising of chickens to a precise art, in which companies such as Tyson's will ship close to 50,000 baby chicks to the door of a farmer, and also provide the food and medicines necessary to fatten them to maturity. Eggs take 21 days to hatch and, eight weeks later, the chickens are ready for stuffing. Thus, the chicken farmer can adjust to market conditions very rapidly, increasing or decreasing his flock according to demand.

The cattle farmer, on the other hand, requires a year or more to bring the meat to the counter, and he has to deal with all the variables—bad weather, bad press, chance and disease. Inevitably, he ends up with a high-priced product when he does finally manage to get it to market, on his allotted and steadily shrinking share of counter space.

Not only must the farmer produce food that is low in all the things that it is supposed to be low in, and high in all the things that it is supposed to be high in—but now there is a new problem to deal with. It must be cut-upable into nuggets, so that it will cook evenly in the microwave oven! Litton Industries alone anticipates that nine million microwave ovens will be sold this year, and more than 40 percent of American homes already have this appliance and use it frequently. The rest heat up their boil-in-a-bag dinners just by breathing on them. They would never admit to using the microwave oven, even when forced to admit that they own one. This is the same body of people who deny ever watching television—except, of course, an occasional bit of Public Television.

We will soon be seeing the same sense of lofty disapproval for what is clearly the imminent arrival of irradiated food. And this despite the fact that irradiation is an accepted medical treatment and without regard to the fact that, during irradiation there is a negligible change in the composition of the foodstuff save that all potentially harmful bacteria are destroyed.

Irradiation is only one part of the new research that is taking place. Much of it continues to come from the military, which has of necessity been in the forefront of new methods of procuring and delivering food. One of their innovations was the idea of reformulation.

Very roughly, this is the principle on which reformulation works. As you know, protein is of the same nutritional value no matter which part of an animal it comes from, and there are a lot of parts that are normally discarded as unusable because they are unsightly or take too long to prepare, or there is just no demand for them. So all these unwanted parts get smashed together, using hamburger extender as a kind of glue, and then this product is frozen. And once it is absolutely solid, it seems you can shave off slices as thin as a leaf of strudel and form them into shapes of familiar food—a steak, or a pork chop, or whatever. Of course, it may be the right shape but that won't convince anyone to actually *eat* it, so in come the scientists to give it the right color, the right taste, the right smell—and *bingo*! If your mind accepts that this is a steak and it looks, smells and sizzles like a steak, then, by heaven—it *is* a steak!

A billion people have been added to the planet in the last 13 years, and another billion will be born in the next 12 years. It will be up to us, and our abilities and advanced technology, to find ways of feeding these new and hungry mouths. It will be American scientists, genetic engineers and food producers, from agronomists to those engaged in aquaculture to giant food processing companies—who will become largely responsible for financing and carrying out the research. They will fall heir to an awesome responsibility: to raise food for the world, and, of equal importance, to develop the means of delivering that food, in eatable condition, to the places where it is so desperately needed.

Vast changes are already taking place, and agriculture is a major user and beneficiary of the high technology that is drastically changing the way food is produced.

Computers, lasers, satellites and infrared technology are among the future tools of farmers and researchers seeking solutions to such critical problems as soil erosion, water loss and the competition for water use.

Lasers, beamed through insecticide sprays, measure the size of droplets, helping researchers to determine the appropriate amount to use for specific pests in varying environmental conditions.

Aerial pictures taken by means of infrared photography and thermal imaging techniques pinpoint problems in irrigation systems.

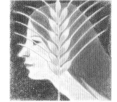

Satellite photos and computer modeling help scientists to predict when and where water runoff will occur, enabling water resource managers to take action to prevent floods.

Computers can program intervals for seed planting. They can also store information about plants around the world, and even be used to create new seeds with genetically built-in insecticides and fertilizers. And, with the use of embryo transplant techniques, genetic engineers can upgrade the physical characteristics of a herd of cattle in a single generation

The technological changes on the farm are immense, and the results far-reaching. Clearly only the largest farms survive, because only they can afford the massive investment that is necessary for funding today's research.

Already—and this is a fact of great significance for a country that was once largely rural and farming—less than three percent of Americans work in agriculture, and the likelihood in the future is that fewer and fewer farms will produce the bulk of our crops.

The ever present yin-yang market forces appear, and some small farmers are becoming solvent again by furnishing fresh ingredients to the growing number of restaurants and markets that call for first-class fresh fruits, herbs and vegetables. Even some local supermarkets are now calling for produce of this quality.

So, on one hand, farming is facing its worst crisis since the Depression. And on the other hand, there is a glimmer of hope on the horizon, as innovative new solutions emerge to supply our diverse and shifting styles of living, and literally dozens of hitherto-unknown fruits and vegetables will be grown here to provide variety for our new craze for fresh produce.

Some small food entrepreneurs will survive and do well, by sheer dint of a combination of hard work, passionate devotion, fear, greed, obsession and obstinacy. But as Gordon McGovern, the president of Campbell Soup, has pointed out, here too the giant companies will be the ones who will prosper.

We are the most fortunate of peoples, living in the richest nation in the world, in a time when our gifts and abilities seem infinite. Our aspiration has always been—and will, I hope, continue to be—to share our technology with the world, so that we all, everywhere on the planet, can eat. ●

July 1986, New York City

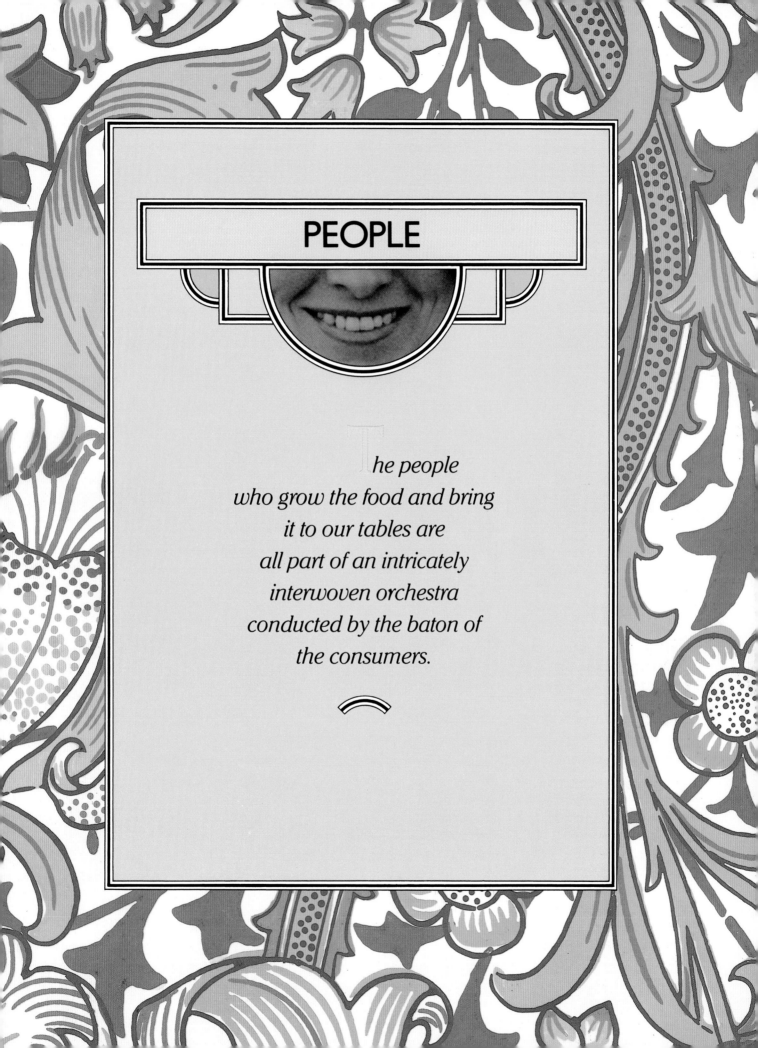

PEOPLE

*The people
who grow the food and bring
it to our tables are
all part of an intricately
interwoven orchestra
conducted by the baton of
the consumers.*

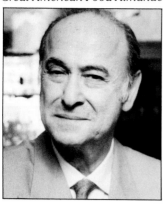

Joe Baum has never flagged in his pursuit of excellence. Creator of The Four Seasons, La Fonda del Sol, Windows on the World, all in New York City, and a galaxy of further brilliant inventions, he has crowned his career with Aurora, and is acclaimed by all as the restaurateur of the century.

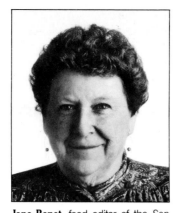

Jane Benet, food editor of the *San Francisco Chronicle*, tells us: "In 30 years, I've watched American eating habits come full circle—we're no longer enamored of modern technology and its convenient, not necessarily healthful, processed foods—it's back to basics and real food. How refreshing!"

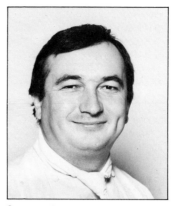

Gerard Panguad, the greatly-acclaimed chef of New York City's Aurora, arrived in America from France with two stars in his hands, and was promptly given another, from Bryan Miller, restaurant critic of *The New York Times*. He continues to dazzle the press and the public with his brilliantly innovative creations.

Author of the *Arcadia Seasonal Mural and Cookbook*, she was named 1985 Woman of the Year by New York University for her innovative cuisine.

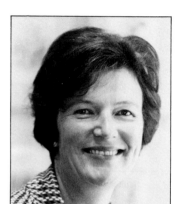

Anne Willan is founder and president of La Varenne Ecole de Cuisine in Paris. Her *Washington Post* food column is widely syndicated and her books include *Great Cooks and Their Recipes*, *French Regional Cooking*, and *La Varenne's Cooking Course*. Her motto: "An apple pie without the cheese is like a kiss without the squeeze."

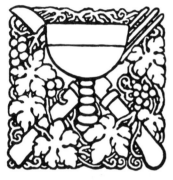

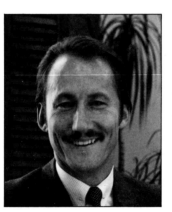

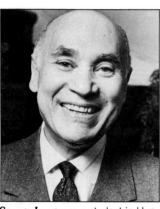

George Lang was a student in Hungary, Austria and Italy; a cook in Europe and the U.S.; worked in the banquet trade and restaurant business; sold the Encyclopaedia Britannica and a few years later wrote for it; penned books on cooking and gastronomy; writes for *Connoisseur, The New York Times Magazine* and other publications, including *Travel & Leisure*, where his column, "Table For One," has appeared for nine years; owns New York's Café des Artistes. For the past 16 years, he and his company have worked as international consultants to the hospitality industry so that over 400 hotel and restaurant owners have someone to share the blame with.

Ferdinand E. Metz is president of the country's leading professional cooking school, The Culinary Institute of America, in Hyde Park, N.Y. He says, "Good cooking, like a beautiful work of art, belongs to those who combine it with feeling, talent and a desire to please others."

Laura Chenel, inveterate dairy goat advocate and dedicated champion of flavorful food, originated American specialty goat milk cheeses. Her commitment to unusual and flavorful quality cheese has encouraged production of an ever-increasing variety of American-made specialty cheeses of all kinds.

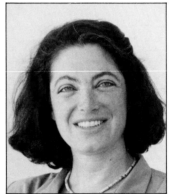

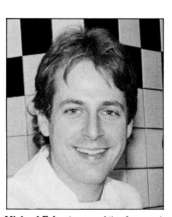

Michael Foley is one of the foremost chefs in the Midwest. The innovative food at his restaurant, *Printer's Row* in Chicago, has set a new standard of excellence for America's Heartland.

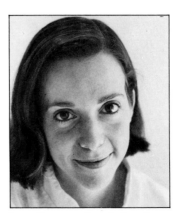

Anne Rosenzweig, chef and co-owner of Arcadia, in New York City, was cited by *Time* magazine as creator of "the most fully developed rendition of new American cooking."

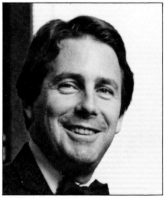

James H. Kabler III is president and chairman of Nikkal Industries, Ltd., the manufacturer and distributor of the Donvier Ice Cream Maker. This ingenious device is changing the ice cream eating habits of hundreds of thousands who now make their own ice cream rather than buy it. "Everybody loves ice cream," he says, and he speaks for us all. . . .

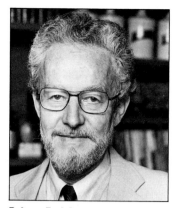

Robert Rodale, pioneer, educator and Chairman of Rodale Press, Inc., is also the editor of *Prevention* magazine and *Rodale's Organic Gardening*. He was among the first to recognize the potential of amaranth and other "lost" seeds. A profound thinker and visionary, he is the sponsor of many innovative food and health research programs.

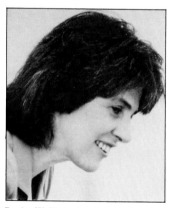

Paula Wolfert, teacher and cookbook author, reports that she loves the old dishes best. "Beef with carrots," she lists first, and afterwards "duck with olives, and *coq au vin*. It's always," she says, "because they include ingredients that work beautifully together, that, in combination, create a flavor different and more pleasing than their flavors on their own."

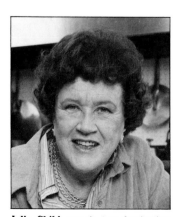

Julia Child reveals two fascinating

facts: First, "I am writing an enormous new How-to cookbook, fully illustrated, including all recipes from our six-hour-long videocassettes and four years of *Parade* articles, plus the other ideas and recipes since my last book, *The Way to Cook* (a presumptuous title but that's the name of the cassettes)." Second, "The way to a long and happy life—plenty ot gin and red meat!" Cheers!

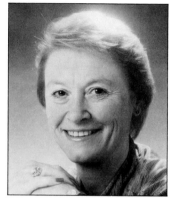

Jean Hewitt is Food & Equipment editor of *Family Circle* magazine. Formerly she was food reporter and critic for *The New York Times*. She has contributed to our increasing awareness of sound nutrition habits and as author of *The New York Times Heritage Cook Book*, published in 1972 (one of ten cookbooks she has written), was among the first to recognize the importance of preserving American cuisine.

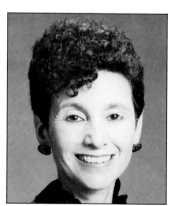

Jan Weimer, senior editor at *Bon Appétit* magazine, reveals that she willingly swallowed 24 scoops of ice cream when judging a competition and "has driven from Turkey to Greece for dinner and to Afghanistan for bread cooked over camel dung." Going beyond her first attempt at cooking (grilled soup bones with ketchup), she has graduated to winning the Maria Luigia Duchessa di Parma journalist award. As they say in the business, it's a tough job, but someone has to do it. . . .

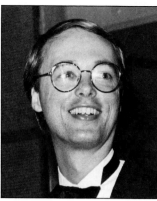

Christopher Kimball is the publisher of *Cook's* magazine. He whispers, "I'm hiding out in my kitchen, waiting for the day that restaurant dining is no longer theater, that renovated diners stop serving garlic custard (just give me Southern fried chicken), and that I can get an honest plate of pasta for under $10 (please, hold the tomatillos)."

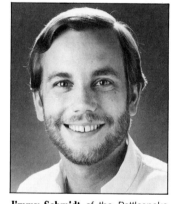

Jimmy Schmidt of the Rattlesnake Club in Denver says: "I would like to see a substantial and meaningful American cuisine emerging from what is currently taking place in this country, executed by the chefs with a true vocation to render their inspirations through the use of sound techniques and knowledge of the chemistry of food."

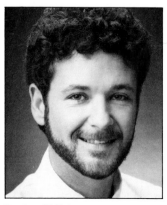

Stephan W. Pyles of the Routh Street Cafe in Dallas is recognized as a ma-

jor influence upon the cooking of the Southwest. About that he says: "My enthusiasm and involvement in the Southwest cookery movement is very natural. The ingredients and flavors behind this exciting food style are those my mother served as I was growing up in West Texas—catfish, quail, duck, venison, a myriad of chilies. . . . My effort at Routh Street Cafe is to preserve the integrity and showcase the splendor of these indigenous ingredients."

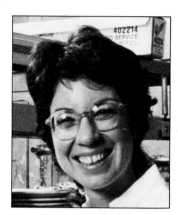

Leslie Revsin, being among the first, stands up for all the many brilliant young women chefs. She tells us, "I picked my first wild strawberry with my father in the Chicago Forest Preserves ages ago! I pushed aside the leaves and was transformed by its complete tinyness, its vibrating redness. I reached out to pick it—the living warmth in my hand. And then the giving juice and sweetness in my mouth." Of such reminiscences are great chefs made. . . .

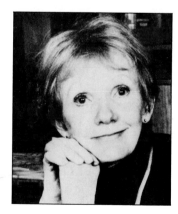

Maggie Waldron is director of the Ketchum Food Center in San Francisco and New York with a roster of clients that reads like a farmer's market of advisory boards, supermarket and food-service chains. "Foodwatching to me is as irresistible as people-watching," she admits. "Nothing is more revealing than the rituals of food, whether one is cooking it, eating it—or selling it."

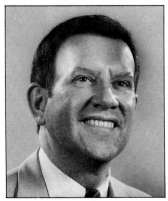

Phillip S. Cooke, creator of the Symposium on American Cuisine, says, "Everything about American cooking has not been discovered. We are still at the threshold of experimentation, and the future belongs to a new generation of young chefs and restaurateurs whose energy and entrepreneurial fervor will amaze us."

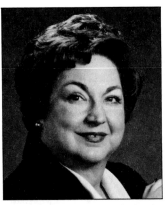

Marian Tripp, well-known for her innovative and creative publicity endeavors, for clients including Kraft, Quaker Oats, Pillsbury, and Uncle Ben's Rice, anticipates trends with visions of tomorrow. She also sometimes wonders if there can possibly be anything new. (There will be.)

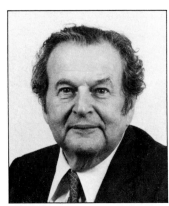

Carl G. Sontheimer is the genius who introduced the food processor to America. "It is true that I generally work seven days a week, ten to 12 hours each day," he acknowl-

edges. "I do that because I am retired. Many years ago, fortunately, I was able to retire from business and was left free to pursue my greatest love of all (next to my family of course) and that was cooking. After a year or so of tinkering in our garage, improving a restaurant model machine we had discovered in France, my wife Shirley and I knew we had a product that would revolutionize the art of cooking here in America. The food processor truly has changed the way millions of people prepare their meals. It saves time, effort and produces better, more consistent results. So each day now I get to spend my life doing what everyone wishes they could do, doing what they love."

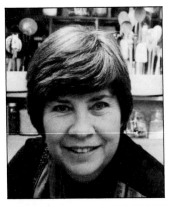

Jean Anderson, who hails from hog-jowl-and-black-eyed-pea country, has not only written three regional American cookbooks but also co-authored the *New Doubleday Cookbook,* which is jam-packed with downhome dishes. "I love everything edible and American," she exults, "from purloo to pine bark stew."

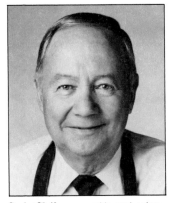

Craig Claiborne, critic and columnist for *The New York Times,* has told us all where to eat, what to eat, how to cook it, what to cherish and what to avoid—and most of us choose to eat from the palm of his hand. His personal journey in life infuses his writing with meaning far beyond the dish and what is on it.

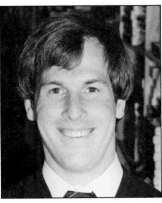

David Strymish created Jessica's Biscuit Cookbook Catalog six years ago. It is now the most complete collection available anywhere and reaches a million people a year. "The cookbook market is changing," he says, "but there will always be room for good cookbooks on good subjects." (He should know.)

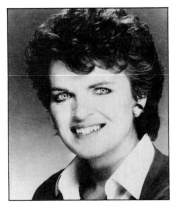

Dian Thomas, a regular guest on NBC TV's "Today" show, tells us the best way to make ice cream is to put the mix in a can nestled in another one, filled with ice. Let two kids kick the can back and forth until they're good and tired, and the ice cream that emerges will taste better than any parlor can provide.

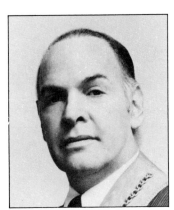

Roger Yaseen is America's preeminent amateur gourmet. As national president of La Chaine des Rotisseurs and the editor in chief of the society's publication, *Gastronome,* he

interfaces with over 6,000 members in 104 chapters throughout the country. "My travel schedule," he reports, "is a ball buster."

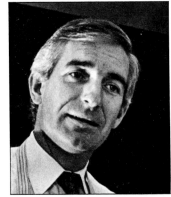

François Dionot is three times a president—of L'Academie de Cuisine, Bethesda; of La Champagne Restaurant, Bethesda; and of the International Association of Cooking Professionals. Of success in cooking, he says, "Whether it is for home entertaining or restaurant work, my four P's for success are Purchasing, Preparation, Presentation and Palate."

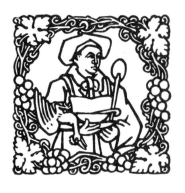

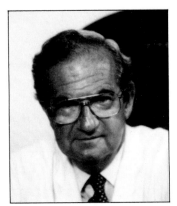

Doctor Isadore Rosenfeld is a world-famous cardiologist, educator, author and television personality. "We used to think," he says, "that anything delicious has to be unhealthy. But it turns out that the major dietary villains are salt, fat and calories. This knowledge, plus culinary imagination now makes it possible to enjoy gourmet cuisine without fear or guilt."

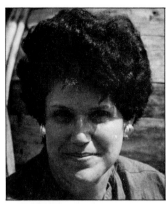

Joan Nathan has been called the Studs Terkel and Charles Kuralt of the food world. A chronicler of American ethnic food, she considers herself "a preserver of an endangered species, authentic American regional cooking." The mother of three children, she is, she says, "constantly searching the meanings behind breaking bread at an ordinary dinner table."

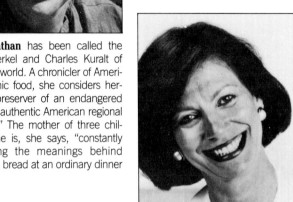

Abby Mandel has taught America how to use a food processor. Her newspaper and magazine columns and three best-selling books, including *Fast and Flavorful*, artfully show that the food processor is the most efficient piece of equipment in the kitchen. Starting with the freshest ingredients, great-looking, great-tasting recipes are easily within reach for anyone who owns a food processor and one of Abby's books.

captain, is a fit representative of our countless entrepreneurs who turn their dreams into flourishing cottage industries. He developed the only mail-order business in the U.S.A. devoted exclusively to selling high-quality milk-fed lambs, raised on his New England farms, and now supplies both restaurants and individuals countrywide.

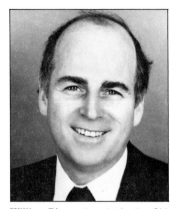

William Rice, columnist for the *Chicago Tribune* and former editor in chief of *Food & Wine* magazine, has identified and encouraged many of the trends, dining places and individuals now shaping today's culinary scene. His forthcoming book, *Feasts of Food and Wine*, links his two favorite hobbies.

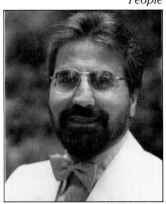

Giuliano Bugialli created Italy's first international cooking school, and today he also conducts classes in America and in many other countries. He is the author of the Tastemaker Grand Prize-winning cookbook, *Foods of Italy*, as well as of *Classic Techniques of Italian Cooking* and *The Fine Art of Italian Cooking*.

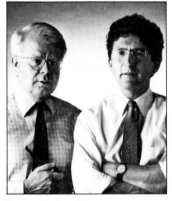

Dean & Deluca is a name on everybody's tongue, recognized as the first and finest of specialty food stores in this country in our time. The men behind the sign are Joel B. Dean and Giorgio DeLuca; they opened their doors upon a delicious enterprise in New York City in 1977, and have amazed our palates ever since, with everything from silken smoked salmon to prosaic pots and pans.

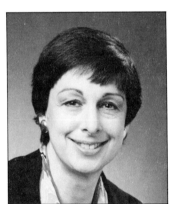

Marian Burros, food columnist at *The New York Times*, recalls her earliest food memories as tapioca and whipped cream and spaghetti and meat sauce, preferably leftover and served for breakfast. Now she would like to be remembered as the journalist who first tried to convince good cooks that healthy food could also taste wonderful. "Exposing the frauds and safety hazards in our food supply is as important as describing the glories of the most decadent chocolate cake."

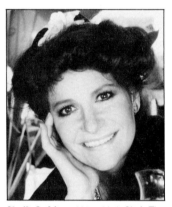

Sheila Lukins of New York City's The Silver Palate says, "So discreet, so delicious and I *still* deliver!—Oh my goodness!!!"

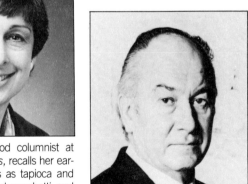

Paul Kovi of The Four Seasons in New York says that a good friend taught him the great secret of restaurateur philosophy, which is: "The guest is always right, especially when he is wrong; because if he is wrong, it is the restaurateur's job to make things turn out the best way for the guest."

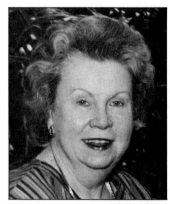

Ella Brennan, the Grande Dame of the Brennans' family of happy restaurants, says "food and fun are what New Orleans is all about. We've given the world Creole cooking and jazz. But the best place to enjoy it all is still right where it all came from."

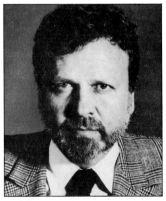

Christopher Idone, food consultant and author of *Glorious American Food*, has decided that "it all boils down to this: The better things in life are fresh. And with a little luck, the farmer will prevail."

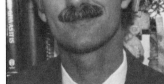

Bill Tuttle, a New York City tugboat

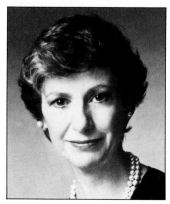

Barbara Kafka is one of the most opinionated and interviewed food writers in the country. An opinion is that recipes for the home must be cookable at home. She wrote *Food for Friends, American Food & California Wine* as well as other books, and writes articles and a column for Vogue. She is also a much sought-after restaurant consultant.

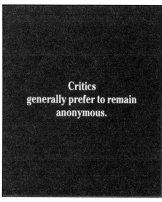

Critics generally prefer to remain anonymous.

Ruth Reichl has been the restaurant editor of the *Los Angeles Times* since 1984; before that she was a freelance food writer. "I feel," she says, "that I've spent the last ten years lurking in kitchens, watching the coming of age of the new American cooking. One chef told me he felt that every time he opened his mouth, there I was with a pad in my hands." (He was right.)

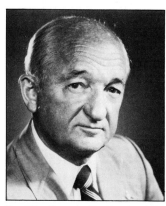

Franklin Parsons Perdue is chairman of the board of Perdue Farms

Incorporated, America's largest regional poultry producer and fifth largest overall. Under his direction, the firm became the first to market brand-name and lower-fat chickens, offer a money-back guarantee of quality, and provide nutrition labeling and in-pack recipes. Frank Perdue, famous for appearing in his company's advertising, is known as "the tough man who makes a tender chicken."

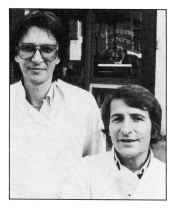

Alain Sinturel (left) and Jean-Pierre Pradie (right) of Les Trois Petits Cochons in New York City could be called the men who created the "pâté phenomenon" in America. Their tiny shop in Greenwich Village grew into a thriving wholesale business in fresh pâtés. Today, Les Trois Petits Cochons pâtés are sold in all 50 states, sales number in the millions and their most popular styles are Pâté de Campagne and Mousse Truffée.

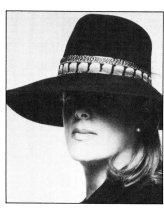

Gael Greene, *New York* magazine's Insatiable Critic (author of two best-selling novels and most recently, *Delicious Sex*), confides that "having dedicated myself to slow death by mayonnaise," she would be willing to pay to do what she does if no one paid her. "I write for sensualists, not moralists," she says. "One raspberry, one kiss, one emerald can never be enough. I'm a fool for *frites, too.*"

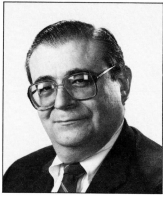

Doctor Sanford A. Miller is the director at the Department of Health and Human Services at the Food and Drug Administration, where his role is to make our food safe to eat. "There is no conflict," he says, "between good food and good nutrition, but if you want to eat like a farmhand, you must live on a farm."

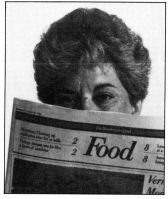

Phyllis Richman, executive food editor and restaurant critic for *The Washington Post*, writes a syndicated column, "Richman's Table." She is author of *Best Restaurants & Others, Washington, D.C.,* and considers the major culinary advancement of the 20th century to have been the discovery of America.

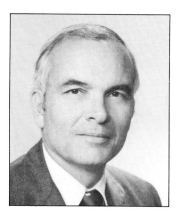

R. Gordon McGovern is the president and chief executive officer of The Campbell Soup Company, where "focus on consumers" is the marketing motto. What's new at

Campbell's? Microwaveable breakfasts and dinners, fresh produce and—in testing—convenience store snacks . . . (and more soup too, we wager).

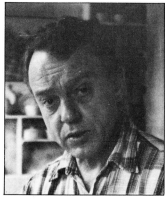

Richard Olney has long been recognized as one of the food world's most distinguished men of letters. It was he who set the standard others aspire to reach. He encourages us "to escape from chic and fashion and rigid rules, to trust our own palates and to think seriously of the wines that best go with different foods to the greater glory of both."

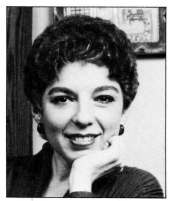

Elizabeth Schneider, author of *Uncommon Fruits and Vegetables, Ready When You Are* and co-author, with Helen Witty, of *Better Than Storebought,* has also written dozens of articles for all the major food magazines. Her fine writing and scrupulous research has earned her the title of the "conscience" of food writers.

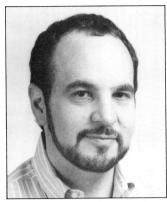

Steve Poses has, since 1973, created a series of unique restaurants in Philadelphia under the banner of Shooting Stars. They include Frog, The Commissary, 16th Street Bar & Grill, the USA Cafe, and City Bites, plus Frog-Commissary catering, and The Market of the Commissary.

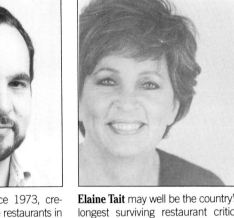

Elaine Tait may well be the country's longest surviving restaurant critic. Her fair-handed assessments have appeared in the *Philadelphia Inquirer* since 1963 and are considered a factor in Philadelphia's emergence as one of America's leading restaurant cities. She once deflated a pretentious restaurant by calling it "Hershey kisses in a Godiva box."

most innovative restaurateurs. He makes dining out fun. As co-founder of the Washington D.C.-based American Cafes, he almost single-handedly created the concept of "grazing" by smiling on those who choose to make a meal of six appetizers or just four desserts. He created the "croissant sandwich" and is cooking up many more surprises.

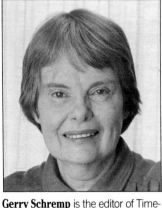

Gerry Schremp is the editor of Time-Life Books' *The Good Cook*—a 28-volume series that explains in words and photographs the techniques needed for producing every kind of food from hors d'oeuvres to desserts. Her personal fascination is American regional cooking — using old-time receipts whenever she can find them.

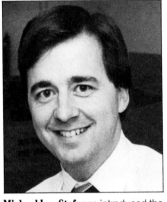

Michael Leo Stefanos introduced the DoveBar—the incredible, hand-dipped ice cream bar—to the nation. The DoveBar, the world's first super premium ice cream bar, has captured Americans' hearts.

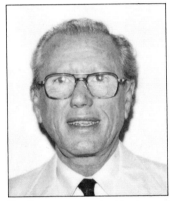

Ted Koryn, specialty food broker and marketer for 25 years, introduced many food products from abroad in the U.S.A. In so doing, he built one of the largest importing and distributing firms in the country, carrying over 1,500 specialty foods from 32 countries. "Sardines," he once remarked, in an unguarded moment, "are not for eating, but only for buying and selling."

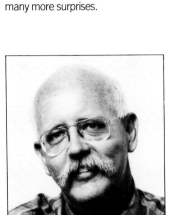

Charles Morris Mount was chosen by McDonald's to design their flagship restaurant in New York's Rockefeller Center. It was an inspired choice. "I grew up," he reports, "in south Alabama and food and eating were important social get-togethers. As a small child I was always fascinated with cooking processes and one of my early childhood memories was putting sheets, towels and my pet cat into the oven. I've come a long culinary road from cats to Big Mac's."

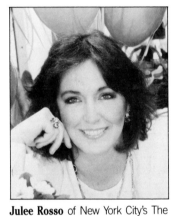

Julee Rosso of New York City's The Silver Palate says, "From meat and potatoes in Michigan to Free Range Chicken and Baby Vegetables in New York."

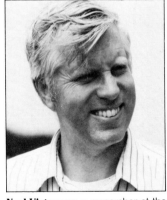

Noel Vietmeyer, a researcher at the National Academy of Sciences, draws attention to the world's wealth of untapped food crops: winged bean, amaranth, "lost" crops of the Incas, quality-protein maize, triticale, the scores of overlooked tropical fruits and more.

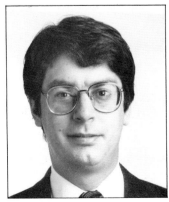

Mark Caraluzzi is one the country's

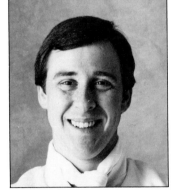

Bradley Ogden of San Francisco's Campton Place believes more and more in the simple, straightforward dishes he learned to love when he was growing up in the Michigan countryside. "Now," he says, "our constant goal is to serve the freshest and finest ingredients money can buy, cooked and presented with infinite pride and care, reminding us all that simple food is the most satisfying."

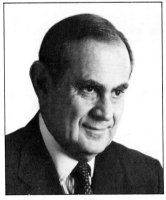

Tom Margittai of The Four Seasons in New York thinks that the restaurant business is "like any business." "It wants," he says, "undaunted professionalism and a constant striving for consistency of performance level. But unlike any other business, there is no shortcut to experience."

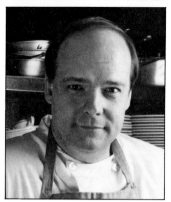

Jack Czarnecki has pioneered the use of over 200 types of wild mushrooms in his third-generation Joe's Restaurant in Reading, Pennsylvania. "Let mushrooms be mushrooms!" he cries. "Don't overdo the ingredients. Keep the preparations simple and natural."

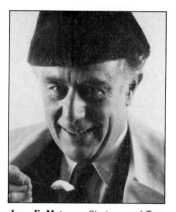

Juan E. Metzger, Chairman of Tomsun Foods International since 1983, is best known as the driving force behind the Yogurt Revolution in America, when he chaired the Dannon Company. He now confidently intends to do for tofu what he most certainly did for yogurt.

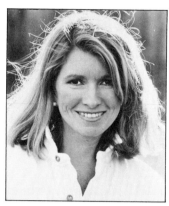

Martha Stewart is both golden girl of publishing and catering and mistress of the art of entertaining. She has influenced thousands of dinner parties with her imaginative, beautifully presented food.

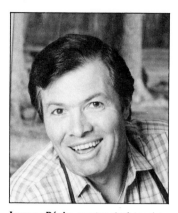

Jacques Pépin, master chef, teacher and author, has been personal chef to three presidents of France: Gaillard, Pfimlin and de Gaulle. He is away from home about 30 weeks of the year, crisscrossing America to share his unique skills at schools, culinary festivals and fundraising events.

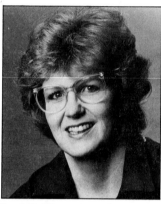

Carol Haddix, as Food Guide editor of the *Chicago Tribune*, leads many in the Midwest to the discovery of new foods and food trends through the pages of the *Tribune's* weekly and widely respected Food Guide.

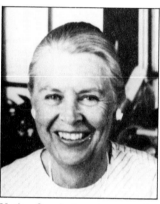

Marion Cunningham is among the most beloved cookbook authors in the country. She thinks that "many of today's chefs and cooks should be in ceramics and painting."

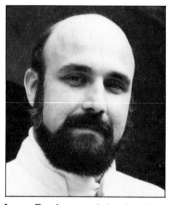

Larry Forgione— of An American Place, New York—though still a young man, could rightfully claim the mantle of being the father of the new American cooking. He was among the first to find the best of our native American ingredients and to cook them with consummate skill.

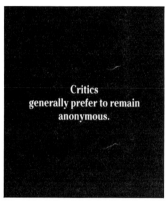

Critics generally prefer to remain anonymous.

Mimi Sheraton, one of the most feared and respected restaurant critics, reports on food for *Time* and is the author of the new *Mimi Sheraton's Favorite New York Restaurants.* "The only ingredient I am allergic to is hype. When I read raves by most other critics, I generally want to ask, 'compared to what?'"

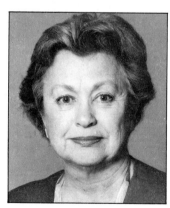

Betsy Balsley, food editor of the *Los Angeles Times*, is a major influence on the eating habits of millions of Southern Californians each week. She and her staff of ten energetically stay ahead of the latest in trendy foods in order to satisfy the restless, eclectic appetites of their readers.

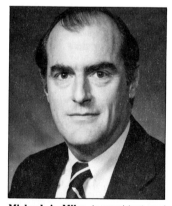

Michael A. Miles is president and chief operating officer of Kraft, Inc., a leading producer and marketer of packaged food products. Under his direction, Kraft is listening to the changing needs of today's consumers and striving to provide high-quality foods and services to feed the nation.

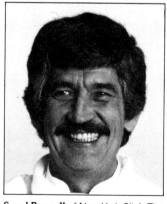

Seppi Renggli of New York City's The Four Seasons says that the reason he enjoys cooking so much is that there is always a fresh challenge. One of those challenges for him, we observe, is to create more and more spa cuisine dishes, a genre he invented himself.

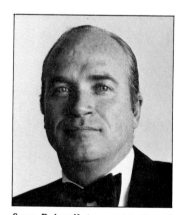

Sean Driscoll is president and founder of Glorious Food, Inc., a catering firm synonymous with elegant and dramatic parties. The company originated in New York but is now also operating in Washington, D.C.

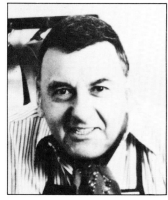

Bert Greene, dubbed "The father of carry-out cuisine," founded The Store in Amagansett in 1966, and hasn't been far from a stove ever since. One of America's more visible cooks, he is seen on TV by over 8 million viewers monthly; his column is read by 25 million readers and his latest book "Greene On Greens" sold 250,000 copies so far.

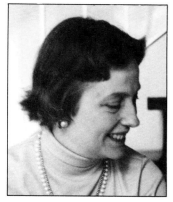

Narcisse Chamberlain has edited cookbooks for 25 years and begs off on counting how many. "Fine new talent keeps appearing, good new books get into print from your desk— and it's a thrill. You wonder why you ever said there are too many cookbooks. The only excess cookbooks are the ones that aren't good enough."

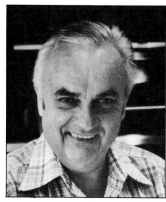

Pierre Franey began his culinary career the hard way—he worked for it.

Starting as an apprentice in his native France at the age of 14, he became the executive chef of Henri Soulé's celebrated restaurant, Le Pavillon, and subsequently was appointed vice president of the Howard Johnson chain. Having seen food from all levels of involvement, he is well qualified to lead us into temptation with his many cookbooks and widely read syndicated newspaper columns.

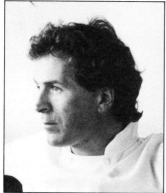

Jeremiah Tower, to quote a recent survey of San Francisco restaurants, is the one who started it all by, instead of imitating classic French cuisine, developing a lighter style using the freshest local ingredients, a style of cooking known as California Cuisine. "Now I look forward to all artichokes tasting as good as the ones in Italy, all chickens as good as French ones, all berries being as perfect as those of the Pacific Northwest, and in the future, nonpolluting waters for fish as plentiful and perfect as in nineteenth century America."

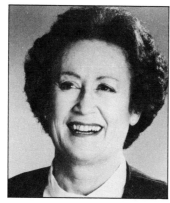

Frieda Caplan first introduced *kiwifruit* to America in 1962. Since then she has added to our consciousness sunchokes, black-eyed peas, spaghetti squash, jicama, cherimoya, Asian pears, enoki and shiitake mushrooms, yellow Finnish potatoes, cactus leaves, Mexibell peppers, tofu—and our own Mother Hubbard is still hard at work.

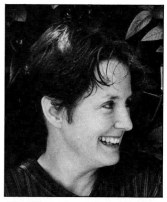

Tim Zagat has brought democracy to restaurant reviewing. Starting in 1979, Zagat, a lawyer by vocation and gourmet by avocation, persuaded 150 fellow food lovers to survey New York restaurants. Today *The Zagat Survey* is the best-selling guide to New York City's restaurants. More guides are under way for four other cities.

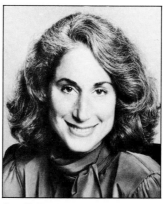

Jane E. Brody has changed the way Americans eat. As author of *Jane Brody's Nutrition Book* and *Jane Brody's Good Food Book*, the Personal Health columnist for *The New York Times* has shown people how to choose and prepare health-promoting, slenderizing, yet delicious food. Diets are her nemesis. "The word diet should be struck from the dictionary," she declares.

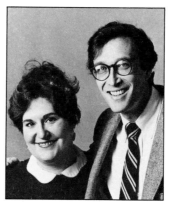

Jane and Michael Stern, the authors of *Square Meals, Roadfood and*

Goodfood and *Real American Food*, as well as the nationally syndicated newspaper column, "A Taste of America," and "On the Road" in *Cook's* magazine, have spent 15 years traveling the blue plate highway in search of honest meals. They are currently writing their memoirs, *Persona Au Gratin.*

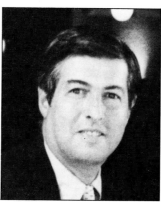

Alice Waters is the owner and chef of Chez Panisse restaurant in Berkeley, California. She opened the restaurant in 1971 offering regional foods prepared with innovation and flexibility in an inviting ambience. Serving one five-course, never-to-be-repeated dinner each night, Chez Panisse menus are planned weekly and refined daily to take full advantage of the most enticing fresh, local foodstuffs available. Drawn from a unique marketplace, a network of special sources developed by and for the restaurant, these ingredients are the heart of the Chez Panisse cuisine.

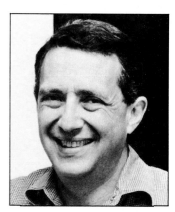

Gordon Segal, president of Crate and Barrel gourmet housewares, Chicago, believes that in the future people are going to continue to want well-designed products for their kitchens and their homes. Those companies that offer selection, quality and design for a fair price will succeed. The cookware industry, in association with the food industry, will continue to flourish.

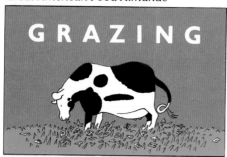

GRAZING

Salad-Bar Popularity Contest

A recent Gallup poll posed the question: If a salad bar offered all the (34) items on this list, which ones would you be most likely to use in your salad?

Tomatoes were the preferred item, by far, and in all parts of the country. Iceberg lettuce and then cucumbers were next, followed by two items of a slightly different sort: bacon bits and shredded cheddar cheese. Raw mushrooms were next. These were followed, in this order, by: fresh fruit, raw carrots, cauliflower, leaf lettuce, hard-boiled egg, croutons, broccoli, celery, sweet onion, coleslaw, cottage cheese, green pepper, black olives, pickled beets, sprouts, green olives, spinach, avocado, seeds or nuts, bread sticks, three-bean salad, grated parmesan cheese, romaine lettuce, chickpeas, small hot peppers, applesauce, sweet and sour red cabbage. At the bottom of the list, for reasons no one understands, were raw green beans.

Back To The Cave, Men! Many people these days prefer to eat with their hands, like our ancient ancestors. As we all know, early man would hunt for food or stumble across it, tear it apart and devour it on the spot. This has its parallel in modern times when we drive in to get hamburgers, fried chicken, doughnuts and the like, and eat them instantly in our hands. When viewed anthropologically, it seems that any food requiring people to sit at a table and eat with a fork has scant chance of long-term success. If a *knife* is also needed, forget it.

How Much Maple Syrup Can One Tree Produce? Would a full quart be enough? It takes four mature (40 years of age or older) sugar maple trees with sap rising, and one whole winter, to produce the 40 gallons of sap needed to make one gallon of pure maple syrup, according to the Vermont maple producers organization.

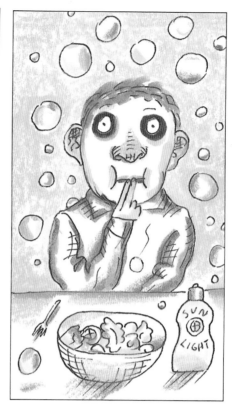

Restaurant Knowledge As Status Symbol In a recent survey, only 31 percent of the respondents thought that being able to prepare a gourmet meal signified a cultivated person, whereas 45 percent said that a cultivated person would know the good restaurants in the region.

Fat Is Fat

Regardless of whether it comes from meat or vegetable or other source, or whether it is in solid or liquid form, fat is worth nine calories per gram. Generally speaking, the saturated fats are firmer at room temperature and unsaturated ones are more liquid.

Contrary to popular belief, the cholesterol content of a food is not directly related to its fat content. For example, shrimp contain very little fat but are high in cholesterol.

The Dimness Of Some Consumers Even experienced marketing experts are sometimes taken by surprise. Lever Brothers' dishwashing detergent called Sun Light was, the company says, squirted into salads or iced tea by at least 1,000 customers simply because the words "real lemon juice" appeared on the container.

The company now has a new shampoo called Dimension which is made of corn syrup, among other things, but that fact is not prominently displayed on the packaging. Maybe they're afraid it would be poured over pancakes.

Give Us This Day Our Jelly Bread And Lead Us Not Into Penn Station Schoolchildren's minds have been known to wander. It is clear from the essays collected by one teacher that in this classroom, at least, their thoughts are firmly on food.

One pupil wrote about a "mackerelbiotic" diet, a second mentioned "fruit compost" and another "canine pepper." "Dessecrated coconut" and "paralized milk" were also touched on. And in a discussion of literary/theatrical history the most startling fact of all emerged, that the greatest achievement of Eugene O'Neill's career was winning the "Pullet Surprise."

Finnish Pasties?

The copper-mining country of Michigan's Upper Peninsula is largely populated by people of Finnish descent. Local restaurants and bakeries feature traditional Finnish specialties such as cardamom bread and rye flatbread. However, the area's best-loved baked goods are not Finnish at all; they are Cornish pasties, savory, half-moon-shaped pies filled with meat and vegetables.

Why are Cornish pasties eaten by Finns in Michigan? The explanation is quite simple: Before Finns arrived, the Upper Peninsula had previously been settled by immigrants from Cornwall, England, who had come to the area to work in the copper mines. When the Finns followed, they tasted the pasties made by their Cornish neighbors, liked them a lot and learned how to make them too. Cornish pasties are now a well-established part of the local cuisine. They are so popular, in fact, that in 1968, Governor George Romney proclaimed May 24 Michigan Pasty Day.

Is An Artichoke A Vegetable Or A Fruit? Neither; it is the flower of the artichoke plant, *Cynara Scolymus.*

Who Was Proclaimed The State Of California's First-Ever Artichoke Queen? Marilyn Monroe, according to the California Artichoke Advisory Board.

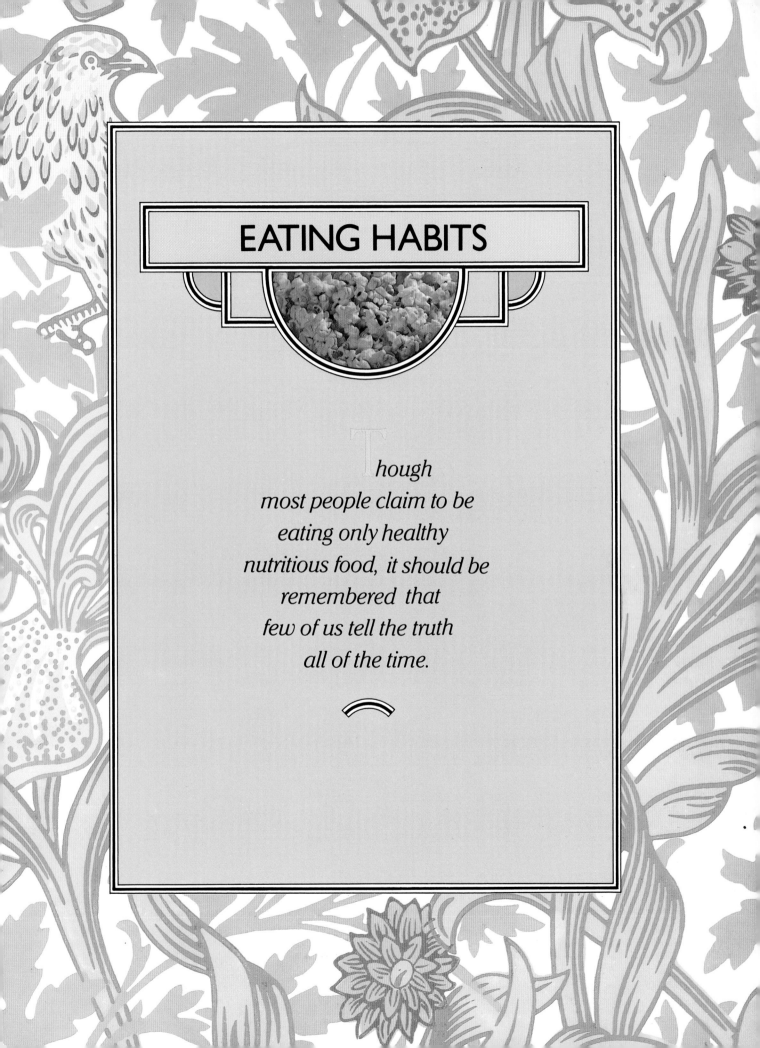

EATING HABITS

*Though
most people claim to be
eating only healthy
nutritious food, it should be
remembered that
few of us tell the truth
all of the time.*

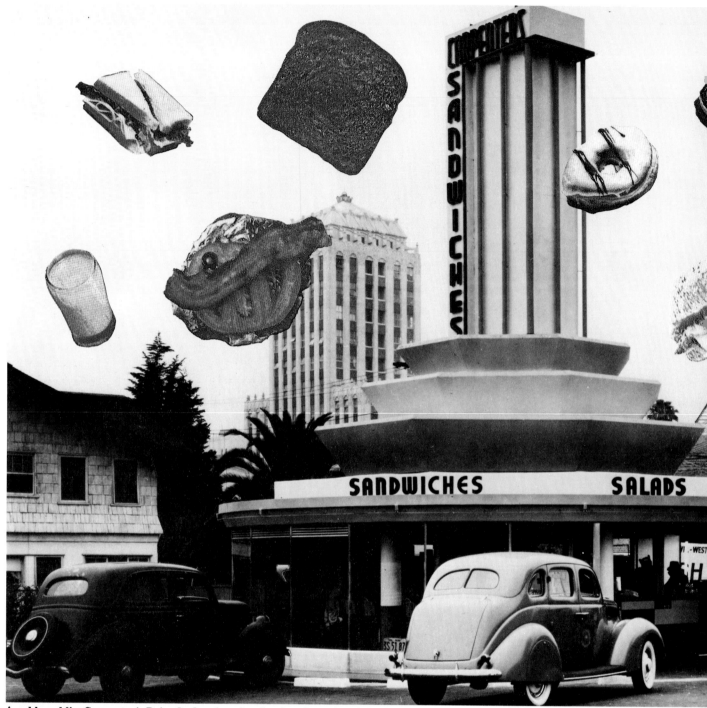

A golden oldie, Carpenter's Drive-In, Los Angeles, inspires fantasies of timeless American fare—donuts, sandwiches, burgers.

What America Eats

Since man is what man eats, or so some say, what Americans eat and how they eat it ought to cast some light on the shape of the nation on the eve of the second Reagan age. Subscribers to the French *Annales* school of history might easily categorise great culinary movements of the American past, from the Pilgrim age (cornbread and waterfowl) through the pioneering (buffalo, beans) to the present (gourmet frozen dinner and Diet-

Rite) and chart the moral fibre accordingly. Thus, in the depression years, people ate casseroles because these were cheap and convivial; in the 1950s, bathed in affluence and ignorance, they dug into steak and milk-shakes in the family kitchen; in the 1980s they are lonely, but healthy, pickers at salad bars and snackers of chocolate-flavored tofu in the street.

The rise of working women, the decline of

family meal-times, the proliferation of places where a meal can be had in a paper napkin and of food to match, have put the moral burden of Eating a Proper Meal on the individual. What is he to do? Perhaps follow the nutritional guidelines issued every decade or so by the federal department of agriculture, which in 1980 recommended that people should reduce their intake of fatty meats, salt and sugar and seek out wholegrains, vegetables and fish; or rely on the statements of increasing portentousness made on their menus by the new army of American chefs, the apostles of the *nouvelle*, who try to

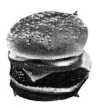

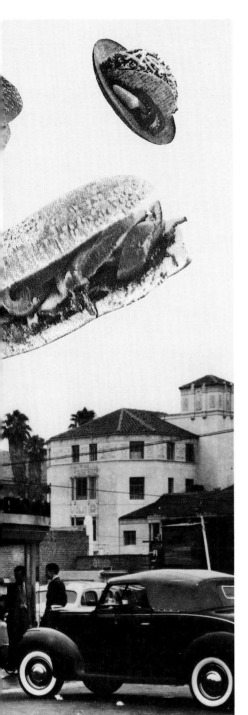

bludgeon the public with their eggwhisks into their own ways of eating and thinking.

Some of this the public has accepted. To paraphrase St. John, what is good is now lite: lite beer, lite hamburgers (as marketed by D'Lites in their greenhouse-like cafés), lite jellies, lite ice cream. Chicken is light, and so consumption of it has doubled in the past 30 years, while consumption of eggs and butter over the same period has fallen by 33 percent and 52 percent. Whiskey, which has a brooding look, has lost market share to vodka and rum; these, in turn, are losing out to mildly sparkling wines; wine sales have

flattened, and it appears to some disheartened brewers and winemakers that the country is tottering on the brink of teetotalism.

Coffee (heavy, expensive and bad in all manner of ways) has now fallen to fourth place in the soft-drinks league, and the first place is held by the great panoply of dyspepsia-inducing drinks in cans. A fifth of these, however, are now diet drinks, and by 1990 it is supposed that half of them will be.

There are limits to this virtue, however. Remove the lite labels, and the food looks much the solid same as it always did. Remove the healthy catch-words, and the diet of most of the people has not greatly changed. Americans eat only half the amount of sugar they ate ten years ago, but that is mostly because their canned drinks are sweetened with corn syrup or aspartame, a chance concoction of two amino acids which has not quite been cleared from suspicions of causing something nasty; they still consumed 113 pounds of sweeteners per head last year, close to the record.

Potatoes, mashed, baked or skins alone, have become good because they are presumed to be healthy and because they are American—patriotism not being confined to foreign policy these days, but rearing its head at the table too. Americans still eat more beef than they eat chicken, and they do not much mind what it has been injected with as long as it ends up tender. Nearly $8 billion was spent last year on crackers, cookies, crisps and the like, and three times as much was spent on "enriched" white bread, limp, sweet, chewy and ghastly as it is, than on all other sorts of bread put together.

None the less, the food companies keep on fussing round, taking out of their products the fat and the alcohol and the salt and the sugar. Two thirds of the public, according to the wheat industry council, now read the labels on food compulsively. They demand guidance, even if it is largely fatuous. Hence ketchup makers, who use scarcely any sugar, now advertise their wares as low-sugar, while soft-drink makers advertise their wares as low-salt. A new range of fruit juices for children is designed, say the manufacturers, to take away the guilt of mothers. Granola bars, by the same token, take away the guilt of people who would otherwise eat a nutritionally useless packet of sweets.

More and more people are now known to the food companies as browsers and grazers. They eat on the hop; they have little or no brand loyalty; they try sashimi one day, radicchio the next, coriander the next; they pick up a trend, such as grilling over mesquite, a shrub which is a dirty word over 55 million acres of Texas, and as quickly discard it again when the next novelty appears (grilling over vines, hot from California); they read up cookery in the Sunday magazines, and they do not spell a profit for any food company that is slow on the uptake. It is for such a market of samplers and tasters, rather than trenchermen, that the companies are producing their multi-flavoured vinegars and mustards and their amaretto-flavoured coffees. "Taste-segmentation" this is called.

The food ethic of the 1980s might be summed up in the national craze for expensive chocolate. This comes in small, exquisite pieces with a foreign label and many flavours; it sells for about $20 a pound and imports of it, helped no doubt by the strong dollar, virtually doubled between 1981 and 1983. Chocolate is scarcely light, but as part of a diet that includes whole-wheat bread, diet Pepsi and tofu ice cream, it may pass. And although it is nice to share it, the signs are that more and more rich chocolates are being bought to be eaten slyly and alone. Thus is the nervous I've-got-mine philosophy of the 1980s writ large across the stomachs of the nation. ● *The Economist*

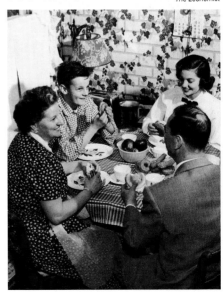

Americans domesticate their favorites.

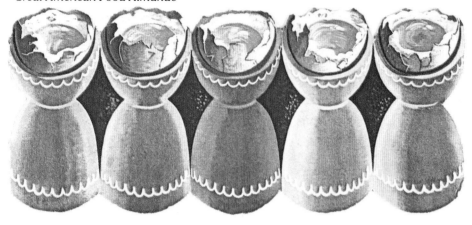

An Early Attitude Of The Mind

Breakfast, a meal long in decline in America, has suddenly become hugely popular again, and for the first time, lots of people are eating their breakfast *out*.

"Breakfast traffic," says the CREST Family Report (sponsored by the National Restaurant Association) increased—between 1978 and 1984—45.7 percent! And this is certainly only the beginning of a phenomenal boom in breakfast business for restaurants.

A matter of opinion

People eat all kinds of things for breakfast. Some clamor for yogurt, some feast on fiber, others still want their steak and eggs. Some yearn for pancakes swimming in melted butter and maple syrup, while others will make do with a cranberry bran muffin or two, and the sissies settle for a bowl of cereal.

There is still a lot of dough in breakfast breads, and croissants have rapidly turned into upscale doughnuts. Now that they are being stuffed with sausage and egg, they have a particular appeal to those who are accustomed to eating an entire meal from a paper bag using only one hand and no utensils. (*Prepared Foods* magazine reports that more than a million croissants are sold in America every day.)

Elegant hotels, such as the Campton Place in San Francisco, and the Regency in New York (which serves 500 early morning meals a day), are hosts to "power breakfasts." Meanwhile, bountiful brunches beckon guests at restaurants throughout the land.

Of course, Brennan's and Antoine's and other palaces of gastronomy in New Orleans have been purveying breakfast for years—but those are breakfasts of a very superior kind. They are leisurely, luxurious breakfasts, sybaritic and splendid, with Sazeracs and champagne and long afternoons of excess and self-indulgence. We will not see their like unless we take time off and go to them.

The big food companies look at all this breakfast business and smack their lips. Not

too long ago, Kellogg's set a task force in motion to see if they had "a breakfast opportunity" in Brazil. The researchers came back with good news and bad. The good news was that Brazil was virgin territory. The bad news was that no one eats breakfast in Brazil. The news is far more promising here at home. MRCA Information Services says that, on a typical day, 89 percent of Americans eat breakfast. No reliable figures are available for atypical days.

MRCA also reports that 23 percent of foods prepared in microwave ovens were served for breakfast. And in the last two years alone, more than 8,000 restaurants started serving breakfast for the first time.

Not surprisingly, McDonald's was the first of the fast-food chains to wake up to the ways in which breakfast can warm up the cash registers. Egg McMuffin made its debut way back in 1972. Where McDonald's goes, the others follow, and Burger King and Wendy's have stepped right up with morning competition for the King of the Road.

There's no saying no to a good idea

American enterprise being what it is, one might have predicted that someone would dream up a restaurant that served *only* breakfast. One Buddy Waldman has, and he calls his place in Denver Le Peep. Already franchisees are lining up to open breakfast-only restaurants under the Le Peep banner. Says Le Peep Director of Franchise Development, Mark Grabowski: "We are projecting that the market will eventually bear 500 to 600 Le Peep restaurants nationwide."

Nor, in the American way, will they restrict themselves *purely* to the eye-opener hour, for after Le Breakfast, they mean to go right ahead with Le Brunch and Le Lunch—and if traffic warrants, Le Dinner and Le After-Theater Supper too. Breakfast, we can reason, is nothing more than an attitude of mind.

So it looks as if the early bird is actually Le Golden Goose, who arrives in our time to lay le golden egg on le bottom line. ●

BRIDGE CREEK'S PEERLESS CORN MUFFINS
A muffin a day keeps the diet at bay.

Makes 12

Ingredients:
1 egg, at room temperature
8 tablespoons unsalted butter, melted and cooled slightly
1/4 cup vegetable oil
1 cup warm milk (about 85 degrees)
1 cup cake flour (not self-rising)
2/3 cup yellow cornmeal
1 tablespoon baking powder
1/2 teaspoon salt
1 tablespoon sugar

Method:
1. Preheat the oven to 400 degrees.
2. Whisk together the egg, butter and oil in a large mixing bowl. Whisk in the warm milk.
3. In a separate bowl combine the flour, cornmeal, baking powder, salt and sugar. Stir with a fork until blended.
4. Add the dry ingredients to the egg mixture, stirring with a fork until just blended into a moderately thick batter.
5. Fill 12 buttered muffin tins three-quarters of the way up with the batter
6. Bake in the middle level of the oven for 15–20 minutes, until the edges are golden brown.

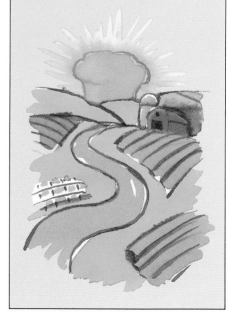

Breakfast At Bridge Creek

Suzanne Hamlin

"*All breakfast restaurants should have sunlight streaming in,*" says John Hudspeth, owner of Bridge Creek, the little corner place in Berkeley, California that may revolutionize America's restaurant-going habits. Right down the street from Chez Panisse, the mecca for new American food, Bridge Creek opened in the fall of 1985 on a wing, a prayer, and a slew of breakfast food recipes that would seduce the most determined "coffee only" curmudgeon.

Greeted by pitchers of freshly-squeezed orange juice, the Bridge Creek customer is given plenty of time to mull leisurely over a menu of such delectables as buttermilk griddle cakes with blueberries, Heavenly Hots (dollar-sized sour cream hot cakes), cornmeal Johnnie cakes served with homemade sausages, French toast with real maple syrup, a Tillamook cheddar cheese omelette draped with apple-smoked bacon, Huevos Bridge Creek (eggs Mexican-style), and fried pork tenderloin with sautéed potatoes, cream biscuits and gravy. Not to mention the basket of homemade muffins and breads, the bacon, ham and egg combos and—this is California, remember—the cut-up fruits so fresh they almost leap out of their bowls. "We go down to the Monterey market every morning and get whatever looks best," says Hudspeth, a cherubic 40-plus former food groupie. "That could be red bananas, or Japanese apple pears or local strawberries, or a gorgeous seasonal melon."

Confronted by the irresistible fruit, along with pots of homemade jam, crocks of sweet butter, and the smell of brewing coffee and a choice selection of teas, most customers find themselves lingering long after the traditional breakfast hour. Indeed, this is not only possible but encouraged: Bridge Creek is open only for breakfast, from 8 a.m. to 2 p.m., every day of the week. Customers during the week tend to be professionals, who come for both early breakfasts and lunch. (Where is it written that hot cakes can only be eaten at 8 a.m.?) On weekends lots of families come to enjoy both themselves and breakfast fare that many feared had been supplanted by instant breakfast drinks, frozen toaster waffles,

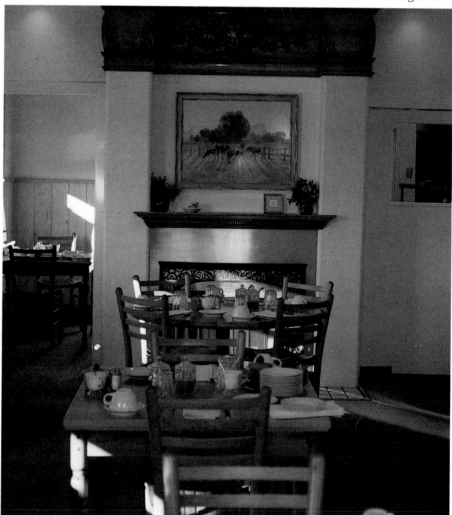

If breakfast is your meal-of-the-day, meet the cozy, sun-lit splendor of Bridge Creek.

and ersatz citrus liquids. "Eating has always been my primary entertainment," says Hudspeth, who volunteers that opening a breakfast-only restaurant was a serious business decision. "I adore breakfast food, and I think most people do, but no one has time to eat it or cook it any more. At Bridge Creek, you can eat a real breakfast for six hours a day."

Hudspeth, who apprenticed in the kitchens of hotels, delis and Chez Panisse, spent a large part of his life contemplating his inheritance, the legacy of an Oregon family. "Then Marion Cunningham changed my life," he says, referring to the distinguished author of "The Fannie Farmer Baking Book." Cunningham, a California neighbor and an indefatigable catalyst for any number of gastronomic enterprises, provided both intense encouragement and the bulk of Bridge Creek's recipes, which were refined, taste-tested and agonized-over for months.

In truth, the food is simply superb. A combination of knowledgeable, passionate cooking and pristine ingredients, the menu reads like a diary of barely-

remembered flavors. Even addicts succumb to Bridge Creek's no-smoking policy when wooed by the pink-cheeked serving staff, the old wooden tables, the prices ($2.50 up to $9), the portions (logging camp size) and, of course, the sunlight streaming into the simple, homey room.

Hudspeth reports that after six months, the restaurant began to break even. "Now we've started to get requests to extend the hours," he says.

Who knows? Maybe breakfast will eventually be served when it could be savored most—at supper time. ●

Suzanne Hamlin is the food critic of the New York *Daily News*.

Who On Earth Would Drink Coke For Breakfast? The experts at the Coca-Cola company say their best estimate for what breakfast consumption is currently worth to them is $237.25 million a year. A trifle when compared to the $7.904 *billion* total annual revenues Coke racks up. But *still* . . .

FUN FOOD: IS IT JUNK?

A nutritionist's definition of junk food tends to be that it is a food with empty calories. But this would not seem to go far enough. A junk food is one with empty calories *which pleases*. Nobody would have bought the first potato chip or Twinkie if it didn't taste good. And it may have been possible to feel guilty about consuming junk foods during the first several years of the concept, but then one day somebody started spelling it *junque* food, and thus the whole genre was lifted onto the plane of social acceptability.

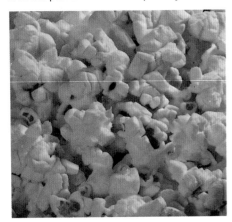

Popcorn plumply popped for the fun of it.

Long before we had the term, we had the thing itself. In the 1930s, a greedy little kid could go to the candy store and buy button candy and little wax bottles filled with colored sugar water. It would be hard to think of anything bearing fewer calories than a wax bottle, but that didn't bother the greedy little kid. When it comes to gob-stopping (the English expression for filling up on fun food), the greedy little kid in all of us is the part of us who rules.

In a recent debate among a few people aged 35 to 40, the following after-school snack, recollected with great nostalgia, was acclaimed the winner: a sandwich of peanut butter, sliced bananas and mayonnaise on Pepperidge Farm wheat bread, toasted, with margarine. The winner is a 37-year-old male, who grew up in Michigan. He was 12 years old in 1960, when he was introduced to this vice by his sister, who was 12 years older.

Today the subject is a businessman living and working in Manhattan. His pleasure today is a cheese pizza with cashews, or peanut butter, or mayonnaise and cayenne pepper, and he specifies that the beverage to be

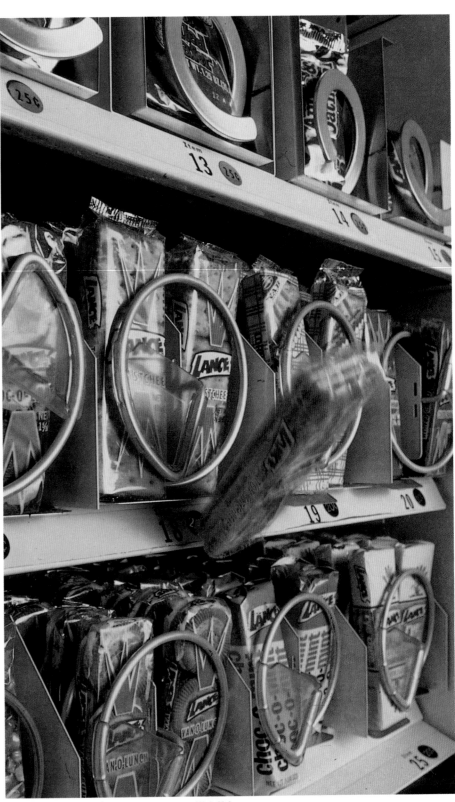

Cheese crackers with peanut butter will fall for you.

drunk with this pizza should be grape juice, never beer.

Because he is on the move during the business week, our subject takes a very spare lunch, consisting of one bag of unsalted peanuts, one bag of popcorn, one bag of crispy Chee-tos, one apple and one Diet Coke. He is pleased not only because the foods please him but because the total cost of his meal is $1.99.

The amount of pizza reckoned to be consumed in America daily would cover 75 acres of farmland. This is a lot of mozzarella, not to mention mushrooms, and hold the anchovies. Pizza is not so much a junk food as a convenience food, but if it were all you ate, it would become junk. It's all a matter of what and how much you eat of a thing.

Raisins, for example, are considered to be a healthy, natural snack food, full of iron, potassium, phosphorus and B vitamins. Yet they have been attacked (by the folks at Hershey, for example) as being devastating for the teeth (Hershey does not use raisins in their concoctions). It's true that, if you ate nothing but raisins, raisins would become a junk food to you.

Popcorn likewise. While popcorn is not nearly so rich in vitamins as raisins, it is a relatively healthful snack food, particularly if you avoid the butter and salt. One advantage is that popcorn is low in calories, and if you use an air popper, rather than cooking the kernels in oil, you reduce the calorie count even lower. But tell that to the people jostling for service at the candy counter in the lobby of your neighborhood Cinema One. They want their popcorn covered in salt, and so copiously slathered in butter that they can drink what remains directly from the plastic bucket. It pleases them.

Before there was fresh popcorn at the movies, there was Cracker Jack, a box of sugar-coated popcorn that made its appearance in 1872. The incentive prize in every box was introduced in 1912. The sale of fresh popcorn forced Cracker Jack well back from its lead in the popcorn stakes, but it still has an edge in the market, its packaging virtually unchanged in more than a century.

Speaking of things traditional, what of Mom's apple pie? Or Hostess's, for that matter? Here's a case where the sugar load is so immense that it cancels out any benefits you might derive from the fruit cut up in the fill-

ing. But who is not going to have some when Mom puts it on the table?

Candy bars? Some people use them to get through the day, because of the quick sugar rush they give. They also give about 13 grams of fat and 270 calories, together with more than 30 grams of carbohydrates. It's well to remember two things (at least) about the candy bar. More than half the calories in many of them come from fat. Try to choose one with nuts in it—they deliver added protein.

The soda fountain may have gone the way of Harold Teen, but not the soda, which is often concocted in the family kitchen. Consider the root beer float. It's a treat that combines the two most popular high-calorie ingredients in America today: soda and ice cream. Both root beer and ice cream are so high in sugar that together they far outweigh the calcium in the ice cream. But no afficio-

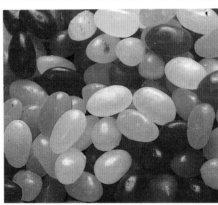

Jelly Beans: Found in all the best places.

nado is going to stop making them. They are as American as Mom's apple pie, mentioned above.

Probably the food most widely deplored as junk is the enormously popular potato chip, which came into being when automatic potato-peeling and slicing devices were introduced in 1925. Production and consumption of potato chips boomed at once, and the American love affair with this ubiquitous snack has never waned. We all know, of course, that the deep-frying adds fat and that, in the thin slicing, many nutrients are lost. We also know that all that salt is not wonderful for us. But we will keep passing the bag because potato chips taste good. Like all of the above, they are a treat. They satisfy. They *please* us. ●

MAJOR LEAGUE STADIUM FOOD SPECIALTIES

Atlanta Braves
Chick-fil-A

Baltimore Orioles
Crab cakes

Boston Red Sox
Pizza

California Angels
Helmet sundae

Cincinnati Reds
Mettwurst

Chicago Cubs
Smoky Link

Chicago White Sox
Tacos

Cleveland Indians
Roast beef

Detroit Tigers
Hot dog

Houston Astros
Nachos

Kansas City Royals
Polish sausage

Los Angeles Dodgers
Peanuts

Milwaukee Brewers
Bratwurst

Minnesota Twins
Bratwurst

Montreal Expos
Pizza

New York Mets
Knish

New York Yankees
Pizza

Oakland A's
Colossal dog

Philadelphia Phillies
Pizza

Pittsburgh Pirates
Roast beef on roll

San Diego Padres
Chili

St. Louis Cardinals
Steak'Umm

San Francisco Giants
Almaden wine

Texas Rangers
Nachos

Toronto Blue Jays
Sausage on bun

It's In The Twist

The first recreational (therefore junk) food to be widely deplored in this country was the pretzel. Its reputation suffered less for its content—baked dough with a liberally salted crust—than from its frivolous braided shapes, unsuited to the family table. It suffered further, of course, on account of its German origins—at a time when immigration to these shores was not popular with already established Americans—and beer; these congregated together in beer halls. (The Moral Majority of the time had the lowest opinion of beer halls, which sprung up wherever the Germans settled: New York, Chicago, Cincinnati.)

Later, of course, the Germans, the beer and the pretzels made their way out to the ballpark, where they all gained a certain cachet in association with sportsmanship and the open air. All of which goes to show that if you make some modifications, and hang in there, almost anybody and anything, even with a twist to it, can make it in America.

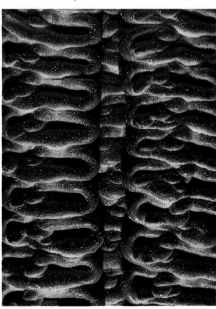

Salty golden braids, to tempt you.

Yes, Virginia, There Is A Twinkies-Taster
A food editor we know passes along the following fragment of a letter she received from a friend keeping her up-to-date on the men in her life: "My latest was very funny but also very heartless. Maybe this was to be expected. His taste was all in his mouth." The man was, she said, "a professional taster of—Can you believe it?—Twinkies."

PASSIONS OF THE KITCHEN FAMOUS

Paula Wolfert
Cookbook Author/Teacher
Fritos

Larry Forgione
Chef and Owner
An American Place, New York
Peanut butter and potato chip sandwich—two chips around the peanut butter

Barry Wine
Chef and Owner
The Quilted Giraffe, New York
Oreo cookies

John Mariani
Food Writer
Vanilla Carvel ice cream with U-Bet syrup

Tom Margittai
Co-owner
The Four Seasons, New York
Kielbasa sausages sautéed in red wine

Jane Kirby
Food Editor
Glamour
Potato chips with ketchup

Julia Child
Cookbook Author
Fritos and peanut butter

Martha Stewart
Cookbook Author
Tomato sandwiches with Miracle Whip and sweet relish on Wonder Bread
Arthur Schwartz
Daily News

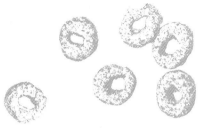

No Accounting For Taste Nothing reveals more strikingly the overwhelming orality of our species than to confirm the heterogeneity of objects recovered from the alimentary tract, during life and posthumously: coins, pens, watches, fragments of shoes and other garments, carpenters' nails, toothpicks, assorted jewelry and astonishing lengths of metallic wire. It would be naive to dismiss the breadth of this inventory on the grounds that such ingestions are accidental or the acts of deranged minds. This would be tantamount to denying the two tenets with which an unbiased student of the species cannot dispense: that there is no such thing as a wholly random human act and that there is much to learn from deviancy.
F. Gonzalez-Crussi, Professor of Pathology
Northwestern University Medical School

Respect For The Kernel

Robert Brucken is an Ohio adman whose enthusiasm for popcorn caused him to bring forth, in 1983, a book with Ballantine entitled *BANG! The Explosive Popcorn Recipe Book.* "The 200 best [recipes]—kitchen-tested and uniformly delicious," include *Popcorn Pizza, Popcorn Meatloaf* and *Popcorn Brownies.*

For *Popcorn Pizza?* Drizzle 3 tablespoons of melted butter over 6 cups of popped popcorn. Layer a large pizza pan with the buttered popcorn. Melt 4 tablespoons of butter and ½ teaspoon of garlic powder over low heat. Remove from heat and drizzle over the popcorn. Sprinkle 1½ cups of grated cheese and some dried hot pepper flakes and place in oven at 250 degrees for 10 minutes. Remove and add salt and pepper to taste.
PresSyndicate

Yum Yum hot dogs had a monopoly as vendors in Central Park and annually paid the city: $80,000.

Because contracts for each of the 58 vending locations in the Park were opened to other bidders last October, the city will get: $400,000.

Manhattan, Inc.

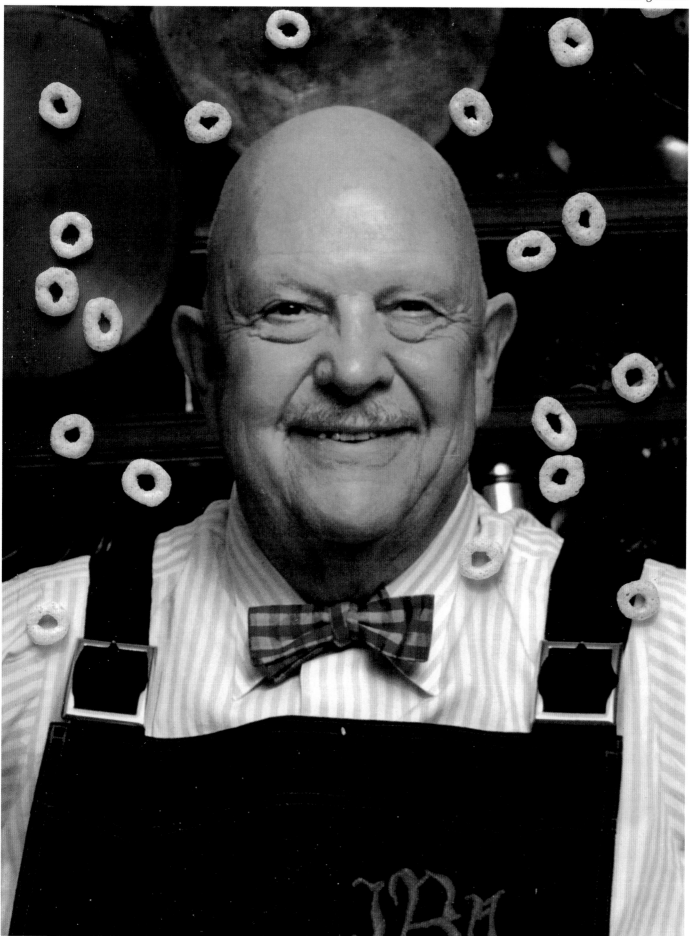

James Beard, revered American cook, author and savant, had a passion for Cheerios by the fistful.

FUN-FOOD FAVORITES OF SOME SOLONS

Senator
Bill Bradley
New Jersey
Wendy's, Pizza Hut and Baskin-Robbins

Senator
Barry Goldwater
Arizona
McDonald's

Senator
Howell Heflin
Alabama
Wendy's, McDonald's, Hardees

Senator
Spark M. Matsunaga
Hawaii
Saimin, udon or a fish sandwich

Senator
Claiborne Pell
Rhode Island
A chicken sandwich on whole wheat bread.

Senator
Alan K. Simpson
Wyoming
A glass of iced orange juice and an Egg McMuffin at McDonald's

Senator
John Warner
Virginia
Colonel Sanders, Golden Skillet and Gino's Fried Chicken

Junk Food

FORBIDDEN APPETITES

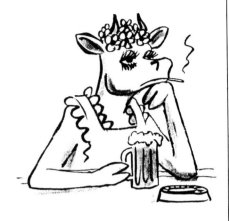
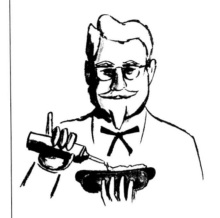
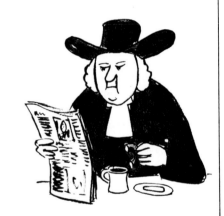
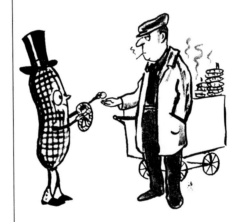
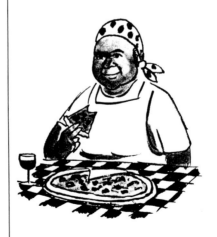
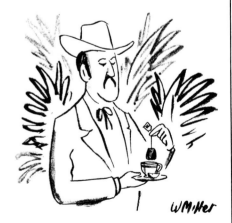

Cake Mix Look-Alike

Good manufacturers are great imitators, and what they see, they do—if it works. Quick now: What popular treat are you reminded of here? Blink and wink and you will see.

The contents of a box of Pillsbury Pudding Pockets Pudding-Filled Cupcake Mix are: sugar, enriched bleached flour [bleached flour, niacin, iron, thiamine mononitrate (Vitamin B1), riboflavin (Vitamin B2)], hydrogenated vegetable oils (soybean, cottonseed, and coconut oil) and/or hydrogenated animal fat (beef fat or lard) with BHA, BHT and citric acid added to protect flavor, dextrose, cocoa processed with alkali, modified corn starch, modified tapioca starch, wheat starch, maltodextrin, nonfat milk, baking powder (baking soda, sodium aluminum phosphate, sodium acid pyrophosphate), cornstarch, carob powder, propylene glycol monoesters, mono- and diglycerides, natural and artificial flavor, salt, sodium phosphate, soy protein concentrate, corn syrup solids, soy flour, calcium acetate, egg whites, xanthan gum, artificial color, lecithin, citric acid, polysorbate 60, sodium caseinate, polysorbate 80, locust bean gum, and guar gum. © The Pillsbury Company. ●

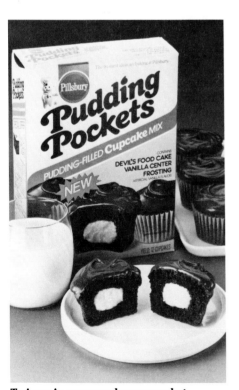

Twins mix: more pudge per pocket.

HORN & HARDART'S BAKED MACARONI AND CHEESE

Nursery foods are still our favorites

Serves 4

Ingredients:
1 cup uncooked elbow macaroni
1½ cups milk
2 tablespoons light cream
1½ tablespoons butter
1½ tablespoons flour
1½ cups shredded Cheddar cheese
⅛ teaspoon cayenne pepper
Salt and white pepper
¼ cup finely chopped canned tomatoes
½ teaspoon sugar

Method:
1. Preheat the oven to 400 degrees.
2. Cook the macaroni, uncovered, in 6 quarts of rapidly boiling salted water for 8–12 minutes until *al dente*. Drain well.
3. Combine the milk and cream in a small saucepan and bring to a simmer over moderate heat.
4. While the milk warms, heat the butter in another saucepan over low heat for 1 minute until foaming. Add the flour and cook, stirring, for 3 minutes.
5. Pour the hot milk into the butter-flour mixture, and cook, stirring with a wire whisk or wooden spoon for a few minutes, until thickened.
6. Add the cheese to the white sauce, about ¼ cup at a time, stirring, until the cheese has melted and the sauce is smooth. Add the cayenne pepper and season to taste with salt and white pepper.
7. Stir the tomatoes and sugar into the cheese sauce.
8. Combine the cooked macaroni with the sauce, and pour into a buttered 1½-quart baking dish.
9. Bake for 25–35 minutes, until the top is nicely browned.

Frito And Lay

Once upon a time, there were no Fritos corn chips in America, nor were there any Lay's potato chips, and darkness covered the land.

Then, one day in the early 1930s, Elmer Doolin borrowed $100 and went into business with Fritos; about the same time, Herman W. Lay also borrowed $100, and went into business with Lay's potato chips.

Abruptly, the American snack industry was born, and the lights came on all over the world.

For snack foods, the lights have never gone out. In a match made in snack heaven, Fritos and Lay's merged in 1961. In 1965, when PepsiCo munched them up into its corporate tummy, their joint sales totaled about $200 million. Today—well, just check the box (overleaf) to see what a business the chip industry has become.

How come all this salty success? Says one Frito-Lay executive, proudly: "We put our money where our consumer's mouth is." And their consumer's mouth is where it has always been: right on the old salt lick.

It has been said that the yearning for potato chips is one of mankind's deepest emotions. This is curious in light of the fact that this yearning lay wholly dormant in the human breast from the beginning of recorded time until 1925, when the invention of the potato slicer changed everything. Since then, the lowly potato has been subjected to indignities beyond common conception, at the loss of all its intrinsic integrity and nutritional value, in the act of dismembering it into a multitude of thin, thinner and thinnest slices of itself. Thus a wholesome but dowdy root undergoes the knife and becomes—but, oh, at what cost—a star.

The poor potato starts its journey to stardom under the ruthless scrutiny of scientists and technicians. If dragooned by Frito-Lay, this means a process of analysis in their research laboratory near Dallas—and as in any such process, many are called but few are chosen.

The thickness of an ordinary potato chip is 55/1,000th of an inch. Your everyday potato chip will be that thick. Ruffles, Frito-Lay's ridged potato chip, is twice as thick. And when Frito-Lay dared to go thicker, in their search for a potato chip that might taste more like a potato, they boldly broke the thickness threshold.

Potato Chip Portraits From Recent Vintages

In this daring, they nevertheless had to respect some immutable precepts. Fracture pattern: When inserted in the mouth, the potato chip must not shatter like a plate. Mouth clearance: When well in the mouth, the potato chip must mash down into a consistency that will chew up quickly; otherwise, people might eat them too slowly and delay, or eliminate, the consumption of additional chips. Replicability: It must be possible to reproduce the same identical chip, unerringly, in each of Frito-Lay's 39 plants.

Think for a moment of the first potatoes that went up against Frito-Lay's efforts, which began in 1984, to find the thicker chip. In a project that was to cost $25 million, those unwitting spuds faced tests their Irish ancestors never knew. They were sliced every which way. They were crushed between steel jaws. They were pierced with surgical devices and fried at temperatures both high and low. Some were soaked in briny baths for hours, days, weeks, before facing the night of the long knives—hurled at force into whirling blades, snicker-snack, as it were.

Nothing worked, until a nameless hero on the spud front suggested that they build into each thicker chip "areas of structural weakness." And that's how O'Grady's, "extra thick and crunchy," was born. "Extra thick" means as much as 210/1,000th of an inch in some parts, alternating with conventional thinness in ridges running parallel on both sides, slightly out of sync. It was a triumph, and Frito-Lay made $140 million off O'Grady's in its first year on the market.

Next time you munch one, spare a thought for the whole potatoes that showed the way, and the steel jaws that came before you, and munched and munched tirelessly, until your potato chip was Just Right. ●

Frito Lay's Seven Sales Leaders	
Doritos tortilla chips	$500 million
Lay's potato chips	$400 million
Fritos corn chips	$325 million
Ruffles potato chips	$250 million
Tostitos tortilla chips	$200 million
Chee-tos cheese-flavored snacks	$160 million
O'Grady's potato chips	$150 million
	Solomon Brothers Inc.

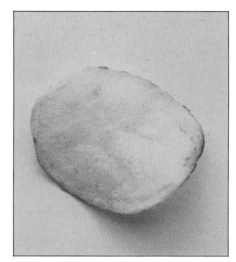
Bachman: bold, rich and assertive

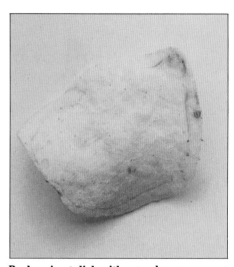
Barbara's: stylish with a good nose

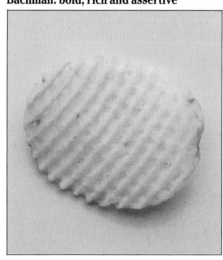
Eagle: immense depth of flavor

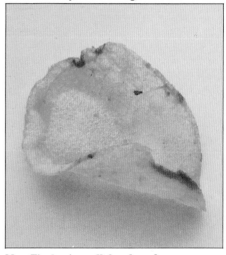
Mrs. Fischer's: well developed

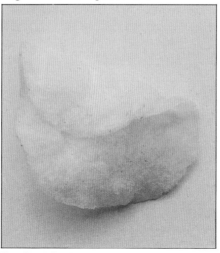
New York Deli: modest and subtle

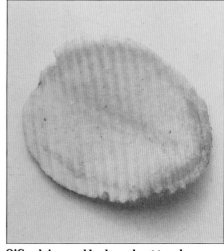
O'Grady's: good body and not too dry

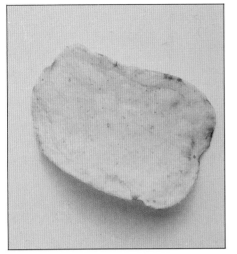

Barrel-o-Fun: excellent dry finish

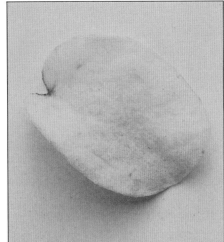

BonTon: glamorous with good breeding

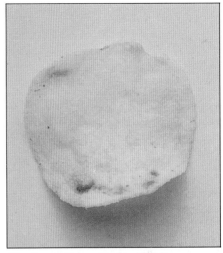

Charles: mellow with depth of flavor

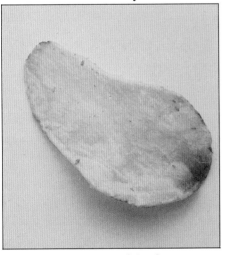

Granny Goose: nicely weighted

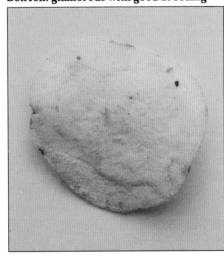

Health Valley: nutty with a hint of oak

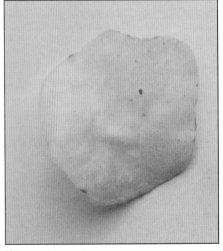

Wise: aging well

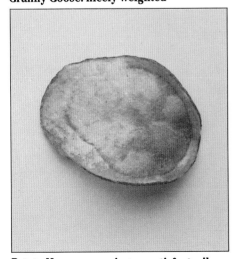

Potato Heaven: opening up satisfactorily

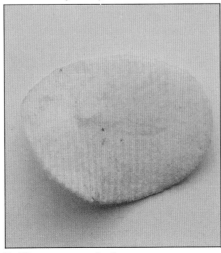

Ruffles: young and crisp

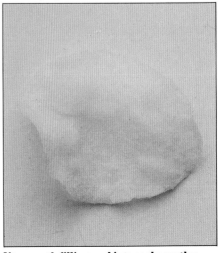

Utz: mouth filling and intensely earthy

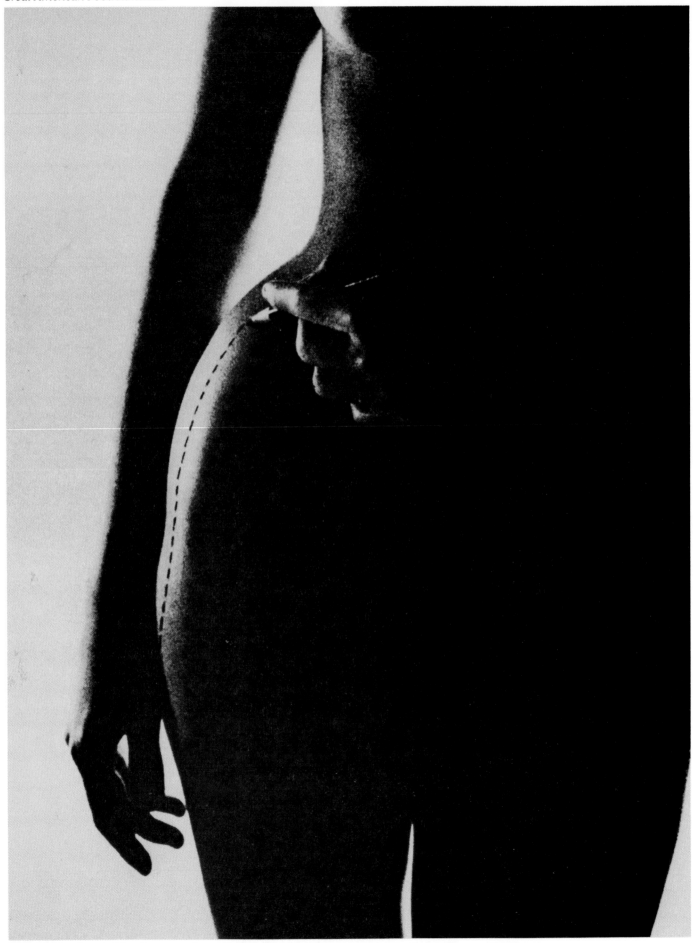

Wishful thinning: waiting for you at the end of the diet, a shape that would make Aphrodite smart with envy

THE SMART MOUTH

If dying young as late as possible has become a national collective goal, so have wise eating habits, exercise and clean living become recognized as the ways to accomplish it.

Not so long ago, eating wisely required no special knowledge. Our species survived in ignorant bliss for eons by eating nature's packaged goods—foods that were whole and entire in themselves. Now it's a different story. The industrialization of food and the infant science of nutrition are besieging us with new food products, new knowledge and new disputes waged with the fervor of religious wars. But though much remains shrouded in mystery, we may be beginning to understand our dietary destiny.

> **"I'm wary of health faddists. When they're done talking, you can't eat *anything*. We need a nutritionist who loves good food."**
> **Julia Child**

One thing is certain. Real food still supplies a better balance of nutrients than do supplements in the form of vitamins and minerals. It's extremely difficult to overdose on food, though easy to cause considerable damage to the body by taking, for example, too much vitamin A, too many calcium pills or whatever is the vitamin of the month.

The craze for single nutrients may be a hangover from the days of the early food scientists, who deprived subjects of one mineral or food factor at a time to learn about nutrition deficiency diseases. As long as ten years ago, those diseases were deemed to have been largely conquered in the U.S.

Ironically, therefore, we still seem capable of depriving ourselves of adequate nutrition, and incurring health risks. We do this principally by eating an imbalanced diet, consisting of either too much animal protein, fat, sugar or salt. This, in spite of the fact that scientists have found that, in general, we do far better on the diet of our ancestors and neighbors in less affluent nations—a diet high in complex carbohydrates. Our digestive and metabolic systems still live in the past, say the savants, and we may pay for our present excesses with obesity, diabetes, heart disease and various forms of cancer, depending on whom you listen to.

> **"People who have little or no knowledge of nutrition will, within a given meal, seek a healthy variety. Animals, children, everyone, seems to have this instinct."**
> **Barbara Rolls**

Our current failings: We should be getting 70 percent of our protein from vegetables. Instead, we choose to obtain them from dairy products and meat loaded with a fearsome 9 calories to the gram of the unhealthiest kinds of fat. We've been taught to eat vegetable oil rather than butter (mono-unsaturated olive oil is the latest favorite), but now we're eating 47 percent more vegetable oil than in 1965, eight times as much as the single tablespoon we need daily. In 1985, we each ate over 50 pounds of fat, which amounts to 40-50 percent of our total calorie consumption. Institutions such as the American Heart Association and the National Cancer Institute recommend that our fat intake provide only 25-30 percent of our calories. In

addition, protein should provide 20 percent of our calories and carbohydrates (mainly complex), 45–50 percent.

It follows, therefore, that moderation in the enjoyment of fat or sugar-loaded comforting foods is recommended by most nutritionists, rather than total abstinence.

> **"If someone told me I could never again have ice cream, or blinis with sour cream, melted butter, chopped egg and caviar, I wouldn't exactly die. But I might want to."**
> **Jane Brody**

We indisputably eat too much sugar, yet at least this substance is not the killer it was formerly made out to be. Salt is the newest villain, linked to hypertension by many scientists, though not by Dr. John H. Laragh, director of the Hypertension and Cardiovascular Center at New York Hospital. He says high salt intake is a problem only for a spe-

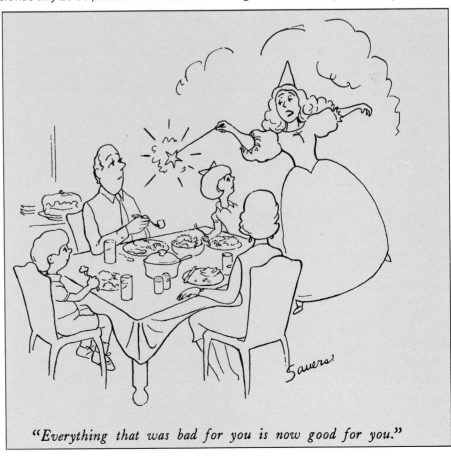

"Everything that was bad for you is now good for you."

cific type of hypertension. Nonetheless, we all consume at least ten times more salt than we need to maintain good health.

"I challenge anyone who thinks differently to spot the absence of salt in a dish skillfully seasoned with garlic and herbs."
James Beard

On the brighter side, there is growing evidence that the cruciferous vegetables—cauliflower, broccoli, peas and dark leafy greens—do a lot to keep us well. And we now know it's butter, not the tempting pasta, bread and potato carbohydrates themselves, that makes us fat. We're permitted to feel full again.

Yet we must stay ever alert to the continuing discovery of new substances in food and theories of nutrition that sometimes seem to go in circles. For instance, we are urged to cut down on our consumption of meat, but iron is generally better absorbed from meat than from other sources. But you should also know that, although fiber is good for us and much touted today, too much of it can hinder the absorption of calcium, possibly contributing to osteoporosis and hypertension.

Fortunately, there are also practical helpers in the form of food processors and packers. Pickle packers are reducing the salt content of their dills, and we can now eat animals specifically bred for their low fat content, such as capybaras—guinea pigs to us. Meat processors and packers are laboring to reduce the fat content in animals, and even cholesterol in egg yolks, through special diets for chickens. There are efforts under way to mimic fats with other substances and to develop non-caloric fats, though some dietitians fear such pampering could lead to inadvertent self-starvation.

However, as Dr. Sanford Miller, Director of the Center for Food Safety and Applied Nutrition at the Food and Drug Administration, has pointed out, the connection between technology and urban culture is inevitably growing stronger and our food is becoming increasingly manipulated. Food preservation has moved from drying and salting to fermentation and fabrication with chemicals, to thermal processing, refrigeration and freezing, to the oncoming phase of irradiation and multipurpose packaging.

The nutritional outlook holds greater promise perhaps than at any other time in history. Though we may not be eating off the fat of the land, we will probably be better fed and be making wiser food choices. Few can any longer doubt that what we eat profoundly affects our health and well being, or that even those calories still consumed in ignorance are being counted and checked against our personal time clocks. ●

Sugar Dread

In the American collective mind, there has always been a close connection between the sweet tooth and an emotion called guilt. It is historically appropriate that this should be so. Sugar came to these shores in the pockets of the Pilgrim Fathers, who encouraged guilt about everything. But this dour sponsorship never did sugar any harm. Nothing has *ever* done sugar any harm—not even when its detractors have cited it as the cause of mass murders and other uncivil behavior. It is estimated that, currently, we consume roughly one and a quarter pounds of sugar each, every week, every man, woman and child of us.

So where's the harm? It makes us fat, we say, though sugar is no more fattening than protein and less than half as fattening as edible fats. Sweets do, however, pack a lot of calories—and little other nutritional value—into a rather meager portion of food, which usually contains fat as well.

"Let's face it," says Rena Wing, a weight control expert in Pittsburgh, who is also an epidemiologist. "No one gets fat from Life Savers, which derive virtually all of their calories from sugar."

Sugar does cause tooth decay, and though we now eat less refined sugar, our consumption of high fructose corn syrup has gone from 7.2 pounds per person in 1976 to 42.7 pounds in 1985. Found mainly in soft drinks, corn syrup accounts for 25 percent of the sweetener in our diet. In 1985, we bought 127.4 pounds of natural sweeteners per person—up from only 109 in 1960.

It won't help just to avoid soft drinks, for the natural sugars in milk and fruit can decay teeth just as quickly. They will also rot infant teeth, if you let your baby go to sleep with a bottle of milk or juice in the mouth. Moreover, sugar calories lurk everywhere. Five figs contain 17 teaspoons of sugar, more than the sugar content of 14 fig cookies, and a single banana contains nearly five teaspoons of sugar, almost twice as much as a Mr. Goodbar. A seemingly innocent Nature Valley Granola Cluster contains 3.3 teaspoons of sugar, more than a Snickers bar.

Only two artificial sweeteners, Saccharin and Aspartame, currently have Food and Drug Administration approval. Saccharin, 300 times sweeter than sugar, causes a bitter aftertaste, yet 3,943 tons of it came to market in 1984. Aspartame (known as "Equal" by manufacturers) is 180 times sweeter than sugar, and leaves no aftertaste. It has found its way into most diet drinks since being introduced in 1981.

In 1984, 3,341 tons of Aspartame were used—the equivalent of 686,000 tons of sugar—and sales totaled $700 million in 1985. Despite Aspartame's wide acceptance, some still question its safety. Recently the Supreme Court refused to review the F.D.A.'s approval of it, though some scientists claim it can cause brain damage.

Will artificial sweeteners help your diet? Russell Lemieux of the Calorie Control Council says, "There have never been scientific studies that show that the use of artificial sweeteners leads to weight reduction. The only way these products can help you is if you eat wisely."

And that's not just sweet talk. ●

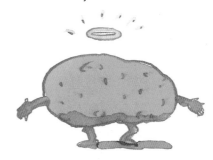

The Indispensable Potato You could almost live on potatoes alone. The Irish used to, and, more recently, a Scandinavian man stayed healthy for 300 days on potatoes with a small amount of margarine. Add a few dairy products and greens, and you're set for life.

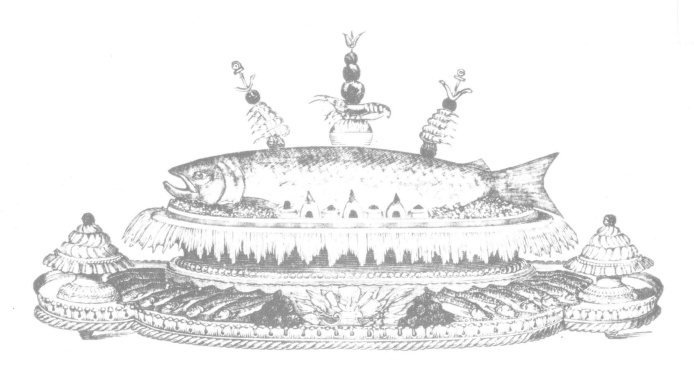

New Facts About Fish

For years, physicians have advised people to eat seafood. And with good reason—it is high in protein, easily digested and low in fat, calories and cholesterol. Even most types of shellfish, once considered inadvisable for those on low-cholesterol diets, are now recommended as part of a healthy diet.

Several significant studies conducted in the past 20 years have indicated that fish oils also have properties that thin the blood, lower cholesterol and can reduce the risk of death from heart disease by more than 50 percent.

Initial research on heart disease began in Framingham, Massachusetts, in 1949. Public health physicians, hoping to discover why heart disease had reached epidemic proportions in the U.S., initiated a survey that followed the habits of a cross section of the town's population for more than 30 years. These physicians established that cholesterol, high blood pressure and smoking were three major risk factors for heart attack and stroke. Recognizing the importance of diet, they recommended an increased intake of seafood because of its healthful properties.

A later study of Greenland Eskimos and their diets raised more questions than it answered. The Eskimos' diets were loaded with fat, cholesterol and protein from seafood and shellfish. Yet they had no cancer, few heart attacks, were not obese and did not get arthritis or diabetes. When fed diets that were high in meat, dairy products and vegetable

oils, however, they became just as disease-prone as Westerners.

In Japan, researchers discovered that fishermen who ate large quantities of fish were far healthier than their counterparts in the farming community. The link between fish consumption and health was becoming clearer. The results of another significant study were published in the May 9, 1985 issue of the *New England Journal of Medicine*. Over a 20-year period, 852 men in the Netherlands were observed by physicians. Those who ate the equivalent of one ounce of fish per day were 50 percent less likely to die of heart disease than those who did not.

Although no one is sure why fish oils seem to prevent heart attacks, certain of their components, eicosapentaenoic acid (EPA) and docosahexaenoic acid (DHA), known as "omega-3 long chain fatty acids," appear to be the best candidates for more research. Omega-3s may help prevent blood clots, a major cause of heart attacks, by thinning the blood. They also may lower cholesterol more effectively than polyunsaturated vegetable oils, and help lower the level of triglycerides, or blood fats, that can contribute to heart disease. They have also been linked to retarding the development of atherosclerosis, a condition in which fats accumulate on artery walls and choke the flow of blood to the heart.

Fresh, fatty fish are the best source of omega-3s, though lean fish are also consid-

ered very healthy food. According to an article in *The New York Times* by Jane E. Brody, some of the best sources are tuna, mackerel, salmon, bluefish, mullet, rainbow trout, lake trout, herring, sablefish, shad, butterfish and pompano. Fish oil supplements containing omega-3s are available from health food stores, but compared with eating the desirable amount of fish, they are not an economical alternative. Canned fish like tuna, salmon, mackerel and sardines are also excellent sources, though if they are packed in oil they should be drained. Fish packed in water are generally high in sodium, so rinsing them before eating may be in order.

Americans eat an average of 13 pounds of seafood a year, compared with 165 pounds of red meat. So eating seafood at least twice a week could have a positive effect on people's health. In most cases, a three-and-a-half-ounce serving of fish will provide half the adult minimum daily requirement of protein, and will contain less than 100 calories. Shellfish, with the exception of shrimp, is low in cholesterol, and is also recommended.

But too much of a good thing has its drawbacks as well. Cod liver oil, an excellent source of vitamin A and D, can be toxic in large quantities. And pollutants tend to be concentrated in the fatty tissue of fish. Nonetheless, though eating more fish may not save your life, as part of a sensible diet and lifestyle, chances are it will do a lot of good. ●

Donna Florio, seafood consumer specialist. *Commentary*

41

Beans Can Do

Legumes, specifically the dry beans and peas, are being hailed as the very latest old but new, do-good food. Their varieties are legion—black beans, black-eyed peas, fava beans, chickpeas and lentils, to name a few—and so are their virtues.

Beans give more protein value to the dollar than any other food, yet lack the artery-damaging fats and cholesterol of most high-protein foods. Eaten with any grain food or seed or small amounts of animal protein, they provide as complete protein as does a hamburger. They keep indefinitely, without preservatives or refrigeration, and can be made into everything from soup to nuts, from milk to ersatz meat. They can also lower cholesterol levels, control diabetes and cure constipation—with more fiber than any food except cereal bran—and might even help fight cancer.

It must be admitted that their fiber and certain sugars cause flatulence. You can't get rid of the fiber, nor would you want to, but you can remove most of the sugars by soaking. On the other hand, maybe you can live with it. Medieval writers like Maimonides and Constantinos Africanos considered gas-producing foods to be aphrodisiacal. The flatulence, they wrote, gave a feeling in the lower body that was very positive. ●

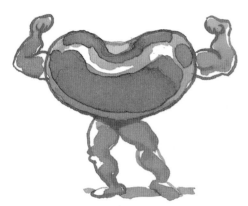

Working Mothers Do It Better Women who work outside the home feed their children more nutritious food and less junk food than do nonworking mothers, according to a study by MRCA Information Services, a Stamford, Connecticut consumer research group. The reason? Mothers who are home most of the day may be more susceptible both to TV commercials for junk food and to lobbying from the kids.

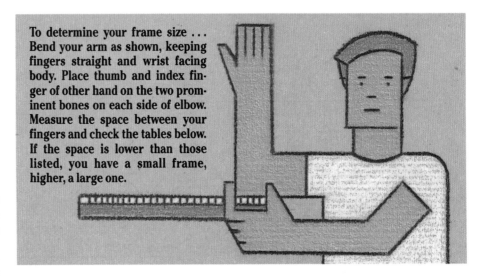

To determine your frame size . . . Bend your arm as shown, keeping fingers straight and wrist facing body. Place thumb and index finger of other hand on the two prominent bones on each side of elbow. Measure the space between your fingers and check the tables below. If the space is lower than those listed, you have a small frame, higher, a large one.

The New Numbers

The U.S. Government now says that a 5′5″ woman can stay healthy weighing between 114 and 146 pounds and a 5′10″ man is fit weighing between 137 and 172 pounds. These and comparable figures for varying heights are based on Metropolitan Life Insurance Guidelines set forth back in 1959. More recent Metropolitan guidelines, issued in 1983 and widely followed since then, were a bit more generous (see tables).

To determine your ideal weight within the new range given, measure the breadth of your elbow, as shown in the accompanying diagram. Then compare this measurement to the figures given on the Frame Size chart which gives elbow breadth for medium-framed men and women. If your measurement is less, you are smaller-framed and your weight should be at the lower end of the ideal range. Conversely, if your elbow breadth is larger, your weight can be in the higher range.

Medium Size Frames

Height in 1″ heels	Elbow Breadth
Men	
5′2″–5′3″	2½″–2⅞″
5′4″–5′7″	2⅝″–2⅞″
5′8″–5′11″	2¾″–3″
6′0″–6′3″	2¾″–3⅛″
6′4″	2⅞″–3¼″
Women	
4′10″–4′11″	2¼″–2½″
5′0″–5′3″	2¼″–2½″
5′4″–5′7″	2⅜″–2⅝″
5′8″–5′11″	2⅜″–2⅝″
6′0″	2½″–2¾″

Metropolitan Life Insurance Company

Height And Weight Table

1985

Men		Women	
5′1″	105–134	4′10″	92–121
5′2″	108–137	4′11″	95–124
5′3″	111–141	5′0″	98–127
5′4″	114–145	5′1″	101–130
5′5″	117–149	5′2″	104–134
5′6″	121–154	5′3″	107–138
5′7″	125–159	5′4″	110–142
5′8″	129–163	5′5″	114–146
5′9″	133–167	5′6″	118–150
5′10″	137–172	5′7″	122–154
5′11″	141–177	5′8″	126–159
6′0″	145–182	5′9″	130–164
6′1″	149–187	5′10″	134–169
6′2″	153–192		
6′3″	157–197		

U.S. Department of Agriculture
U.S. Department of Health and Human Services

1983

Men		Women	
5′2″	128–150	4′10″	102–131
5′3″	130–153	4′11″	103–134
5′4″	132–156	5′0″	104–137
5′5″	134–160	5′1″	106–140
5′6″	136–164	5′2″	108–143
5′7″	138–168	5′3″	111–147
5′8″	140–172	5′4″	114–151
5′9″	142–176	5′5″	117–155
5′10″	144–180	5′6″	120–159
5′11″	146–184	5′7″	123–163
6′0″	149–188	5′8″	126–167
6′1″	152–192	5′9″	129–170
6′2″	155–197	5′10″	132–173
6′3″	158–202	5′11″	135–176
6′4″	162–207	6′0″	138–179

Metropolitan Life Insurance Company

Nature And Nurture Obese people—20 percent over their ideal weight—are either pear-or apple-shaped, according to Jonathan Kurland Wise, M.D. He and his wife, Susan Kierr Wise, a dance therapist, run a comprehensive weight loss clinic in Boston.

Pear-shaped obesity, in which most of the weight is concentrated on the buttocks and thighs, is hereditary. It's harmless but impossible to get rid of except through a new technique that suctions fat out of the thighs.

The much more common apple-shaped obesity, though not necessarily hereditary, is a health risk associated with diabetes and high levels of cholesterol. It can be dieted off, but not easily. Ninety percent of those who lose weight regain it, warns Dr. Wise, since the ability to burn calories is genetically related.

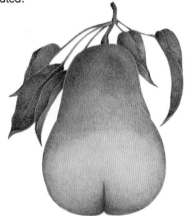

Dieting is fruitless for pear-shaped people.

The 7,000 Calorie A Day Diet You might be able to eat all the fat you want, up to 75 percent of your diet, when you're near the North Pole, with only body heat to keep you warm. The seven human members of the 1986 Steger International North Pole Expedition did just that. They subsisted for two months on two bland meals a day of butter and peanut butter, fatty meat pemmican, noodles and oatmeal. The 50 dogs on the 500-mile trek may have eaten better, on a special diet of dry meat rations.

Walking It Off A pound of fat equals 3,500 calories. Walking an extra 15 minutes a day burns up 450 calories a week, five pounds in a year.

Boring Yourself Thin We generally crave variety more than any particular food, says Barbara Rolls, an associate professor in psychiatry and behavioral sciences at Johns Hopkins School of Medicine in Baltimore. This inborn drive helps to regulate our diets. It also makes us eat more than if we were to eat just one food.

Yet cutting down on variety doesn't necessarily reduce the appetite—boredom brings it quickly back. Learn "how to eat normally," advises Rolls. Eat a variety of foods, without eliminating any particular category, but restricting foods *within* categories. Keep only one flavor of yogurt in the refrigerator, and choose only one kind of cheese from the dessert tray.

A Prayer For Dietary Moderation

I dare not taste one drop of oil
For if I do, my health I'll spoil.
I'd spread my bread with gobs of butter
But that would set my doc aflutter.
Don't serve me poultry, pork or beef
Or I will surely come to grief,
And that fine fish just from the sea
Would, fried, become the death of me.
At breakfast I must never poke
My fork at any golden yolk,
And salt, to which I was a slave
Now lures me to an early grave.
Sugar, friend of childhood, sweet,
Is now a rare, forbidden treat.
A shot of gin, a glass of wine,
A vermouth cassis—sins times nine,
For Nathan Pritikin is my guide,
And by his Law I must abide.
Farewell to all the eats I love.
Farewell, so long, to all the above.
But as I chomp through fields of green
And shrink each day to sinewy lean,
Teach me, Lord, not to wish each
　course
Was rare roast beef with béarnaise
　sauce.

Workout, Pig Out We're exercising more—79 percent of us according to the latest Gallup Poll—yet candy and cheese sales are booming. Some say we've set up "Diet Bank Accounts" in which we hope celery sticks and the gym will compensate for the ice cream we have after our workout. Dart & Kraft, one of the largest U.S. food manufacturers, has capitalized on this paradox by buying both Frusen Glädjé, a premium grade ice cream, and Borg, a manufacturer of bathroom scales.

The Ultimate Diet Aid

Newsweek informs us that if all else fails, dieters can now resort to the Gastric Bubble, developed by gastroenterologists Drs. Lloyd and Mary Garren. The Garrens' soft polyurethane sac is the first device of its kind to have obtained the approval from the U.S. Food and Drug Administration.

For around $2,000, your doctor will insert the uninflated sac into your stomach via a plastic tube. When the tube is withdrawn, the sac inflates to a free-floating cylinder the size of a small juice can that lets you feel pleasantly full without overeating.

The Garrens caution that the bubble must be removed every four months and should only be used as an adjunct to a medically-supervised weight loss program. In tests on 400 patients, gastrointestinal discomfort was the most common side effect; however, seven patients developed ulcers.

Dr. John B. Kral, director of surgical metabolism at St. Luke's-Roosevelt Hospital Center in New York, says, "It's going to be one more diet. And like other diets, people could go on the bubble diet again and again."

But some users are already happy. One satisfied patient has lost 83 pounds during nine months with her Gastric Bubble and plans to lose 60 more. "The balloon makes me feel cozy and comfortable," she reports, "and it has given me time to deal with my emotional reasons for overeating. My satisfaction with food, compared with before I had the bubble, is like night and day." ●

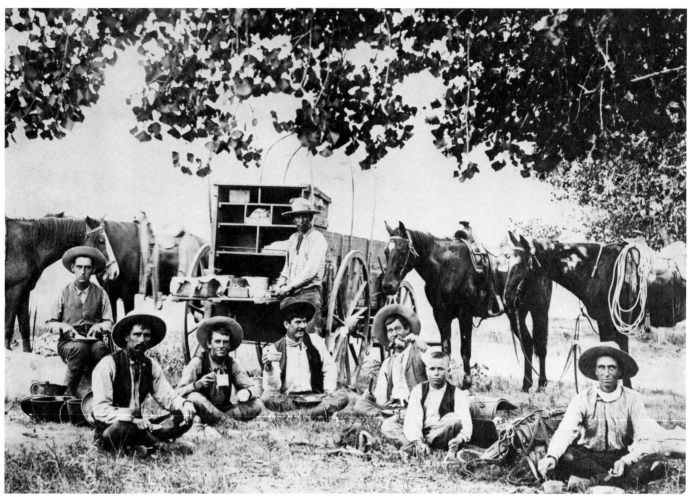

Home on the range, cowboys gather at the chuckwagon and tuck in. But the dish was probably not chili; more likely, son-of-a-bitch stew.

Grease And Gladness

John Thorne

Chili, chili con carne, Texas red—whatever you call that savory concoction of meat, grease and fire—is the natural child of the arguing state of mind. There's no recipe for it, only disputation, and almost anyone's first thought after a taste of somebody else's version, no matter how much it pleasures the throat, is that they could make it better.

Chili naturally brings out that attitude. There's something contentious about Texas red, something so restless, rootless, and just plumb wild, that you never come to terms with it for long. Even your own chili—however good it is—keeps you wrangling.

Chili's restless, ornery nature is why men have made a special effort to claim it as their own. Until recently, it was men who wrote about it and mostly men who made it—or argued their women into fixing it for them. The word itself calls to mind army camps and cowboying and oil-town chili joints crowded with hurried men pouring coffee into their saucers to

blow it cool. This isn't to say that women don't like chili or that they can't make it as good as any man—only that there is something about chili that draws men to it, especially men who otherwise don't have much interest in cooking at all.

These men, at least the ones who first claimed chili and made it their own, did not much agree on anything. They recognized in chili their own fractious nature—and this is why it is its essential character, not any specific ingredient, that makes a real bowl of red.

The great-grandpappy of the chili bowl was the buffalo roast, a great, greasy orgy that was—apart from the yearly drunken sprees at the trader forts when he sold his pelts and restocked his supplies—the mountain man's premier social event and his only contribution to American cuisine.

This gluttonous gorging sprang from more than simple hunger. These men saw themselves as the royalty of the prairie; they claimed their meat to be the best there ever was. Like those who came to

play this same role after them—the cowboys—the trappers rarely had any money. The emblems of pride for these men were their free ways and free meat, a diet half due to craft and half to the sheer boldness of the taking.

None of the earliest authentic cowboy narrative mentions chili, and it is unlikely that this omission was accidental. Chuckwagon cuisine was so strictly codified that every food the cowboy ate can be itemized in a single exhale: chicken-fried steak, beans cooked with fat pork and lick (the cowboy tag for molasses or corn syrup), sourdough biscuits, and, if they were lucky, vinegar pie or a sourdough cobbler of stewed fruit for dessert. With this came all the coffee they could drink, brewed strong enough to chew.

This isn't to say that the early cowboy never ate chili, but when he did, he probably felt mistreated. Anglo cowboys thought Mexican seasoning was generally low class and an insult to good chuckwagon cooking. Also, chili con carne is made with tough, cheap cuts, and cowboys, like the mountain men before them, claimed all the fresh, choice meat they could eat as their natural due. And, except on the poorest ranches, they got it.

Unlike the mountain man, however, the cowboy could not claim his own cow. The closest he came to the conspicuous consumption of the buffalo feast was in the chuckwagon specialty that provides the evolutionary link between buffalo hump and the chili pot—son-of-a-bitch stew. Euphemized as son-of-a-gun or 'that gentleman from Texas,' cowboys reminisced about it with genuine relish long after they had savored their last bite. It and not chili would have been the cowboy's symbolic dish right to today, if civilization hadn't caught up with them first. But, as ranching modernized, the smaller ranches were driven out of business and the larger ones needed less manpower. And, once a cowboy was laid off, he wasn't a cowboy anymore to anyone but himself. To his employers and the world at large, he was a drifter and a boomer and no longer welcome. He had no choice but to head for town and the bigger the town the better. In Texas, one of the towns was San Antonio—where the cowboy was to discover chili and eventually make it his own special brand of grease and gladness.

In the second half of the last century, San Antonio was a wide open town: a cattle town, a railroad town, and an army town. It was the natural focus for sundowners, drifters, loungers, and hangers-on, a significant segment of the population and one always on the lookout for entertainment and ladies of the evening. Their hangout was Military Plaza—just then "the liveliest spot in Texas."

Because he was chronically broke, a cowboy could only enjoy the company of real, card-carrying prostitutes on the rare, bust-out occasions when he rode into town with a pocketful of pay. Once that was gone, and it went quickly, the best he could hope for was to enter into a temporary alliance with a woman who—given her alternatives—would find him an acceptable catch. With her he found shelter, food, and as much company as he cared

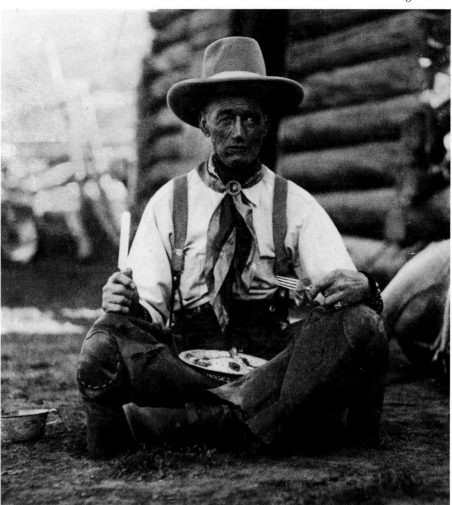

After a day punching cows, this good ole boy knows what's good to the last bite.

for until the ranches were hiring again. And, at least in the early years of cowboy life, it is unlikely that was an Anglo woman, but a Latino-Indian one.

Surely it is in households such as these that the original stew of chilies and chicken or pork was made over into the dish it now is. The woman adapted her cooking to the pleasure of her man, who himself was just prosperous enough—especially in a cattle town—to afford the cheap cuts of meat the dish required, and who had little tolerance for the inexpensive but foreign dishes his woman would otherwise be inclined to make . . . always discounting beans, already familiar cowboy fare.

Texas red, then, began its life as the natural child of a cowboy father and a Latino-Indian mother, and this scandal is why the families of both parents have kept the child at arm's length. There is a common suspicion that there is something unrepentantly vulgar about chili, something stubbornly low class. Its parentage was too clearly displayed to be missed and too scandalous to be admitted. Chili has always been the one Tex-Mex dish that refused to know its place. It

wouldn't pretend to be Mexican nor would it adopt good Anglo manners. It was what it was, and when it grew up and found no welcome on either side of its heritage, it headed straight for the honkytonk side of town.

The chili joint appeared in Texas sometime before the turn of the century and gradually spread across the nation. By the 1920s, it was a familiar if seedy sight just about anywhere west of the Mississippi. It gave the nation a taste for chili and at the same time gave chili the status of ordinary American chow. Nobody who ate a bowl of red in a chili joint ever had the illusion he was eating Mexican food—here at last is chili as we know it, chili peppers and herbs no more than seasoning; the meat everything.

The chili joint itself was no more than a shed or room with some minimal improvement: a counter put up and some stools knocked together, a blanket hung up to privatize the kitchen—which consisted of a wood stove and, most likely, no sink. No need even to hang a sign outside: "Chili 5¢" hand-lettered on a piece of cardboard and propped in the window would bring the customers drifting in.

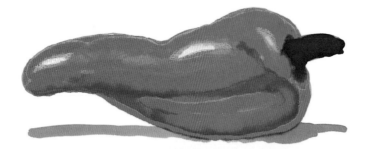

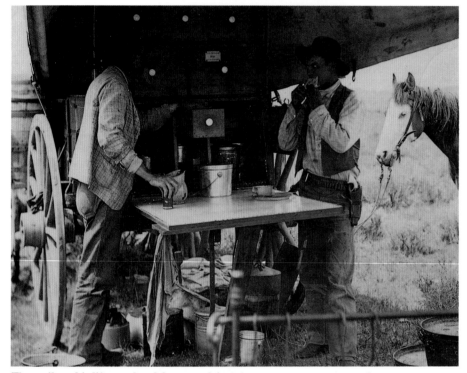

The trail cook's life was hard, but on a drive, there was no one more welcome.

Most likely, the owner was also a cowboy who at one point or another in his career had turned to trail cooking. Unlike the regular ranch cook, the trail cook's position was temporary. He was laid off with the rest of the boys when the year's work was done. The only trade he was qualified for—apart from washing dishes—was running a chili joint. Since he ate in them himself when he was at loose ends, he knew what was required and—even more important—how to handle the clientele.

These were generally a low bunch. Reputable restaurants didn't serve chili in those days any more than did respectable homes. The men who frequented chili parlors were not only hungry but also attracted to chili's wrong-side-of-the-tracks reputation. What that meant was that a chili joint was a man's place, like a pool hall or a saloon, and so eaters could consider themselves "sports" for going to one, and not the almost-paupers they generally were.

Later, when the Depression hit, a man with a nickel would rather go to a chili parlor than a soup kitchen—if there was

one—because it saved him his self-respect. For his five cents, he got a bowl of red, with or without beans, a double handful of crackers to break over, and hot coffee.

He also got companionship. Not necessarily company . . . that depended on the circumstances. He found companionship in the chili. Unlike the usual stew, half-decent chili held its own kept hot on the stove all day; it relished abuse. Because of that, there was no constant reminder in it that the best you could do was second-best. On the contrary, unlike the usual lunch-counter item, chili had the stamp of individuality about it. Each bowl was different and worth contemplation. And, finally, the stuff had some fire to it. A man could mutter to himself that he might take it twice as hot as this, and that gave him a good feeling. It reminded him that he was a cowboy. And if that was the best feeling he was going to get that day, it would do. ●

John Thorne is the writer and publisher of the *Simple COOKING* letter.

HUNTLEY DENT'S TEXAS CHILI
Chili warms the soul.

Serves 8

Ingredients:
2–3 pounds boneless beef chuck, trimmed and cut into ¹/₂-inch cubes
3 tablespoons vegetable oil, approximately
1 pound onions, chopped
¹/₄ cup flour
2–4 cloves garlic, finely chopped
5 cups beef broth
6 tablespoons ground red chilies
2 teaspoons whole or ground cumin
1 teaspoon dried oregano
¹/₂ teaspoon freshly ground pepper
2 teaspoons salt
3 tablespoons cider vinegar
1–2 canned chiles chipotles, chopped

Method:
1. Heat half the oil in a large skillet over moderately high heat. When the oil is hot, brown the beef in 3 or 4 batches to avoid crowding the pan. Add more oil, if needed, to keep the meat from sticking. Transfer each cooked batch to a heavy 4- to 6-quart pot.

2. When all the meat is browned, add more oil, if needed, to make 2 tablespoons of fat in the skillet.

3. Reduce the heat to low, stir in the onions, and cook, covered, for about 5 minutes, until they soften slightly. Uncover the pan, raise the heat to moderate, and cook, stirring frequently, until the onions are lightly colored.

4. Sprinkle the flour over the onions and cook, stirring, for 1 minute, until thoroughly blended. Transfer the onions to the pot with the meat.

5. Add the remaining ingredients, stir, and place over moderate heat and bring to a simmer; reduce the heat to low. Cover the pot and cook, stirring occasionally, for about 1¹/₂ hours. Check the chili during cooking: if too thick, add up to 1 cup water.

6. If you are serving the chili immediately, degrease it first; otherwise, let it cool, refrigerate it, and degrease before reheating.

7. Serve with sourdough bread, flour tortillas, biscuits or cornbread.

Ins And Outs

Potato pancakes and cornmeal crepes with crème fraîche and three different caviars are *in*. Aunt Jemima is *out* to lunch.

Blackened redfish is *in*. Blackened catfish is *in*. Squid ink is *in*. Bluefish is *out*.

Black ravioli with piquant lobster and scallops in a sharp champagne curry sauce is *in*. Fettuccine in Cajun sauce served Japanese Style is *in*.

Red and white radishes are *out*. Black radishes are *in*. Black eggplants are *out*. White eggplants are *in*. White potatoes and white eggs are *out*. Blue potatoes and blue eggs are *in*. Green, red and yellow peppers are *out*. Black peppers are *in*. Black pepper however is *out* and white pepper is not being sneezed at.

Dark and white chocolate are still *in*. So are chocolate pasta, chocolate terrines, chocolate fettuccine and chocolate sushi. Chocolate cheesecake, chocolate bread pudding and chocolate croissants have arrived. Chocolate popcorn, chocolate peanut butter and chocolate potato chips are galloping over the horizon.

Chocolate mousse has been taken off the menu and instead we are combing our mousse into our hair.

Alcohol abuse is *out*. Chocolate abuse is the newest social disease.

Tapas are *in*. So are the nibbles of many other countries. Even if they don't actually exist, we will cheerfully invent them and give the words the right-sounding ethnic endings.

Littlemeals and macrobiotic epiphanies are *in*.

Range-fed chickens are *in*. Wild mushrooms have been tamed and the deer and the antelope are now home on the range.

The alligator that has been around for 130 million years is staging a comeback.

Duck breasts are *in*. Duck legs are nowhere to be found.

Duck sausages are sizzling. Pork sausages are long gone as is the whole idea of heating high on the hog.

Tofu pasta with all-bran Parmesan cheese is *in*. Fiber is moral. The cachet of calcium is incalculable.

Nasturtiums are blossoming in our salads. Nasturtium and cream cheese sandwiches have replaced the heros of yesteryear. Squash blossoms stuffed with goat cheese have found favor with the steak and potatoes crowd. Lemon is the grass of the day. We are

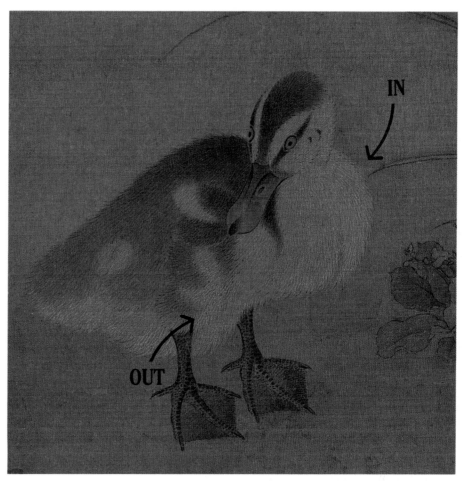

now frolicking to our neighborhood florist for lunch.

Look too on the menus of the *in* restaurants for such delights as caviar on a country biscuit, foie gras on a raisin muffin, brains with pinto beans, sweetbreads with black bean cake and quail eggs on a whole wheat crouton. Steak tartare has been replaced with tuna tartare. Dinner is a bay scallop tied with a very thin, very pink trash fish and garnished with a violet.

Under the influence of the Japanese Empire, all our vegetables are being bonsaied. We are already seeing that a fully grown turnip, once as large as a small pumpkin, has shrunk to the size of a green grape, seedless. Watermelons have been dwarfed to the dimensions of a cherry, pitless. Eggplants have dwindled to the contour of the index finger. Heaven knows that zucchini, which becomes smaller by the season, will either disappear altogether or simply be painted onto the plate as part of the pattern.

Salad dressings and mustards come in more flavors than Baskin-Robbins ever

dreamed possible.

Figs are *in*. Passion fruit is *in*. Fig leaves are *off*.

DoveBars are *in*.

The handmade cheese from the strong-tasting milk of very large, lumbering buffalos is *in*.

The triple-cream, buttery cheeses made from the rich milk of plump cattle grazing in lush green meadows—cheeses that are the glory of France—are *out*.

The food of almost all third world countries is *in*, unless they are unfriendly nations. The Russian Tea Room stands as an exception to the unfriendly nation rule.

Ethnic food is *in*. But couscous goes against the grain. Sushi is *in*. Mexican food is *in*. Tex-Mex is *in*. Mex-Mex is *in*. Arizona-Mex is *in*. Pacific Rim food is *in* though no one knows quite what that is.

Cooking in store windows and in the middle of tiny restaurants is *in*. Cooking in the kitchen is no longer *cool*.

All food that ought rightfully to cost less than $5.00 but is actually priced closer to

HOT HOT CHOCOLATE

$50.00 is much in favor. The noise in the restaurants covers the pain.

The New Young American Chefs are taking courses in public speaking along with lessons in sauce and pastry making.

Waitpersons are competing for the Service Oscar—to be awarded for the most stirring soliloquy in the form of the dramatic reading of the evening's specialty. Those wearing sneakers or nurses' shoes start with a competitive edge.

Liteness has largely replaced cleanliness as being next in line to Godliness. Instant Gratification is our immediate goal.

Rabbits are *in*. Fertility is *in*. The Diet of Denial is *in*. Red meat is *out*, except when it comes in the form of Tex-Mex, Mex-Mex, Arizona-Mex, etc. etc. It is all right to eat red meat as long as it is brown when it is cooked.

Onion marmalade is *in*.

Homemade ketchup is *in*.

Homemade everything is *in*, especially if it comes from the local *take-out* store.

Smoked lobsters are *in*. So are smoked tuna, smoked scallops, smoked oysters, smoked eel and 12 kinds of smoked salmon. Smoked cigarettes are *out*. The idea of smoke-free zones in restaurants is rapidly catching fire.

Gourmet meals in Cryovac packages are very *in*. Lean Cuisine is *thin*. Everything you can cook in a microwave oven is *in*. Microwave ovens however are still *out*, though long range they will be *in*. The idea of radiation is so unpopular the name will soon be changed to 'Cosmic Processing.'

White bread is *out*. Brown bread is *in*. White rice is *out*. Brown rice is *in*. Croissants are still *in*. But croissants filled with hamburgers, hot pastrami, corned beef, bacon, lettuce and tomato and peanut butter are *out*. Snails on a strudel are *in*. Muffins are *in* but only if it takes two hands to lift them from the plate.

Chili is *hot*.

Cranberries and pumpkins are *in*. Star fruit is *in*. Decaffeinated herbal tea is *in*. Double espresso is also *in*.

Fortunes are being made in afternoon tea.

No-oil salad dressings are *in*.

No-lettuce salads are *in*.

Breakfast is *in*, but only if it is eaten *out*. Eating *out* is *in*. Eating *in* is *in*. Eating *take-out* food is *in*. Eating *outside* is *in*. Eating Real Meals is, however, quite definitely *far out*. ●

Linnaeus, that long-ago Swedish botanist who spent his lifetime giving Latin names to plants (and to himself as well—he was born Linne), chose an especially apt one for the cacao tree. *Theobroma* he called it—food of the gods. The name was at once a tribute to the chocolate it produced and to the history it carried with it, for the Aztecs reserved the drinking of chocolate for their godlike royalty. The emperor Montezuma was served his 50-cup-a-day ration in golden goblets. Each goblet was thrown away after a single use, thereby sustaining the emperor in style and anticipating the disposable drinking cup by about 400 years.

Chocolate has been praised as an aphrodisiac, denounced as a narcotic by the city fathers of Bayonne, viewed with indifference by the Spanish court upon Columbus's fourth return from the New World, dumped as worthless cargo by pirates preying on trans-Atlantic shipping, rejoiced in by Quakers who regarded it as a substitute for gin, and recently touted as a replacement for the feeling of being in love because one of its components called phenylethylamine is produced by the human brain in increased quantities when it considers itself in love. Eating or drinking it undoubtedly leads to chocophilia, of which there have been three large-scale outbreaks.

The first global epidemic can be attributed to the conquistador Hernando Cortes, when he brought the cacao bean back to Spain in 1528. The chocolate Cortes tasted in Mexico had been a thick and bitter brew, but with

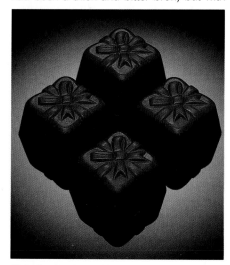

Four to go . . .

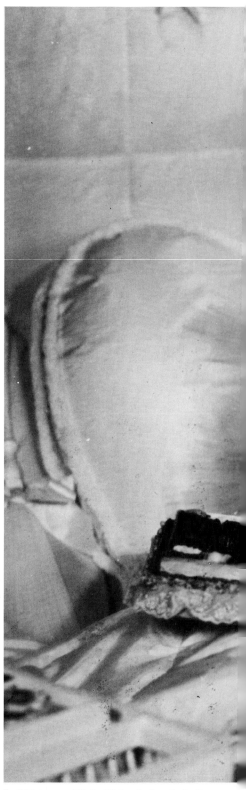

In "Dinner at Eight," blonde bombshell

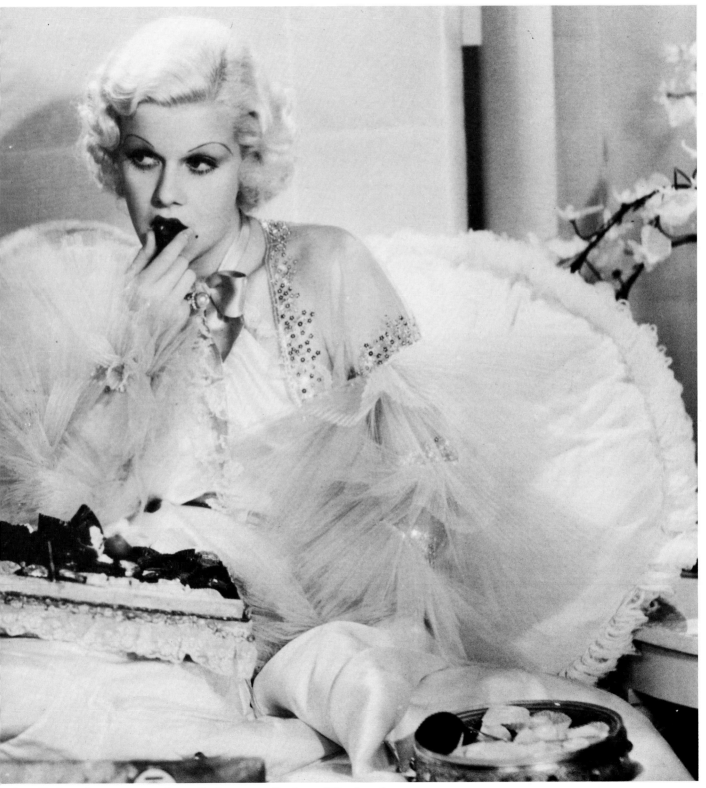

Jean Harlow plays a pampered poopsie, here consoling herself the American way.

the addition of vanilla, sugar and water by the Spaniards it was transformed. (So, too, were the teeth of the Spanish court.) They also added chili peppers, anise, powdered roses, nuts and cinnamon on occasion. Despite the additives the drink swept the country, or at least the nobility who could afford it. Somehow Spain managed to keep chocolate both a secret and a monopoly for almost 100 years.

And then word got out. Before long, the drink had warmed the hearts of French courtiers and chocolate fever spread across the continent. Dentistry was the result.

The first advertisement for "this excellent West India drink" appeared in 1657 in England, where chocolate was selling for half its weight in gold. The ad established London's first chocolate house (and quite possibly the pricing policy of "continental" restaurants). Finally, in the year before the Revolutionary War, cacao beans returned to their native continent with the opening of the first chocolate factory in the colonies, now known as Baker's Chocolate. The American drink was similar to the one mixed in Spain, but it was diluted with milk instead of water, and it was served hot. During all the time of the first chocophilia epidemic, chocolate was served only as a beverage, and so things remained until 1847.

In England, the 19th century was the hey-day of the gentleman-scientist, the naturalist, the back-yard inventor. And someone at the firm of J. S. Fry and Sons (now merged with Cadbury's) combined these pursuits and what he came up with was . . . the candy bar. Simple, really, when you think about it. All that was needed was to add some extra cocoa butter (extracted in the process of making cocoa) back into the paste of ground and roasted cacao beans, to mix in a little sugar, and to cool the chocolate in a mold. Early candy bars were rough-textured and crude, but once the second chocophilia epidemic got under way and improvements came thick and fast, chocolate became thick and smooth.

Soon the Swiss got into the act, inventing machinery to knead the chocolate paste until its flavor was intense and its texture that of a baby's skin. Thus encouraged, an Alpine baby food maker named Henri Nestlé developed a method for incorporating condensed milk into the candy, creating milk chocolate and Switzerland's reputation as a haven for foreign money seeking chocolate. Back in the United States Milton Hershey took out the condensed milk and put in fresh whole milk and the Hershey Bar was born. Another U.S. landmark was the Goo Goo Cluster, a melange of marshmallows, caramel, peanuts and milk chocolate, the world's first combination candy bar, introduced in 1912 and still being made today. ●

Ruth Epstein, editor, *The American Festival*

Never Say Americans Don't Have Their Priorities Straight Last year $4 billion was spent on chocolate in the U.S., which is a bit more than the amount spent on personal-computer hardware and software put together.

She Oughta Know According to Helen Gurley Brown, "Chocolate goes very well with sex: before, during, after—it doesn't matter," though it has been reliably reported that she herself does not like it (chocolate).

Does Chocolate Contain Caffeine? Yes. An ounce of chocolate has 5 milligrams of caffeine. By way of comparison, one cup of coffee has about 100 milligrams and a cup of tea about 35.

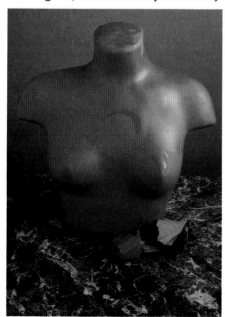

A chocolate anatomical delight.

IRENA CHALMERS' CHOCOLATE TRUFFLES
Virtue exults in excess.

Makes about 4 dozen

Ingredients:
1/2 cup sugar
1/2 cup whole almonds
1 tablespoon vegetable oil
6 ounces semisweet or bittersweet chocolate
4 tablespoons unsalted butter
2 tablespoons Grand Marnier or rum
The grated zest of 1 orange
2 tablespoons heavy cream
4 ounces semisweet chocolate
1/2 cup unsweetened cocoa

Method:
1. Put the sugar in a small heavy saucepan over low heat and cook until it has melted into caramel.

2. Add the almonds and cook until the mixture turns a rich dark brown. Be careful that the caramel does not burn.

3. Pour the hot mixture onto an oiled cookie sheet and spread with a metal frosting spatula to form a thin, even layer. Leave to cool, then grind to a fine powder in a blender or food processor. This is the praline powder.

4. Melt the 6 ounces of chocolate in the top section of a double boiler set over hot water. Stir in the butter, Grand Marnier or rum, grated orange zest, cream and praline powder. Chill for 1 hour.

5. Shape the mixture into balls about 1/2 inch in diameter and freeze until firm.

6. Melt the remaining 4 ounces of chocolate in the top section of a double boiler set over hot water. Cool to lukewarm. Roll each truffle in the melted chocolate. This is best done by putting a little of the melted chocolate in the palm of your hand and rolling the truffle in the chocolate until it is thinly coated.

7. Spread the cocoa powder on a sheet of wax paper and roll the truffles in the cocoa.

8. Store in an airtight container and use within a week; otherwise, the truffles may be wrapped, first in plastic, then in foil, and frozen.

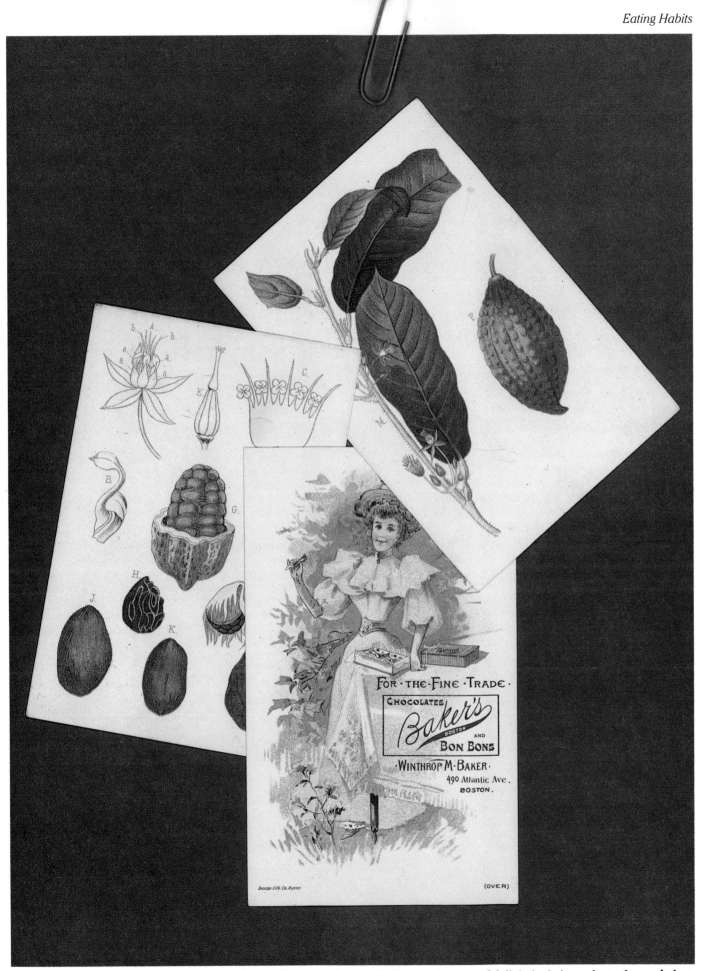

Promoting chocolates in Victorian times, Baker's trading cards featured both cocoa beans and delight in their product—the candy box.

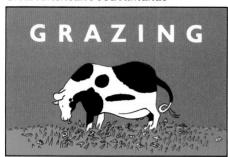

GRAZING

Table Of No Contents

In the first seven months of 1985, the A.J. Canfield Company of Chicago sold 101 million cans of a new drink they developed called Diet Chocolate Fudge Soda. How can anything with chocolate fudge in it be a "diet" drink? Here's how. This drink contains *no* chocolate fudge and not much else either. It is 100 percent artificial, with the aroma and simulated taste of chocolate, and it delivers four calories per can.

New entries in the No Contents Sweepstakes:

- Diet Shasta Chocolate Fudge
- Diet Nehi Chocolate Soda
- Yoo-Hoo Diet Chocolate Fudge Soda
- Famous Amos Diet Chocolate Sundae Soda
- Famous Amos Diet Chocolate Soda
- Famous Amos Diet Chocolate Rocky Road Soda.

Other manufacturers are looking now for an upscale No Contents chocolate beverage with "snooty appeal."

Something with truffles, we wager.

Virtuous Oil

The International Olive Oil Council wishes the world to know that olive oil is:

1. of all oils, the one best absorbed by the intestines;
2. an enemy of ulcers and gastritis;
3. consumed the most in two places where cardiovascular fatalities are rarest: Greece and Crete;
4. an impeder of the blood platelet aggregation which can cause arterial thrombosis;
5. helpful in preventing the wear and tear of age on the functions of the brain, and on the aging of tissues and organs in general;
6. of an ideal chemical composition.

In short, the oil of the olive is just about perfect in every way.

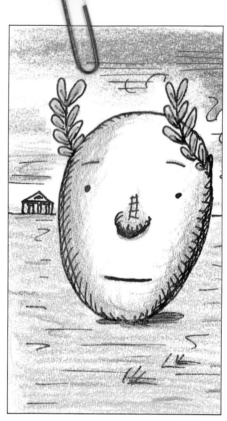

Garbage Significance William Rathje is professor of anthropology at the University of Arizona, where a study called the Garbage Project has been going on for 13 years. Says Rathje, "The food that we throw away can be very revealing." Among the study's findings:

¶ Halloween garbage contains candy wrappers but no candy, while Valentine's Day garbage contains both wrappers and candy. "On Halloween what's important is the candy; on Valentine's Day what's important is the gesture," Rathje concludes. (One could also conjecture that children do not throw away candy, but some adults do.)

¶ The more repetitious a family's diet is, the less food they throw away. (They keep buying the same limited number of foods and eating them up without wastage.)

¶ Paradoxically, there is more discarding of foods that people think are in short supply than those they see as abundant. This is basically because they tend to overbuy the "scarcer" foods, which then go bad before getting eaten up.

¶ Buying of processed foods such as TV dinners does not mean that other foods won't be thrown out. TV dinners are completely eaten—in preference to fresh food that requires work to prepare. More fresh food is thrown out—eventually. ●

Kool Kids Fifty-nine-year-old Kool-Aid is reaching for a new lease on life with ads pitched to children, designed to show adults as fools. "Make adults into bumbling bozos and the kids will love you," says an ad agency spokesman.

Food Flies

Pick an airline meal, any airline meal. George Honchar has eaten it.

Airline food is a subject near and dear to the heartburn of Honchar, president of Miss Universe Inc.

He began taking pictures of airline meals five years ago and has amassed six folders stuffed with airline entree slides.

His worst meal: spinach quiche. The best? "I don't think I've had a memorable *good* meal," he says.

A jet peeve: harried attendants.

"I've seen every sort of accident," Honchar says. "I've seen flying chateaubriand."

During one "food caper," whipped cream squirted over the front of a passenger's blue suit.

"While he was cleaning that mess," Honchar says, "another stewardess lost control of a ball of ice cream and it plopped into the guy's open briefcase."

Honchar once ordered a Piedmont optional breakfast recommended by his sister.

"She got a cheese omelet and braised tomatoes, as opposed to the little hockey puck steak and weird scrambled eggs," Honchar says.

But an attendant presented him with a bowl of puffed rice. Initially taken aback, Honchar decided "puffed rice would be sort of enchanting," he says. "I tried to peel off the Saran Wrap, but all the puffed rice kept clinging to it because of the static electricity."

As soon as Honchar removed the seal, realization struck—his overhead air vent was blowing full force.

"That finished emptying the bowl," he says. "Puffed rice was all over the plane. It just blew away. I didn't get a picture of that meal."

USA TODAY

Potato Chips The average American consumes a total of 17 pounds per year, which is 110 calories for every single day for every single—*or* married—person, who is thus adding annually over 40 *thousand* calories to his or her intake of food, truly a staggering (or should we say waddling) total.

How Many New Food Products Are Launched Annually In This Country?
Currently about 2,000—and the number rises by about ten percent each year.

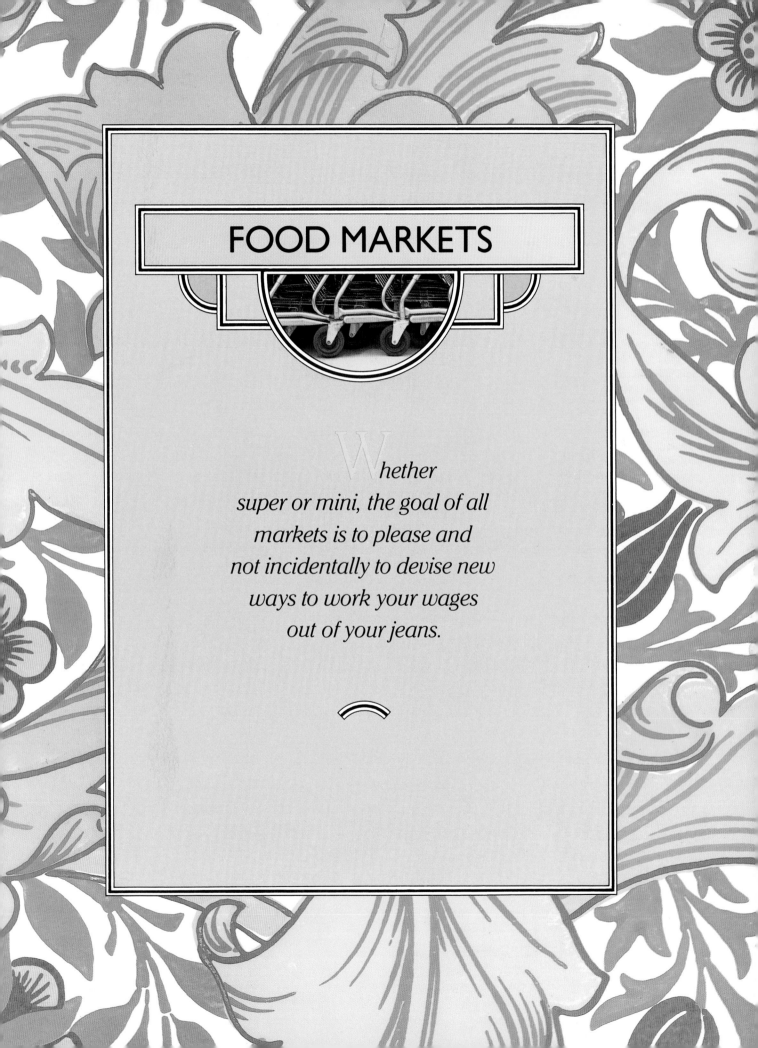

FOOD MARKETS

*Whether
super or mini, the goal of all
markets is to please and
not incidentally to devise new
ways to work your wages
out of your jeans.*

TO MARKET, TO MARKET

Once upon a time, not very long ago, everybody shopped for their groceries at Mom-and-Pop's corner store. And a few Mom-and-Pop shops still exist and even thrive. But for nearly 40 years now, it is the supermarket that has held sway over the American landscape. It draws the local crowds, and draws to itself, as well, strings of satellite shops, banks and gas stations which nestle at the edges of its vast parking lots. In the lots are gaggles of empty, abandoned shopping carts, rolling aimlessly across the macadam or resting, temporarily, against any convenient bumper.

Chains and changes

There are now just under 30,000 supermarkets in the United States, ringing up over $200 billion in annual sales. But the profile of the typical supermarket customer is no longer the housewife 18 to 49 years old with 1 husband, 2 to 3 children and 1 dog at home. For one thing, the dog has changed into a cat, as it is less trouble to look after a cat. And because traditionally, the dog and cat food aisle has been the most profitable one in any supermarket, expect to pay more for your salami when the dog food profit center is lost!

Today, new categories of customers have center stage in the minds of supermarket magnates. Bolder managements are moving "upscale" to cater to the youth market which, in five years, will represent 50 percent of the entire customer headcount. The demand here is for convenience, value, new products and one-portion packages. Other managements spy upon comparably specific communities. The over-55 group is one: It will total over 63 million people in 1990 and represents 30 percent of the customer count; another is the Hispanic population—it will grow to 25 to 35 million people in the next half-decade.

As a result, the supermarket industry is in a fine state of turmoil, confusion and change. Some chains are being redesigned and drastically rethought, as in the case of Grand Union.

Others are expanding, either growing

1930 This radically new store created a revolution in the American food market.

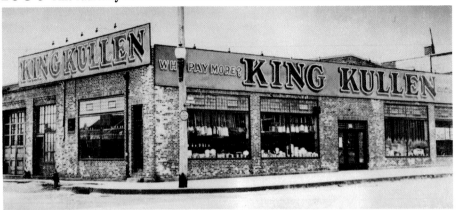

Smart copy caught the mood of the time; people felt that Kullen was on their side.

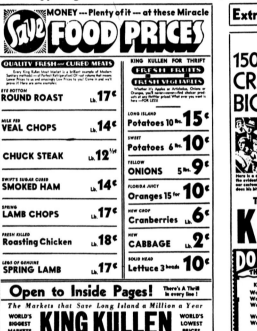

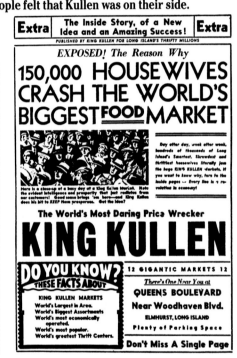

Precursors abounded: Down South, cash 'n carry was a Piggly Wiggly rule by 1918.

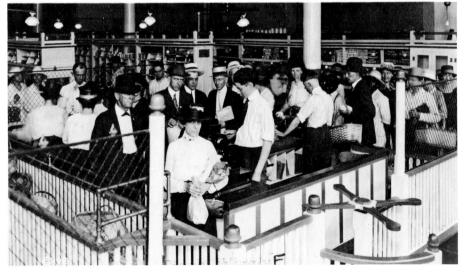

1986 Milton Glaser's facade design for Grand Union functions too as a billboard.

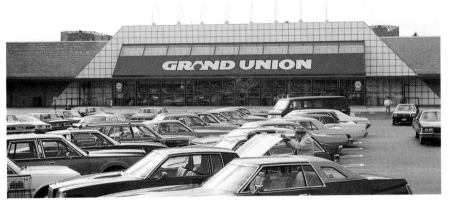

Charming graphics coax the folks into a sense that Grand Union is on their side.

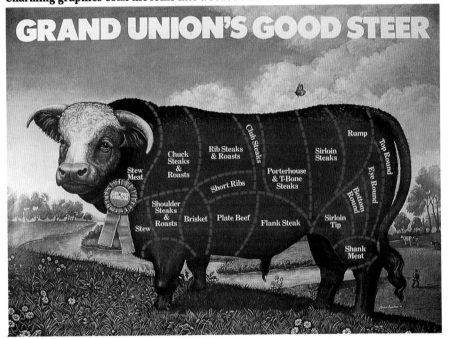

Checking out in style: egress is sleek, polished; terms, still cash 'n carry.

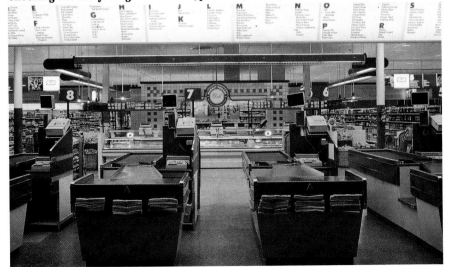

into huge so-called hypermarkets where you can buy everything from hair spray to Harlequin novels and videos to violets (a must to decorate the warm goat cheese salad), or turning into warehouse shopping barns that are largely self-service, with huge bins filled with everything from carrots to cognac.

New products for new buyers

Surprisingly, many large food industry manufacturers have been slow to respond to the changing panorama of supermarket customers. But the very large supermarket chains are joining with each other to bring greater pressure on the mammoth food processing companies such as General Foods and General Mills to provide them with lower prices, deeper discounts, more advertising dollars, more food for sampling and more efficient computer-to-computer ordering.

Service: the latest frill

In-house nutritionists and in-house chefs for the take-out department mark the leading edge of the new competition in special customer services. The established super-supermarkets are competing against each other to obtain the largest possible volume of customers in a given neighborhood. And in a concerted effort to win customer loyalty, today's weapons are the subtle seduction of amazing services and luxurious convenience.

Already we are seeing that the largest and most profitable stores are offering such amenities as baby care, insurance sales and tax advice, travel planning, mail service, hunting licenses and bill-paying for utilities, along with an ever increasingly dazzling array of fresh fruit and vegetables from local farmers, and more and more exotic specialty foods.

In yet another form of service, supermarkets are trying to make it *fun* for people to flock to them and to make it *easy* to prepare the food that is bought there. Chains in Washington, D.C. and New Jersey and many other states are concentrating on so-called "value-added" products. If you crave a Chinese meal, you can buy neatly cut-up vegetables, sauces and chicken or beef—packaged together with a recipe. A pork roast can be bought with a ready-made stuffing, and the Caesar salad is sold along with the dressing. Choices are almost unlimited: You can cook a meal yourself, buy it from the take-out section, opt from the deli counter or pluck it from the freezer and deposit it into the microwave oven. And while you're right there, you can buy the paper plates, the candles, the flowers, the wine glasses and the wine cooler—an entire meal service at your fingertips.

As eating out for every meal becomes more and more costly and food shopping becomes easier and easier, there is going to be a swing to "back home" for dining and entertaining. And eating at home is good news for supermarkets, hypermarkets, folksy warehouse shopping barns and even for Mom-and-Pop. The shopping cart won't be rolling into the Smithsonian any time soon. Look for it now in your local supermarket parking lot. ●

Old Fashioned Service

By 1934 the grocery store was no longer the haven of the idle male. It had become the hangout of the women: air-conditioning, rest rooms for women customers, chairs for youngsters . . .

Of course, the store became a super social institution, where ladies made appointments with each other to visit, drink a "Coke," and buy their bags of groceries. Clerks were dressed down for failing to dress up; ties were compulsory.

The positive approach was the thing, and butcher Clarence Hall once overdid it, when late on a Saturday evening a lady came to buy a chicken. Hall reached in the case and brought out his last chicken. He showed it to the lady, but she characteristically wanted to see a larger one. Hall put the chicken back in the case, bent over, moved his arms about, rattled the ice a little—as if looking for the right sized one—and ceremoniously came back up with the same chicken. The customer replied with a very satisfied smile: 'Yes, that one is just fine. I'll take both of them.' ●

William Henry Holman

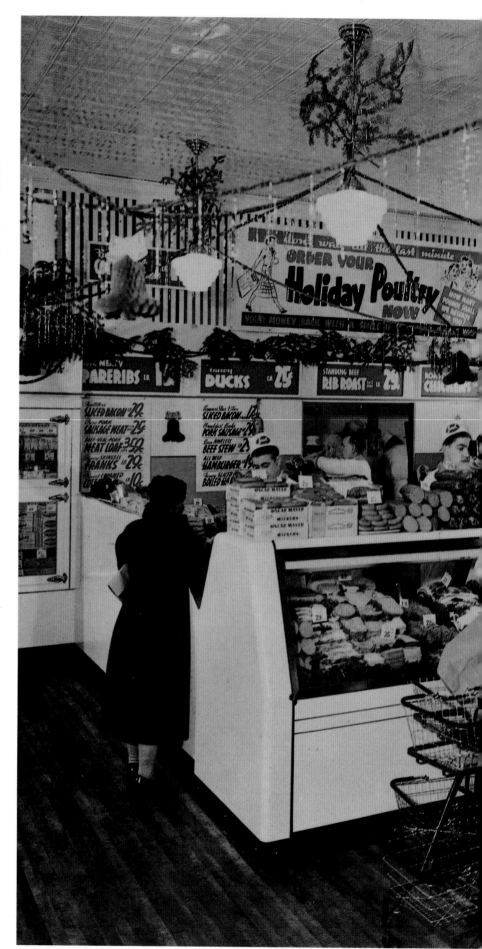

At Christmas in 1938, fancy ducks were going for 25 cents per pound. Note, too, the gleamin

Conversation With a Grocer

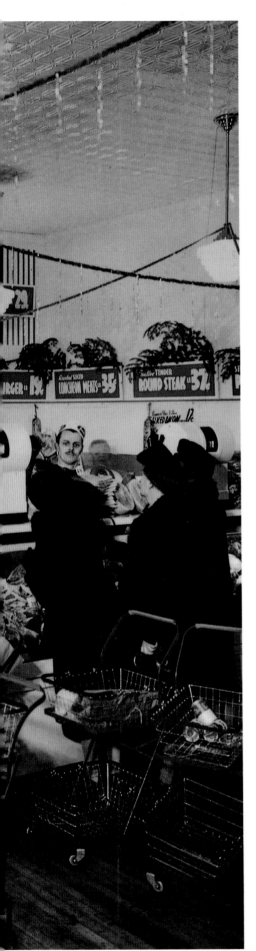

When I was a teenager, I ran from the family grocery business. I went off to Georgia Tech, but I dropped out and took off for Florida. I sold numbers for mailboxes, door to door, and when that failed, I cleaned restaurant kitchens for a while. I wanted in the worst way to hop a freighter for Cuba, but there weren't any at that time, so I worked construction to get the plane fare over there. I never could find steady work in Havana, and I lost 25 pounds just trying to earn the fare home. I went back to Tech and graduated, and then I went into the service during the Korean conflict. After all that, I was darn glad to come back home to the business.

So, Mr. Holman, how does it feel to be a grocer, after all these years?
The grocery business is people, dealing with people—it's the most exciting job there is. And each week, you know, I can look and see how I'm doing. The rewards are immediate and the customers will keep you on your toes.

At first, I thought I couldn't do anything better than my father; maybe that's what made me leave in my early years. But then I realized that our business was small—smaller than A & P, Kroger, or Safeway—and that we had room to grow. Once I realized what I could do for the company, I got over my fear. And I know, now, that if my father were to see me, he would be pleased. Sure, many people could have done better. I probably should have done better. Yes, I should have. But then, this isn't an easy business—a lot of people over the years have gone broke.

Do you ever miss the days when the business was smaller, Mr. Holman?
Of course. When we were small, things were fun. You knew everyone and you had your hands on every decision. I guess, compared to New York, we are still small; $400 million a year *is* small compared to the market giants. But still, I can't have my hands on everything anymore.

When your business is small you can tell everyone what to do. Even now that is one of my greatest temptations. But that is not my place anymore. As we've grown, we've had to make some management changes. If you don't change you'll fail.

Mr. Holman, does that keep you up at nights?

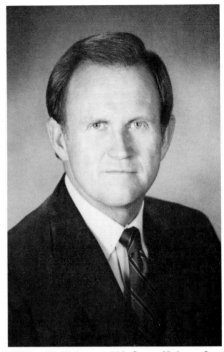

William H. Holman of McCarty-Holman Inc.

No, what keeps me up at nights is a resignation by a member of our staff, or even the possibility of a resignation. It really grieves me when there is a problem within the ranks. You know, this business can be like a ministry, if you let it!

Would you wish this business on your son? Would you like to see him assume leadership?
I would hope this to be so. He loves people. He would have a wonderful opportunity here, but of course there are other children, too, and you can never tell.

The world is so complex now: There are legal deals, computer deals and all manner of other deals to handle. I went up to Harvard not long ago, along with 40 other company presidents, and I found out that there are a lot of smart men and women in this grocery business. Most are much smarter than I. So whoever runs this business in the future will have to be smart. But that person will also have a wonderful opportunity. ●

William Henry Holman has led his Jackson, Mississippi-based grocery business from a $17 million business in 1967 to a $400 million business in 1985. He now serves as the president and chief executive of McCarty-Holman Co., Inc. His company has also seen an increase from 38 stores to 51 and an increase from 1700 employees to over 3500.

Holman is now the chairman of the board of the largest food buying co-op in the world, TOPCO. Their retail sales exceed $18 billion every year.

stamped ceiling and polished hardwood floor.

How May I Help You?
Whirr, Click, Beep

Never heard of J. Bildner? Well, look out, because he's heard of *you*, and he's coming at you right now with what he calls "the high-tech end of food."

Bildner opened his first J. Bildner & Sons in Boston in 1984; by the end of 1986 he will have 20 stores and 18 "gourmet boutiques" in various parts of the country. "We see ourselves," he says, "as a unique microchip rushing to market."

One of the store's most appealing offers is "dinner with a movie," in which you get a rental VCR and the cassette of your choice along with the meal. And if there's something you forgot to pick up on your way home, your Bildner deliver-

person will collect it en route to you.

The exciting new word for all this micro-chippery is "service." It's synonymous with J. Bildner & Sons. It's also what Mom-and-Pop stores offered long years ago, before the rise of supermarkets drove credit and carryout and delivery and "thank you" out of the marketplace.

All this proves that there's nothing new under the sun, and nothing that can't be revived with the right economy and the right technology. And the right timing.

Look out for Bildner. He's determined to give us what we want . . . now that we know what that is. ●

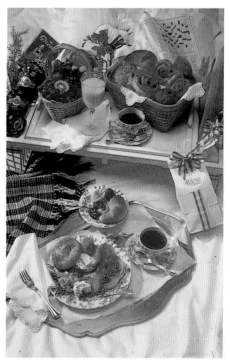

Breakfast as delivered by J. Bildner & Sons

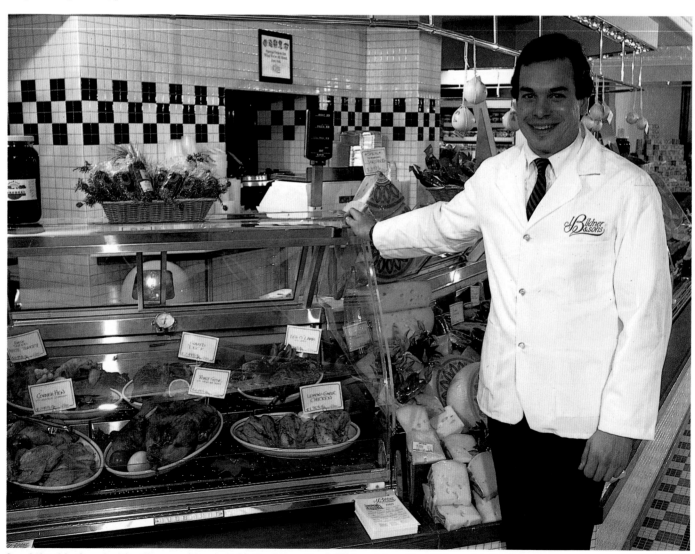

Sparkling black and white tiles provide a suitable backdrop for J. Bildner himself and his sophisticated wares.

Cashing In On The Wow Factor

Leslie Wells's recent expedition to the new Cub Foods store in Melrose Park, Illinois, was no ordinary trip to the grocery store. "You go crazy," says Ms. Wells, sounding a little shell-shocked.

The difference between Cub and most supermarkets is obvious the minute a shopper walks through Cub's doors. The entryway aisle, called by some "power alley," is lined two stories high with specials like bean coffee at $2 a pound and half-price apple juice. Cub's wider-than-usual shopping carts, which are supposed to encourage expansive buying, fit easily through Cub's wide aisles, channeling shoppers toward high-profit impulse foods.

Cub didn't invent the warehouse store, and it's far from the only company in the business. But since 1968 when "Jack" Hooley opened the first store in the Minneapolis suburb of Fridley, Cub has worked on perfecting its own formula: low prices made possible by rigidly controlled costs and high-volume sales, and exceptionally high quality for produce and meats.

A Cub store stocks as many as 25,000 items, double the selection of conventional stores. This leads to overwhelming displays—including 88 kinds of hot dogs and sausages. And the assortment is sprinkled with gourmet items, exotic fresh seafood, like octopus and rarities like banana blossoms, cactus leaves and fresh sugar cane.

"I laughed all through the store, it was so much fun," says Sheila Williams, another shopper. Ms. Williams's enthusiasm was also expressed in dollars: she spent about $40 more than she had planned. ●

The Wall Street Journal

Why The Super Warehouse Store? "The supermarket is sort of like an old DC-3 airplane," says Michael O'Connor, a Chicago-based food industry consultant. "It's been great to fly, but we can't afford to pay the pilot, the co-pilot and the guy who waves the sticks. It doesn't go fast enough."

The Wall Street Journal

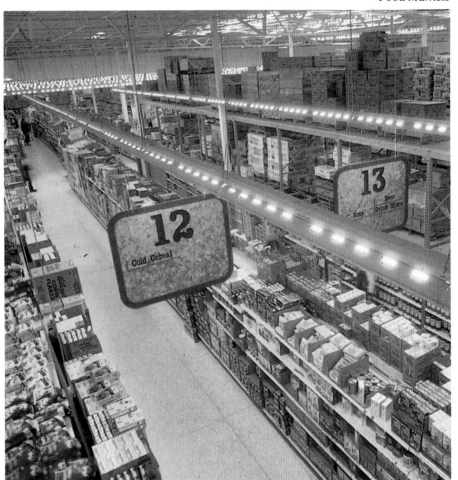

Cereal by the mile, warehouse style, lining the aisles of a Cub store.

Cannery Woe

As the passion for fresh produce has grown exponentially, so dust has slowly settled over the canned goods sections of America's supermarkets. Recent sales of canned peas were down 27 percent, corn down 17 percent and snap beans down 9 percent—and these are the Big Three, accounting for over a third of all canned vegetable sales. Only canned tomatoes (for pasta, presumably) are on the rise. Canned asparagus is down 53 percent and leafy greens are down 61 percent. Efforts to combat this downward trend have met with some success. For example, Del Monte found that when they packed vegetables without added salt, they won 23 percent of the market share—their largest ever.

Meanwhile, Continental Can has developed the revolutionary Veri-Green process to stabilize the chlorophyll in canned green vegetables, giving them a better color, texture and flavor. Introduced coast to coast in 1985 by S & W, Veri-Green is still proving out. "We did substantial research," said Jack Miller, Continental Can spokesman, "and discovered that most people achieve a balanced diet by choosing colors. In vegetables, the brighter the green color, the greater the perceived vitamin content of the product. So we set out to develop a process that would make canned vegetables more green." The result: a 40 percent increase in the sale of peas.

Stokely's of Oconomowoc, Wisconsin is also involved. They are now marketing Veri-Green peas, and beans may be introduced in 1986.

"Eventually," says Miller "all vegetables that were green to begin with will be Veri-Green." ●

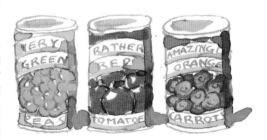

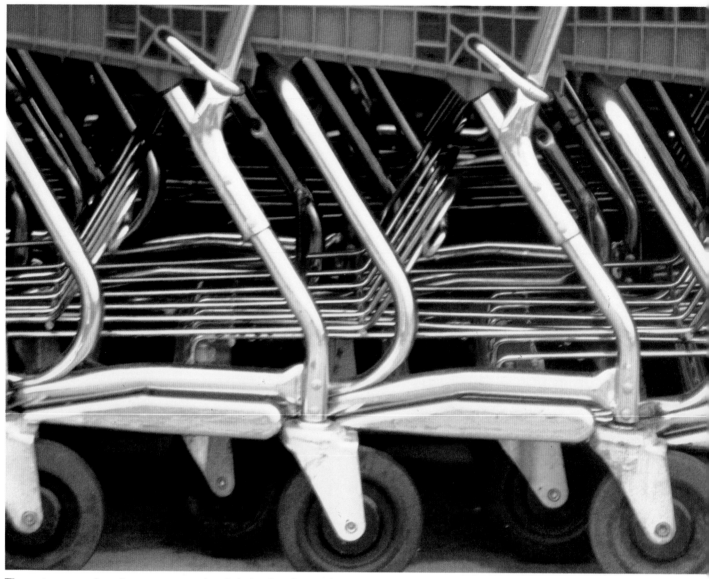

The carts are coming, the carts are coming, in knitted ranks, ready to go.

Cart-Ography

The unsung inventor of the supermarket cart is Sylvan N. Goldman, an Oklahoma City grocer who noticed, way back in 1937, that shoppers tended to stop buying when their shopping baskets weighed too heavily on their arms. An electric light bulb labeled *shopping cart* flashed on above his head, and he proceeded to invent one.

Goldman's first fantasy was of a kind of armchair on wheels, but his scheme went through many collapsing prototypes until it emerged as two wire baskets on four flexible tires.

Proudly, Goldman introduced his invention into his store. Coldly, shoppers rejected the outlandish thing. Shrewdly, Goldman took a notion: he hired attractive people of both sexes to push the carts along his aisles, "shopping" casually.

Monkey see, monkey do. And we have all been doing it ever since.

¶ The classic supermarket cart that we know and love today costs anywhere from $70 to $90 brand-new.

¶ Every year, some 12½ percent of all existing carts are "lost," and must be replaced. To avoid this expense, managements have hit upon the idea of creating blockades at their doors, to prevent egress and vagrancy of carts. Others have found it to be more cost-effective to employ low-cost bag boys, who deliver groceries to shoppers' cars. (This is a coveted job, as it is the only one in the supermarket that warrants tips from grateful customers.)

¶ The Minyard supermarket chain, based in Dallas, has given thought to the cart needs of the handicapped shopper. Each of its stores is now provided with one or more wheelchair-adapted carts (see photo). These cost twice as much as ordinary carts, but the cost may well be offset by increased patronage and good will from customers.

¶ Because the aisles of supermarkets are thoroughfares for carts, and speeding cart-pushers are a constant hazard, some managements now provide seat belts for babies and other tiny cart passengers.

¶ In some supermarkets, carts are used for delivering commercials as well as groceries. Colorful boards, slotted into the sides of carts and in constant view of shoppers, advertise products available and "specials of the day."

¶ Carts to come will be highly sophisticated versions of the Model T's we know today. Visionaries expect that the cart of tomorrow will be equipped with a small video screen which will chat to the customer as the cart rolls down the aisles, perhaps extolling the goodness of soups in the canned-food section or demonstrating how to stuff a turkey during a visit to the poultry counter. The shopper's video friend may also have a good

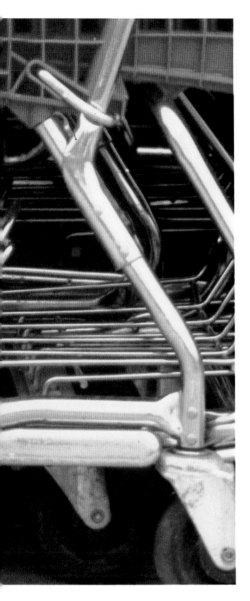

Checking Out

¶ *The Wall Street Journal* reports this story: As a grey-haired woman buying groceries at a supermarket here walked down the checkout aisle, a buzzer sounded and a red light blinked on. Other shoppers turned and stared. The woman's face turned red. She pulled out two rib eye steaks, then paid about $6 for them. The manager doesn't think she will ever shoplift again. ''The embarrassment was punishment enough,'' he says.

¶ Then there's the one about the woman who hid a frozen chicken under her hat. All might have been well, except that she had to wait so long in the check-out line that she fainted from rapid heat loss. As she slid to the floor, the chicken fell from its roost and rolled out into plain view. She had inadvertently cooked her own goose.

The jig is just about up for the shopper who drops a package of steaks—absentmindedly, of course—into the folds of a voluminous garment. More and more, supermarkets are wrapping tiny electronic tracking devices inside expensive items. If the item is borne past the checkout stand without being registered and paid for, the device will emit a piercing wail, and a heavy, restraining hand will fall upon the shoulder of the bearer thereof. ●

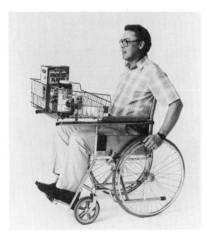

For the disabled shopper, an enabling cart.

word to say for in-store services such as banking and travel booking and will urge the shopper to dial advice from the in-store home economist. What these carts will cost has not been determined, but their re-sale value is expected to be high. ●

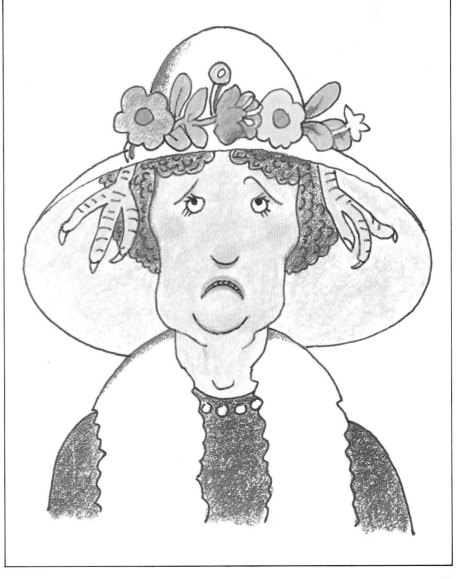

Cassettes To Keep Kids Safe

The Stop & Shop Supermarkets Co., based in Boston, has introduced a free video-cassette lending library to teach children how to protect themselves. The tapes are geared to youngsters between the ages of 5 and 18.

Entitled "Kids, Drugs and Alcohol" and "Use Your Smarts—Don't Go With Strangers," the tapes are being made available on a one-day loan basis in all Stop & Shop supermarkets located in Massachusetts, New York, Connecticut and Rhode Island.

"Parents, community leaders and educators are being challenged to teach children how to protect themselves at younger ages than ever before," says Christine Filardo, Director of Consumer Affairs for Stop & Shop Supermarkets. "We want to make the tapes available to as many families, community and educational groups as possible."

Stop & Shop's free videocassette lending library was introduced in March 1985 in the Massachusetts stores. The response to the first tape, "Use your Smarts—Don't Go With Strangers," was so positive that the chain decided to open up video libraries in all 118 Stop & Shop units this past summer. ●

Progressive Grocer

Young And Contradictory A recent poll among girls aged 13 to 19 found that 60 percent of them do much of the family shopping and an additional 28 percent do some of it. (Also, an amazing 72 percent of them do much of the cooking.) These young shoppers are very responsive to food advertising, and they buy at both ends of the nutrition scale, from calorie-controlled boil-in-the-bag meals to calorie-catastrophic binge or junk foods. As an example, due to the impact of youth, annual sales of diet dinners recently passed the $1 billion mark, while at the same time, ice cream sales were pushing two billion.

Now You See It, Now You Don't The dyes used in some product packaging have been developed to change color as time goes by, so that staff will know how long a given item has been on the shelf. Only the staff knows, however, where the rainbow ends.

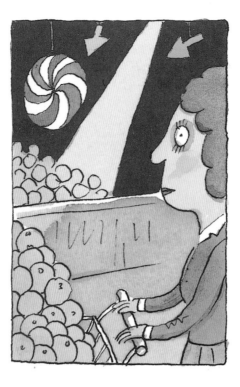

East Is East And West Is — Different Nancy Arum, cookbook author and food writer, and a New Yorker born and bred, has sent the following dispatch from Los Angeles:

"There is a different cuisine culture here. It's obvious from the calls a local radio food show received just before Thanksgiving.

"The first caller wanted to know if she could defrost her turkey in the sauna.

"Another called to say that the turkey prepared according to a recipe hadn't browned properly. This one wondered if a few minutes under the sunlamp might do the trick.

"This is:
C*A*L*I*F*O*R*N*I*A C*U*I*S*I*N*E
Regards,
Open-Mouthed."

There's Gold For "Frequent Buyers" Food World has come up with a "frequent buyer" plan modeled on the airlines' very successful "frequent flyer" programs. The plan allows customers to accumulate valuable "checks" proportionate to the dollar amount spent in the chain's stores. The checks can be redeemed at Pizza Hut, Eckerd Drug, Frenchy's Creole Chicken, B.F. Goodrich, The Men's Warehouse, Cineplex movie theaters, One Hour Martinizing Cleaners and even Eastern Airlines. A check is worth $1.00 to $15.00, depending on where it is redeemed.

Unbeknownst To You

Behind the scenes, grocery planners are busy night and day to devise new ways to work your wages out of your jeans. Are the lights turned way down low in the produce section of the market where you shop? And is the fruit back-lit? Planners call that effect "romance," and it's meant to woo you into buying more of that luscious-looking fruit. Has the bakery section been moved up front, near the door? That's so you'll smell the fresh-baked bread and salivate.

Do you notice that you have to roam all through the store to find an item you want? And that you sometimes see that item in two or more different places? That's so you'll make a personal appearance in every aisle ... be tempted to forget your list. ●

"Help Yourself" CheckRobot, Inc., of Deerfield Beach, Florida offers an automated self-check-out system for supermarkets. A customer can run purchases across the scanner, which reads the UPC-coded price bars, get a bill from the CheckRobot and pay the cashier. He or she may also have the dubious privilege of bagging the order.

Supermarket Expeditions

Instead of canned goods, meats and cheese
  they smother us with expertise;
    floppy disks and salad bars,
  computer papers, caviars,
    Adidas sneakers, in some states
  wines.
    Yuppies stand in check-out
  lines with mung beans, video
    tapes and Gouda.
  What next? Pickled barracuda?
    Items French, Italian, Greek, the
  General Store has gone boutique
    and markets once called merely
  super have been upgraded to
    superduper.

Beatrice H. Comas, freelance writer.
The New York Times

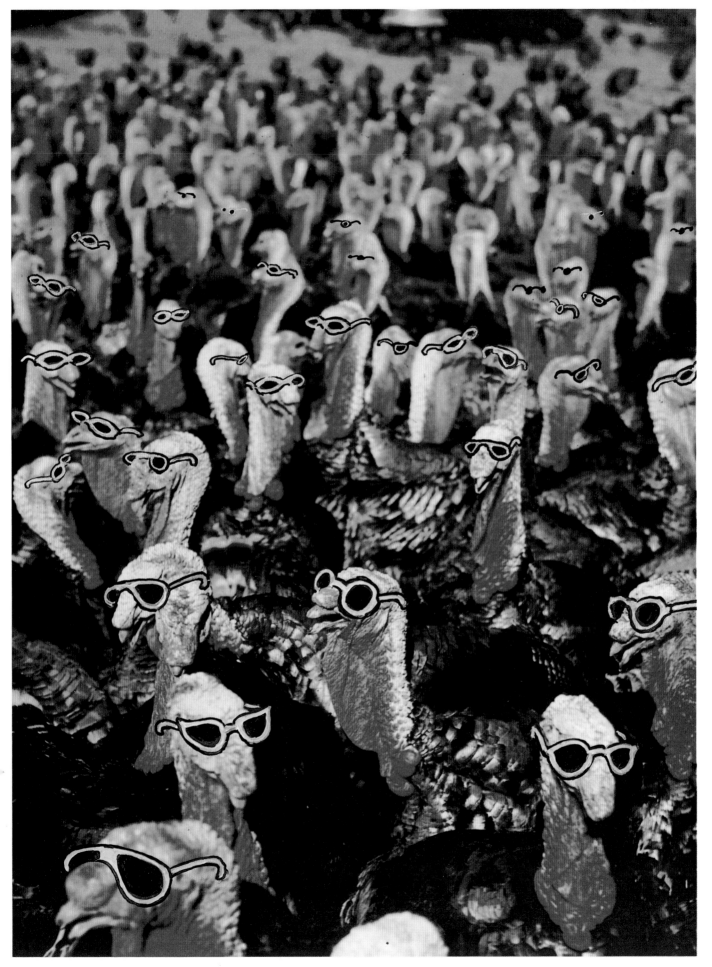

Korean Grocers

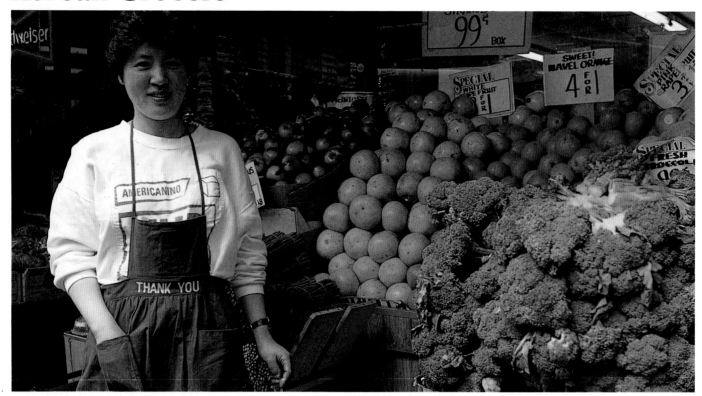

A Green Miracle in Manhattan: Seeing the need and the opportunity, Korean immigrants have moved massively into the retail produce business, bringing leafy green freshness to city streets. To many, "Korean" is now synonymous with "greengrocer."

Making Megabucks The Natural Way

It all started in the psychedelic 60s, with funky little stores on side streets in the wrong part of town. There would be bins and barrels full of mung beans and garbanzos, strings of dried chilies and garlic hanging from the rafters, and dazed shop girls in long skirts who would invariably remark, upon hearing of any natural phenomenon, "Oh, *wow,* man!"

Nature was a trip then, right up there with acid and the sacred mushroom. A natural high could be had from any organic pea or piece of carrot cake, and carob was king. And it all had to be talked about, endlessly, right there in those little stores. With their beat-up wooden furniture, and the encouraging welcome extended by their impoverished, patched proprietors, health food stores became the clubhouses of the freaked-out generation.

Are you ready for this?
Times have changed. Total sales of natural foods in independent health food stores alone reached $2.14 *billion* in 1985. Put that together with sales of the same in supermarkets, natural food chains, drug and other mass marketers and you get an industry total of $3.4 billion overall for last year.

High hopes dashed
Even Colonel Sanders would have thought that business in the billions was pretty good pickins' any time, but the health food folks are disconsolate. According to their trade tabloid, *Natural Foods Merchandiser,* they had their sights set a smidge higher for 1985 than what the year delivered. It seems that back in 1981, a market research outfit called Business Trends Analysts predicted 85's total sales at $5.3 billion, en route to a 1990 sales prediction of $12 billion! So you can at once see the problem. It's not just coming up short a couple of billion in 1985; it's wondering how much short they're going to come up five years from now, with all their investors and bankers standing around wondering just the very same thing. Is it back to funky stores on the wrong side of town? Back to patches and poke bean salad with tofu? And all those garrulous customers? Mebbe so. Mebbe not.

The bright side
There are those who feel that a two percent increase in sales over 1984 isn't shabby. Says Doug Greene, publication director of *NFM,* "Regardless of the exact sales figures, the natural foods industry had a suc-cessful year of advancing its goals. The food industry overall, from grocery manufacturers to fast food restaurants, continued to introduce healthier and more natural products. When you look at the entire specialty foods market, you see an arena that is very aware of the concepts of natural foods. We see the natural foods industry undergoing a transformation that merges with and influences other specialty and commercial food areas."

Simply stated
That is the long way of saying that, predictions and prognostications aside, the health food business is in good shape. Meanwhile, *NFM* itemized some new behavior in certain product categories.

"Produce sales jumped 22 percent. Food service absolutely exploded, up 67 percent over last year with the addition of delis in many stores (which countered the decline of sit-down cafés in others). Frozen foods jumped 28 percent, attributable to the increasing number of non-dairy frozen desserts. Refrigerated foods were up 17 percent, with the growth coming in cheese and beverages."

Frozen desserts in Mamacita's Whole Earth All-Organic Nature Palace and Bean

Sprout Center? Are you kidding? Well, no, they're not. And change is not simply in the air, it's here.

Snobbery is bad business

"In its early years," says *NFM,* "the industry struck an irreverent pose, defining itself as totally different and separate from everything else. With maturity that attitude has changed." Echoing that sentiment is Stan Amy, president of Nature's in Portland, Oregon. "We used to sell our products on the basis of fear and guilt," he says. In his first store (he now has three), which he opened 16 years ago, strict macrobiotic principles ruled. "We used to define ourselves," says Amy, "by what we didn't carry—no white sugar, no preservatives." Amy would not even carry natural vitamins.

Today Amy's stores carry a full range of grocery items, including vitamins. And according to *NFM,* the majority of his new store's sales "will come from items not currently provided by traditional natural foods suppliers—produce, meat, fish, poultry, beer, wine, coffee, imported cheese and a host of deli foods made in the store's own kitchen."

"Now," says Amy, "we define ourselves by what we emphasize, which is the best quality products in each category."

An impending market merge?

And what other kind of business defines itself that way? Why, the gourmet foods business, of course, which does, overall, about $4 billion a year, which puts it right in the same ball park with health food stores.

So what lies ahead for nature's own food entrepreneurs? Patched, empty pockets and longwinded customers? Or will it be bulgur pâté, cold sturgeon over organic fennel and a nice, iced, natural Dom Perignon?

We rather think the latter. ●

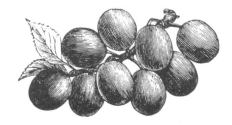

The Rising Sun

According to a study conducted by the Business Communications Company of Stamford, Connecticut, sales of Oriental foods in this country are expected to rise to $1.2 billion by 1990.

Most of these foods and food products are imports from Japan, and fall under the macrobiotics banner. Until recently, that's where they've been positioned in American health food stores. However, the customer base in this category has now widened significantly, beyond strict macrobiotic dieters, and many storekeepers are now dispersing many of these items and allying them with domestic items in a reach for double sales: Such combos as Japanese pasta and Italian tomato sauce are no longer unholy alliances.

Macrobiotic staples such as miso, tamari, seaweeds, rice and pasta are the leading products in this category, with noodles—such as whole wheat, udon and soba—at the head of the pasta pack. And storekeepers report that more unusual pickled items—ginger, daikon and umeboshi plum—are rapidly picking up in sales. But nothing can beat soy products for recent growth. "Tofu and tempeh have really skyrocketed," says Sandy Pukel of the Oak Feed Store in Coconut Grove, Florida. And soymilk sales lead all.

Basically, storekeeper strategy now is to move macrobiotics from the realm of esoterica into mainstream grocery shopping, and let the dried seaweed chips fall where they may. ●

Whither Mom & Pop?

Something there is in the corporate soul of some husbands and wives that causes them to dream of having a nice little store somewhere, someday, where they can work together, serve their customers in a neighborly, personal way and accumulate a little nest egg for their golden retirement years. Generations of Moms-and-Pops have

realized this dream in times past, when the economy provided the independent businessman with a chance to make a decent buck in a modest way.

The rising tide of giantism in the world of American food retailing would seem to dim that dream in the souls of modern Moms-and-Pops. However, while complete independence may be unfeasible for most, there does still remain a way to realize something like the old dream. It lies in a trade that calls itself "the convenience store segment" of the grocery business. Its estimated real growth for 1986 is 5.6 percent, a greater rise than that predicted for any other category in the market. And while it's true that the general public wouldn't know a "convenience store" if it saw one (aren't supermarkets convenient?), everybody knows what a 7-11 is, or depending on what part of the country you live in, a UtotM, a Little General, a Circle K.

Circle K, a major acquisitor, has grown in the last five years from 1,194 units to 2,650, largely from having snapped up UtotM and Little General; meanwhile, "C- stores," as they are abbreviated in the trade, have moved beyond grocery items into fast food of a particular kind: fresh sandwiches, fruit, beer and wine. And they can furnish this food to customers faster than a fast-food counterperson can say, "What'll it be?"

According to the trade magazine *Restaurants & Institutions,* "Convenience stores are looking to establish a reputation as fast-food restaurants that happen to sell other products," rather than the other way around. But what, you may ask, has all this to do with Mom-and-Pop?

Simply put, Mom-and-Pop can buy a franchise for one. *R&I* suggests that they can "put in some individuality and obtain a much better quality of product because of the sophisticated distribution system of large chains." And there you have it—a chance to do your own thing in a small way, as neighborly as you like, with back-up that only a large chain can provide.

Current industry figures show that most consumers make a couple of trips to convenience stores every week. And we all know that a little TLC from some dedicated Moms-and-Pops could run that figure right on up the flagpole. ●

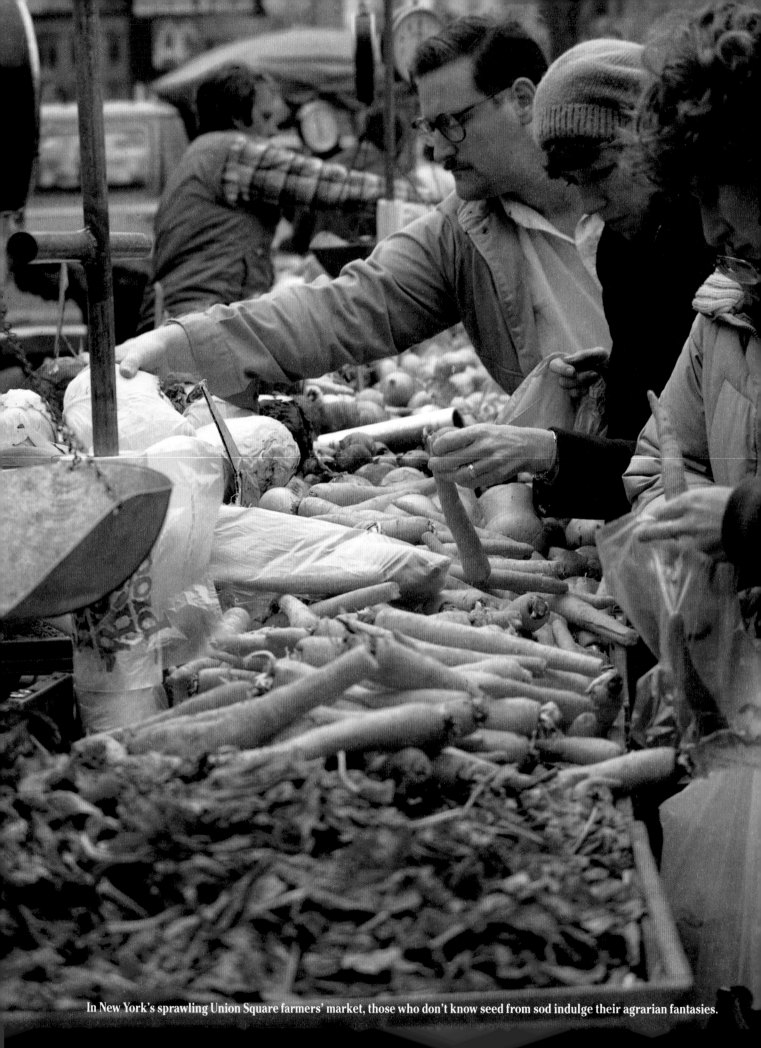

In New York's sprawling Union Square farmers' market, those who don't know seed from sod indulge their agrarian fantasies.

When The Farmer Leaves The Dell

The American Dream, however painted or advertised, has always had a certain bucolic flavor about it, as if to suggest that truly we are just a gentle nation of noble farmers, shoulder to the plow in honest expectation of God's own harvest. It's not surprising that this association with the moo, the oink and the cluck-cluck should cling to our fantasies into the present, because the fact is that we were—once—just that: a small, agrarian people. In 1820, when President James Monroe was in the White House, three-quarters of the entire population of this country lived on farms. The dream lingers even when there are none left alive to tell us how it was then. It lingers even in a time when less than 3 percent of Americans live on farms, and that percentage is being whittled away all the while.

Memories and make-believe

Americans are, today, preponderantly an urban people. We learn about the moo, the oink and the cluck-cluck at nursery school, and millions of American kids will never see a cow or a pig, or a chicken not dressed by Perdue. This is one reason, perhaps, why we have such an on-going affair with the farmers' market—there's at least one in every American city of any size—for we take to our pavements in huge numbers every week, to whatever place where farmers come with their produce, and we eagerly buy whatever is farm fresh really, and not a label. We wander there, among the stalls heaped up with God's harvest, and visit our genetic memories.

Richard Sax, in his new book *From the Farmers' Market* (Harper & Row), evokes the romance of that experience in this description of his visit to a farmers' market in New York: "We see the bushel-baskets filled with ripe tomatoes, vine-ripened and full of flavor. Loose tender heads of butter lettuce share space with cucumbers, red and white radishes, bunches of spring onions with the moist earth still clinging to them, garlic and shallots, and bouquets of fresh chives, thyme, tarragon. The effect is of a colorful seed catalog come to vibrant life."

Interesting, isn't it, that the simple recitation of all these good things from the farm sings to us like a kind of poetry, almost every word a picture and a taste on

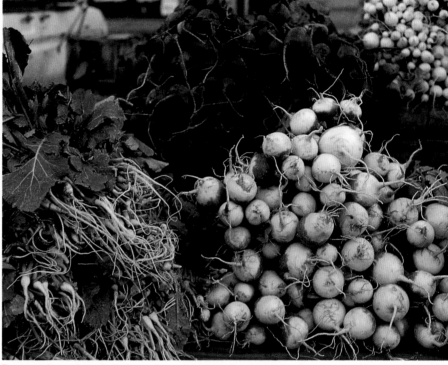

Beets and turnips of all sizes glow with dewy freshness.

the tongue, swirled together with the times we've tasted these things, and the aromas then, and who was there to share them. Visiting the farmers' market is no mere shopping excursion, and it is about a lot more than food for dinner. It is much more about food for thought.

Meetin' time at the carrot basket

Of course, we have had farmers' markets ever since there were farms. In bucolic America, market day was party day in any town. And once a week, the dreariest little courthouse town in Georgia, the most sun-baked little farm corners in Oklahoma, would come alive with a crowd to beat Sunday. It was a social boon for farm families because they lived all week in such isolation; they were as tickled to come as the townsfolk were to see them coming. And only the circus could make any hearts beat faster.

Today, of course, in our great cities, we have circus every day, and the farmers' market works a kind of antidote to that on urban dwellers. Deep in the stalls, sniffing up that indescribably pure smell of ozone that seems to arise from fresh vegetables,

we seem to have a chance to revive. Oddly, the experience is as refreshing to the farmers as to city customers.

Richard Sax quotes Helen Kent, a farmer from Milton, New York, who comes into the city to the market: "I enjoy it most for the people," she says, "because I talk to them as I sell. We've met some fascinating people, and I've learned a lot about cooking and about recipes."

Dorothy Lokey, who takes truckloads of cantaloupes from her farm in north Texas to the Dallas farmers' market every week, says the same. "I love to sell, " she says. "I never knew I would. I was a legal stenographer in Houston before I married a farmer. I never knew I could do this. But now I *sell.* I say, 'Hey, looky here, lady, isn't this the sweetest, best-looking cantaloupe you ever tasted?' She'll take a taste and say, 'Well, I do believe it *is*,' and the next thing you know, I've made a sale!''

James Monroe is long gone, and so is anybody and everybody who ever shook the great man's hand. But the farmers' market we have still with us, needed now more than ever before to help us to keep cultivating our noble dream. ●

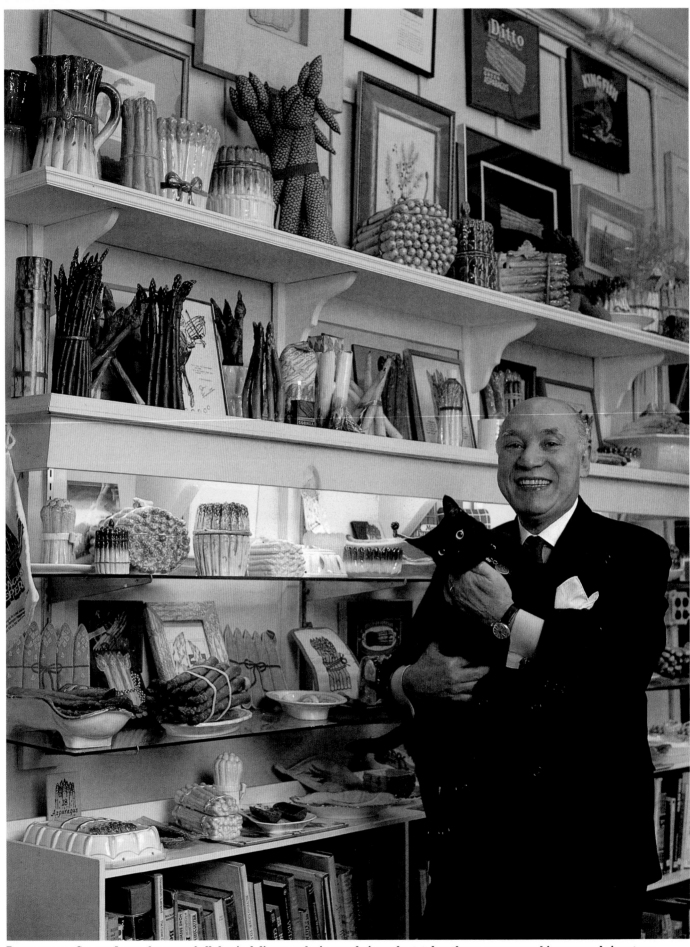

Restaurateur George Lang, devotee of all that is delicate and winsomely impudent, takes the asparagus as his personal signature.

Asparagusto

By George Lang

S ome of the most discriminating people believe the world is conditioned by love, supported by half a dozen or so lively arts, and succored by foods which are just as exquisite to behold as they are satisfying to eat.

Truffles contribute impeccable aroma to our taste experience, but they are ill-shaped; goose liver is one of the few sensuous flavors, but its richness almost evokes displeasure, and even the most delectable caviar looks like an ungraceful lump of compressed BB shots.

Only the asparagus has the stunning artistry as well as all the other elements we require from the perfect food.

Asparagus has the correct shape for the human mouth and hand. If an industrial designer were assigned to create the perfectly shaped food, it would probably end up as an asparagus.

As beautiful as a flower, asparagus officinalis, in fact, belongs to the lily family.

Eating asparagus is the earthiest experience, and an obscure nineteenth century source lists 23 ways of doing so. One of the best-known methods, apparently, was to suspend the asparagus on pulleys about three feet off the floor and approach them with open mouth lying on one's back.

Asparagus is also good for you. We must have grace to conceal our enjoyment of magnificently fattening foods, but asparagus is lean and healthy and you can be overwhelmed by quantities of it without serious consequences.

Asparagus is one of the best sources for folic acid (a B vitamin) which is vital to the formation of red blood cells. It also contains rutin which is a factor in preventing small capillaries from rupturing.

Last but not least, asparagus' priapic columns contain lust-provoking qualities—or, so it is said in Hindu amatory treatises. And, on the flip side, Greek mythology associated it with cuckoldry. However, according to a noted Swiss psychologist, eating asparagus will help to develop a sense of responsiblity.

I must caution impatient "Type A" people about growing asparagus: it takes about three years before one can cut the first spears. If you take care of the bed, however, it will yield for 10-15 years

thereafter.

I am not sure if we should call it a curiosity, but asparagus plants do have sex, and the female ones grow plumper stalks—make what you want out of this bit of intelligence. The male flowers contain a rudimentary pistil and the female flower has stamens. One spear can grow as much as ten inches in a day and it is this rapid growth that accounts for the vegetable's tenderness.

Asparagus can be white or green, and there is as much controversy about which is better as—let us say—about the qualities of Sir Georg Solti vs. Herr von Karajan.

The white, often with a pale purple point, is grown and appreciated in Belgium, Holland, Germany and France; the green or the purple in England and Italy. The U.S. grows and enjoys the green variety almost exclusively.

The two most popular varieties in the U.S. are the Connover Colossal, an old American variety, and the dark green Mary Washington. Our production figure of 170 million pounds per year comes mostly from the El Centro and Sacramento River Delta sections of California. The state of New Jersey's production is, however, declining because of high labor costs and, to keep up with demand, Mexico has become our principal outside supplier of fresh asparagus.

I am relieved to report that Thomas Jefferson—who by now is credited with just about every invention and import of note—did not bring this plant to the New World, though he did experiment with growing it from seeds at the end of the eighteenth century.

According to some reports, the first settlers did find wild asparagus in America along sandy coastlines and riverbanks but, to the best of our knowledge, asparagus was brought into New England by 1672 and a Dutch consul began its systematic cultivation in the mid-1700s somewhere in Massachusetts.

Ideally, asparagus, like corn on the cob, should be cut, cooked and served without dilly-dallying on the way to the dining room. If this is not possible, at least choose young asparagus with straight tender stalks and petals that are

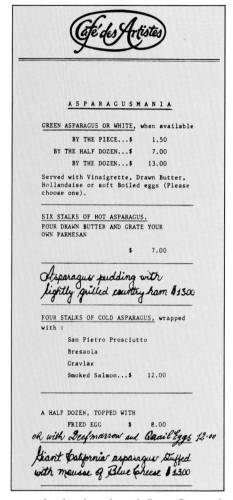

completely closed and firm. Cut ends should be fresh looking and approximately even in thickness; they should also be smooth and a rich green color.

The world is divided into people who cook asparagus standing upright with the tips out of the water and the others who believe in the normal law of the universe and place the neatly-tied asparagus bunch horizontally in a frying pan of water for a short period of time. I definitely belong to the second category and cannot understand why anyone would submit poor asparagi to the stand-up torture, especially since one must peel asparagus stalks, at which point the stem becomes just as tender as the tips.

Asparagus must be slightly crunchy, and a couple of minutes' cooking time makes an enormous difference in its texture. Unfortunately, there are two things impossible in life: to put toothpaste back into the tube, and to fix overcooked asparagus.

Whether you'll try to duplicate Apicius' recipe in his Ars Magirica (written

GEORGE LANG'S CLASSIC ASPARAGUS

Life is measured by such simple joys as a plate of perfectly prepared asparagus shared with a perfect person.

Serves 4 to 6

Ingredients:
1½ pounds large asparagus spears of approximately the same size, with tightly closed tips
Coarse salt and freshly ground black pepper
2 three-foot lengths of butcher's twine

Method:
1. Rinse and drain the asparagus and cut off the woody ends of the spears. Peel each spear, beginning just below the tip and cutting downward with a vegetable peeler or paring knife.

2. Divide the spears into two bunches.

3. Hold one bunch of asparagus upright with tip ends down, making sure all tips are even and touching the work surface. Tie securely with twine in the middle of the bunch.

4. Using a sharp knife, trim the stalks with a single stroke, if you can manage it, to make the asparagus all the same length. Repeat steps 3 and 4 with the remaining bunch.

5. Bring an 8-quart pot with 7 quarts of salted water to a rapid boil. Lower the asparagus bunches into the water. After the water returns to a boil, cook uncovered for approximately 6 to 8 minutes, or until the stalks are tender when pricked with a fork.

6. Using a wooden fork, lift the bunches from the water by slipping the fork underneath the twine. Drain well. Cut the twine loose with a scissors and discard.

7. Arrange the asparagus in a preheated platter lined with a napkin dipped into the asparagus cooking water. Serve at once with coarse salt and freshly ground black pepper and any sauce you desire.

between the first and third centuries A.D.) in which he grinds up asparagus with spices and raisin wine and makes a kind of hollandaise out of it using it as a sauce for roast warblers, or just serve it with melted butter, depends on your personal relationship to this wondrous vegetable. If you want to get off the gastronomic-missionary position, you can find well over 500 recipes in current cookbooks, ranging from Asparagus-Stuffed Eggs; Tagliatelle with Asparagus Sauce; Asparagus with Mustard Dressing, Japanese Style; *Jane Grigson's imaginative* Asparagus Soldiers; Asparagus Salad with Mussels; Asparagus in a Blanket; *or in a* Crab Sauce, Chinese Style.

It helps to have a catchy name if you are a hurricane or a new dish. Ambushed Asparagus, *in which the spears are placed vertically in a hollowed-out slender loaf, first appeared in Mrs. Marion Harland's* Common Sense in Households, *published in New York in 1885, which in turn is copied from Mrs. Hannah Glass's celebrated* The Art of The Cookery *(1753) as* Asparagus Forced in French Roll.

Which brings us to our recipe which might just bring you to such excess. ●

George Lang is an international restaurant consultant, journalist and owner of Café des Artistes. His interest in asparagus goes beyond reasonable boundaries.

Way Out West I

Richard Atcheson

On my first trip to California, I stayed in LA with my friend Steve. And the first place Steve took me was the supermarket.

I had never seen such ravishing, backlit fruits and vegetables, and I had never seen such ravishing shoppers—every one a movie star.

"Steve," I said to him, "All these people are gorgeous."

"I know," he replied.

"But this is a grocery store," I complained.

"No, Dick," he replied. "For all these people this is a media event. They are not here just to shop. They are here to make a personal appearance."

I quickly saw that this was so. Well-muscled young men in tank tops and shorts posed at the deli counter behind their market baskets. Beautiful young women in halter tops and shorts nonchalantly picked up grocery items and absent-mindedly slipped them into the baskets of the young men. They were all burnished to a silver tan and each one had a broad white smile to dazzle the eye. I couldn't believe it. They were in the supermarket to be discovered.

Later, when I lived in LA, I found myself a part of this life, found myself dressing carefully for even my next appearance at the 7-11 for bread and cigarettes. And I met southern California women who admitted to spending half the morning getting ready to go grocery shopping. In main part it's because in the vast new faceless towns such as Irvine and Laguna Hills there isn't anyplace else to go. When you need to see other human beings, there's no use going into the streets and parks. Nobody is ever there. They are all at Albertson's and the Alpha Beta.

It has always been true, of course, of every culture, that people gather in the marketplace. The marketplace is where it's happening. But no culture has ever seen so lush a marketplace as Alpha Beta on an "off" day, where perfect fruits are not so much piled as "architected" into place, where the lighting is designed to bring out the blush on every peach and the pregnant suggestion of nectar on the slick skin of every bulging grape on the stem.

Down wide aisles lined with polished cans of processed food we stroll. We amble. We are dressed divinely, but casually. It is useful to look as if we had just come from tennis or sailing, though we neither play tennis nor sail. The look is the thing. Because around the next aisle may come the man or woman of our dreams, with practically nothing on. Will it be in Dog Food? Will it be in Dairy?

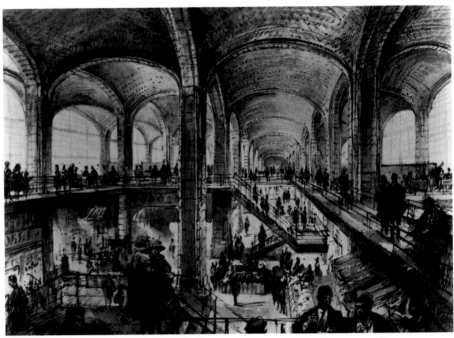

In this artist's rendering, New York's proposed Bridgemarket teems with life.

There is no way to know. There is only to be at the ready.

There is also aggression. Some women I know are not above ramming a man's cart, then whispering apologies while batting their eyes and distractedly fondling the Miracle Whip. Sometimes it works.

One woman I know drops things in the cart of any man she admires, so as to be able to say, "Oh! Did I do that? I'm so sorry."

Nor are men above these strategies, though their approaches are usually based on helplessness. "Gee, I don't know which salad dressing to get. Have you tried the Paul Newman? Do you have any advice?" Boyish laughter. Sometimes it works.

Another one, of course, is "Here, let me help you with that," as a woman sags under the weight of her bag while trying to heft it into her car. But this is primarily a parking-lot ploy; bush league. The main event is in the marketplace itself, on the terms of the marketplace.

It's an old story. There's nothing like groceries for bringing people together. There never was and there never will be. Witness a sight I saw at Albertson's in Dana Point one day, when I pushed my cart into the parking lot under a brilliant sun and saw a large bus humming and sighing and disgorging a hundred or so Japanese tourists strung with cameras. They were crying out to each other, and pointing at Albertson's and at me, and taking pictures of us. Then they passed in a wild dither and rushed into the store.

They had experienced me, in my tank top and shorts. Now they were going to experience Albertson's in all its lush opulence, with its gorgeous fruits and vegetables and people. They were, I realized, to experience America as we are now. ●

Richard Atcheson is a freelance writer.

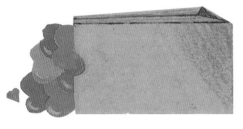

A Shell Of Dreams

In the heart of the Upper East Side of Manhattan, beneath the Queensborough Bridge, lies an empty shell. In 1914, this space was a simple walk-in farmers' market with strong pillars and a beautifully tiled arched ceiling. In the 1930s, when hard times fell, it was abandoned to be used as a garage for city trucks, highway signs and other odds and ends from the four corners of New York City.

Now, 56 years after the demise of the original market, Harley Baldwin, a real estate developer and restaurateur, dreams of turning this empty shell into a futuristic computer-operated market.

When it is completed, area residents will be able to phone in an order that will start computers whirring and, from the more than 50 stores within the market, the items ordered will be selected, placed on a circling conveyor belt and deposited in a space reserved for outgoing deliveries. If the mainframe computer fails, there will be no delays; a second computer will serve as a backup.

In some ways, Mr. Baldwin's market will look much like the farmers' market of earlier days. But it will be modern technology that will enable him to recapture those once-lost nineteenth century qualities of goods and services, and to add contemporary updates as well.

Plans call for a three-level indoor market covering 120,000 square feet, the largest international food complex in the world. In addition to fresh produce, meat, poultry, game and fish galore, there will be prepared foods organized by nationality: Russian, German, Middle Eastern, British, Oriental, American, Italian, French and Scandinavian to name a few. Customers who so wish will be able to order these dishes after consulting Baldwin's forthcoming international cookbook. A working bakery and a demonstration dairy that includes a cheese-making section will be additional features, as well as a cook's center offering pots and pans and a bookstore. All shops will be run individually but they will be designed more like departments in a large store than separate shops in a mall.

Outside, visitors will find a farmers' market, a three-tiered Greenhouse Restaurant and a pedestrian park. Valet parking will be provided.

Mr. Baldwin has fought an uphill battle to translate his dream into reality. It has been a tough fight but the $23 million project *is* scheduled to begin construction in 1986, and *is* scheduled for completion by November of 1987. ●

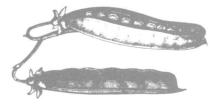

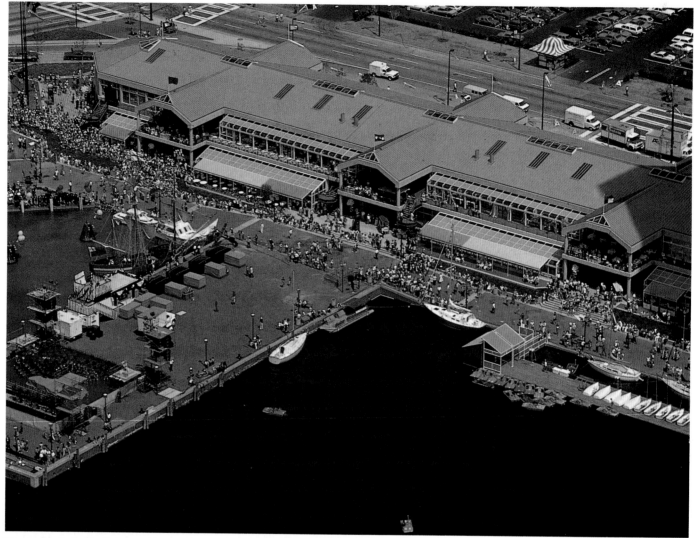

Every day is festival day at Harborplace, a Rouse complex of shops and restaurants in Baltimore's financial district.

A Rousing Cheer For Rouse

It would be difficult to praise too much the work that the Rouse Company, of Columbia, Maryland, has done to bring light and cheer and pure fun to the revival of so many city centers in America. With the Faneuil Hall Marketplace in Boston, the South Street Seaport in New York and Harborplace in Baltimore, they have seen the way to take a tired setting and turn it again into the teeming hub it once was—and that is to name only three of the stars in its portfolio of glittering retail centers. They dot the country, and every one of them acts on the populace like a magnet on iron filings. We are drawn, inexorably, to where it's happening, and it's happening wherever Rouse has put its stamp. It is as if this wily company actually knows what the marketplace means in our genes—since time immemorial, *the* place where everybody wants to be, trading goods and glances, with good things to eat and drink, an exotic swarm of sights and sounds, laughter and music and the eternal promise of surprise. Without

that, our ancestors would never have gotten out of bed to go to market.

The marketplace is the lifeblood of civilization. In Marrakech, you go to buy tangerines and to watch a fellow stick a sword through his cheeks; in Iquitos on the Amazon, you shop for seared monkey meat and buy a potion guaranteed to keep your sweetheart faithful. In the Viktualenmarkt in Munich, you squeeze the victuals and think very seriously about squeezing the girl in the apricot velvet coat. To us all—though Americans forgot it for a long, long time—the market is life.

Back to Rome

Rouse has brought back to us the meaning of the Latin word *mercatus*—a place of contact for buyers and sellers. That's what it meant in Imperial Rome, and that's what it means today. In the Rouse approach, it also means re-creating the setting where buying and selling, and all the colorful commerce surrounding that, can take

place. Seventeen years ago, Boston's old Quincy Market lay dying derelict, in a dangerous part of town where nobody of any probity wanted to go any more. It lay there in despair, until Rouse.

Romance on the half-shell

The company took this area and made historic Faneuil Hall, which stood at the head of the sheds, as its focal point. It restored the long market sheds and filled the cobbled walkways with the stalls of merchants—sellers of flowers, books, amusing trinkets. It leased space to restaurateurs of the seafood persuasion, calling on Boston's romantic relationship with the sea. And it provided space to small, ethnic food operations along the sides of the sheds, so that the air was always aromatic with curry and spice, and everything nice. To the multitudes, it proved irresistible.

The same applies, and more so, to the moldering Fulton Street Fish Market in New York. Fulton Street had never been fancy, but it had been real, much like Les Halles in Paris. At the turn of the century, people of the most elegant reputation had thought nothing of going to a Fulton Street café after midnight for a couple of dozen oysters and a pint of ale.

By the 1960s, it was defunct. The covered wharfs extending into the East River were still busy enough, but crime and the crust of time had taken the glamor off the neighborhood; nobody wanted to go there any more. Rouse invented the concept of a South Street Seaport, and things began turning around. With the city's enthusiastic cooperation—as in lining up a few old tubs at quayside, their masts gleaming silver in the crystalline moonlight—some atmosphere was restored. Rouse dressed up the old market to yuppie taste, with 20 or more food emporia to a single floor, the aroma of ethnic foods cooking and lots of neon—and the market came alive again.

A poem grows in Baltimore

Rouse's work with Baltimore's Harborside is identical with the above, but most succinctly described by certain journalists. Said Wolf Von Eckardt, that most trenchant critic of American architecture, in *The Washington Post,* "A remarkable feat, as significant to the recovery of our cities as the invention of the pedestrian mall . . . a triumph." A less romantic observation was made by Michael Olesker of *The Baltimore Sun:* "They have taken what once was a sewer and ringed it with a poem."

In a sense, Olesker's barbed praise is correct; a sewer ringed by a poem is no less a sewer. But there is no way to restore to these once-natural sites of commerce the conditions which accounted for them when they sprang up. All that is lost to us in the passage of time and the movement of essential commerce to the unseen marketplace of the telephone and the computer. But it is no less noble to make what Rouse calls "adaptive use" of the temples of an earlier day—to save our past from the wrecking ball and to give us a glimpse, at least, of the rowdy world that once was.

And the fact remains that nothing is really changed at the Quincy Market. It's still a place for buyers and sellers, winks and glances, a half dozen oysters and a glass of champagne—and wonderful surprise. ●

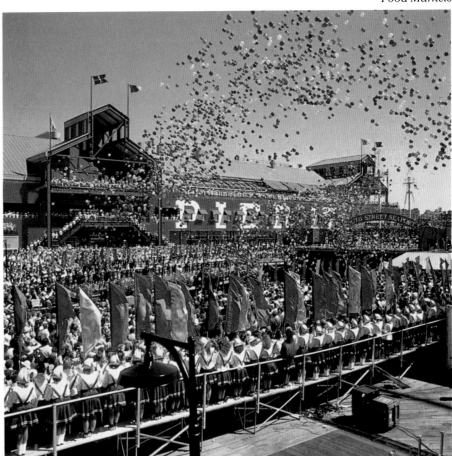

Festivity at South Street Seaport, a mecca for Wall Street shakers and movers.

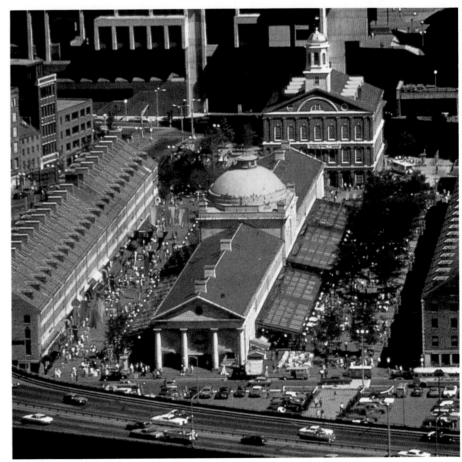

Cobblestone streets fan out from Faneuil Hall in Boston's rejuvenated Quincy Market.

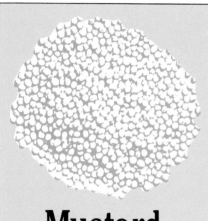

Mustard, Anyone?

A sampling of flavors offered by the specialty food industry

Champagne Mustard
Banana-Hot Pepper Mustard
Raspberry Vinegar Mustard
Sweet Mustard with Venetian Herbs
Lime Prepared Mustard
Mustard with Violets
Mustard with Olives and Anchovies
Hot Mustard with Roses
Pineapple Prepared Mustard
Sweet and Rough Mustard
Green Peppercorn Garlic Mustard
Emerald Herb Mustard
Smoked Barbecue Mustard
Dill Mustard Sauce
Russian Style Prepared Mustard
Spicy Basil Prepared Mustard
Beer Mustard
Scotch Mustard with Whiskey and
    Herbs
Mustard with Truffles
Chinese Hot Mustard Sauce
Honey Mustard
Sherry Mustard
Piccalilli; Chow-Chow
Creole Mustard

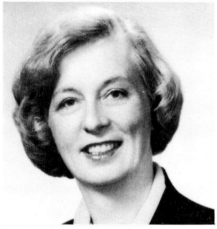

Elaine Yannuzzi, Expression unltd.

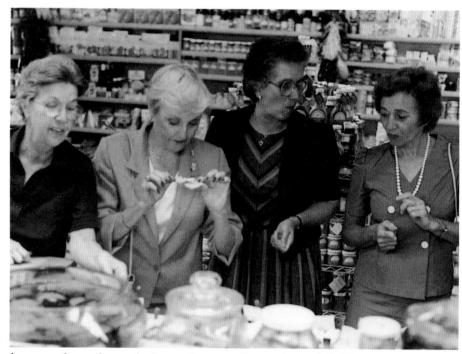

An array of rare cheeses invites customers at Expression unltd., Warren, New Jersey.

The Groundbreakers

Six or seven years ago, specialty foods meant the ethnic groceries and neighborhood delis that you find in most cities of any size. That was the specialty food industry. You know—the sort of place where you'd walk in, and, over to the left of the door, covered with dust, you'd find six jars of olives stuffed with anchovies, eight tins of crab legs, three tins of reindeer meatballs and two of escargots. These items remained there for years, because nobody thought to buy them. The bulk of the business in these places was whatever their main line was: provolone cheese, etc.

Then one day somebody—we don't know who, we don't know where, maybe in New York—actually *bought* one of those items. Shock waves rippled through the industry and before you knew it, somebody bought something somewhere else, and a ripple effect began. Next thing you knew, little cheese shops and gourmet specialty stores opened everywhere.

Then the supermarkets, who never sleep, saw what was happening and they licked their chops. "Here's a nice little pearl," they said. "Let's give it eight feet of shelf space and dust the jars." And they did. And as soon as they did, the specialty food people had to run out and find some goods that were even *more* special than anything the supermarkets had taken to their bosoms.

This business is very young and you have to be fast on your feet to keep up with it. Specialty items operate like waves that crest and break on the beach. Consider Jarlsberg: That was a special cheese once

upon a time. It crested, it broke and now you find it in the supermarkets with the Velveeta. Brie, which was once only very "high end," is breaking now. Another wave cresting fast is exotic French cheese—the triple creams, also the chèvres—they're still special at the moment but it won't be long before they join the Jarlsberg at the supermarket.

"Special" is the word to underline in this business; when a thing ceases to be special and is widely available to the general public, it has no place in a specialty food store. We carry the rare, the unusual, the unique. If you can't get it anywhere else, try us.

Gene Bennet, public relations director of the National Association for the Specialty Food Trade, says that we gross $3 to $4 billion annually—that figure based on a close study of the overall market. More specific figures, however, are hard to find. We know, for example, how many tons of cheese are sold annually in this country, but what kind and where? We don't have those figures.

All we know is that the industry is made up entirely of small business people—no major movers. The big boys touch specialty foods only as a department, whereas— for us—this business is our lives. It's been said that we've changed the palates of America; I prefer to say that we've worked with the American palate and we've learned in the doing.

Yesterday, there wasn't a specialty food industry. Today there is. Tomorrow? Well, speaking for myself—there'd better be! ●

Elaine Yannuzzi, specialty food store owner

Food By Mail

Mail-order food has come a long way since the early 70s, when the *piece de résistance* of a "gourmet" food catalogue was, more often than not, a huge gift basket filled with foil-wrapped processed cheeses in various flavors, smoked salamis chock-full of preservatives and artificial flavorings, tinned pâté that tasted more like dogfood and impressively large, totally tasteless fruits.

In just the last few years, the mail-order food business has grown in leaps and bounds, with sales estimated to be in the billions. Today's catalogues include an extraordinary range of products—preservative-free buffalo meat sausages, extra-virgin olive oil from France and Italy, salsa from Arizona, Chinese sesame oil, homemade berry jams from the Pacific Northwest, fresh wild mushrooms and more.

What follows is a list of mail-order food purveyors that should give you an idea of the enormous variety of resources available to us today.

Good Overall
These companies have a wide variety of products, with an emphasis on French and Italian foods.

Balducci's
424 Avenue of the Americas
New York NY 10011
(212) 673-2600

Dean & DeLuca
110 Greene Street
New York NY 10012
(212) 431-1691/(800) 221-7714

Convito Italiano
11 East Chesnut
Chicago IL 60611
(312) 943-2983

C. Steele and Co.
1628 West Camelback Road
Phoenix AZ 85015
(602) 266-5797

Indian
Spice and Sweet Mahal
135 Lexington Avenue
New York NY 10016
(212) 683-0900

Indonesian
Mrs. De Wildt
R.D. 3
Bangor PA 18013
(Unlisted phone)

Latin American
Casa Moneo
210 West 14th Street
New York NY 10011
(212) 929-1644

Bueno Mexican Foods
P.O. Box 293
Albuquerque NM 87103
(505) 243-7477

Middle Eastern
Sultan's Delight
25 Croton Avenue
Staten Island NY 10301
(718) 720-1557

Oriental
Uwajimaya (Chinese, Japanese, Thai, Vietnamese, Filipino)
P.O. Box 3003
Seattle WA 98114
(206) 624-6248

Caviar
Caviar Direct (Russian, Iranian and American)
524 West 46th Street
New York NY 10036
(212) 757-8990/(800) 472-4456

Cheese
See Good Overall

Coffee And Tea
Schapira Coffee Company
117 West 10th Street
New York NY 10011
(212) 675-3733

Freed, Teller, and Freed
1326 Polk Street
San Francisco CA 94109
(415) 673-0922

G.H. Ford Tea Company
P.O. Box 3407
110 Dutchess Turnpike
Poughkeepsie NY 12603
(914) 471-1160

Health Foods
Walnut Acres
Penns Creek PA 17862
(717) 837-0601

Herbs
Fox Hill Farm (fresh)
444 West Michigan Avenue, Box 7
Parma MI 49269
(517) 531-3179

Select Origins (dried)
Building 139, Sulfolk Cty. Airport
Westhampton Beach NY 11978
(516) 288-1381

Meats—Fresh
Irving Levitt Company (meats, poultry and game)
34-36 Newmarket Square
Boston MA 02118
(617) 442-6700

Pine Ridge Farms (free-range chicken)
P.O. Box 98
Subiaco AR 72865
(501) 934-4565

Glen Echo Farm (baby lamb, seasonal)
P.O. Box 2
Wendell NH 03782
(603) 863-6780

Meats And Poultry—Cured
Menuchah Farms (preservative-free, applewood-smoked meats and poultry)
Route 22
Salem NY 12865
(518) 854-9423/(800) 621-6030

Gwaltney of Smithfield (Smithfield ham)
P.O. Box 489
Smithfield VA 23430
(804) 357-3131 .

S. Wallace Edwards & Sons (country-cured Virginia ham, bacon and sausage)
Box 25
Surry VA 23883
(804) 294-3121/(800) 222-4267

Harrington's (smoked hams, bacon and poultry)
Main Street
Richmond VT 05477
(802) 434-4444

Fred Usinger, Inc. (sausages and wursts)
1030 North Third Street
Milwaukee WI 53203
(414) 276-9100

Specialty Produce
Flying Foods International
43-43 9th Street
Long Island City NY 11101
(718) 706-0820

Seafood—Fresh
Legal Seafoods Market
237 Hampshire Street
Cambridge MA 02139
(617) 864-3400/(800) 343-5804

Smoked Fish And Seafood
Murray's Sturgeon Shop (smoked salmon, sturgeon, whitefish, sable, pickled herring)
2429 Broadway
New York NY 10024
(212) 724-2650

Ducktrap River Fish Farm (smoked fish and shellfish, smoked seafood pâtés)
RFD 2, Box 378
Lincolnville ME 04849
(207) 763-3960

Sweets
Corné Toison D'Or (Belgian chocolates)
Trump Tower, 725 Fifth Avenue
New York NY 10022
(212) 308-4060

Mother Myrick's (hand-made American confections)
P.O. Box 1142
Manchester Center VT 05255
(802) 362-1560

Arnold Reuben Jr's Cheesecake
15 Hill Park Avenue
Great Neck NY 11022
(516) 466-3685

Neal's Cookies (freshly-baked chocolate chip and other cookies)
423 Southwest Freeway
Houston TX 77002
(713) 520-6602

Sweet Things (brownies, carrot cake and other baked goods)
1 Blackfield Drive
Tiburon CA 94920
(415) 388-8583

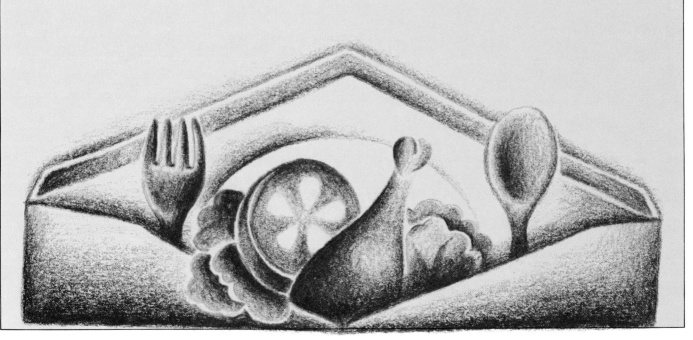

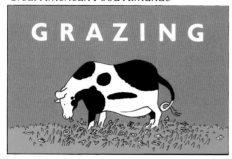

GRAZING

Needs Hitherto Unnoticed #1

Hungry people desiring to know just how hungry they are will be able to find out easily whether their food craving is a) Low, b) Moderate, c) Strong, d) Intense, if they are carrying Craving Indicator Cards. The hungry person whips out the card, presses one thumb on the card's color patch and then watches as the patch changes color to answer the burning question. The card was developed by an organization that calls itself the American Leadership Group, and they say the card will be a boon for dieters; precisely how is not clear.

I'll Worry Tomorrow The commodity brokerage firm Man Producten Rotterdam BV has a real world-shaker to pass. "We believe," the firm's latest annual report says, "that the availability of pepper will decline to an all-time low in the coming six months, which in turn will create a potentially explosive situation in the world market." Exportable production of 100,000 tons will not be adequate for consumer demand for 132,000 tons.

The New York Times

On A Wistful Note In the account books of one thirteenth century household in Tudor England, expenditures for seven to ten gallons of mustard a month were listed. On the continent, in the following century, when the Duke of Burgundy entertained his cousin Philip, the King of France, 70 gallons of mustard were consumed by the guests at a single state banquet. These facts are brought to us through the courtesy of the Grey Poupon Mustard company, accompanied by the following understatement: "Generally, people used to consume a lot more mustard than they do today."

Which Age Group Eats More Ice Cream In The Home Than Any Other? It's not the kids, but rather the over-55 age group. The latter eat ice cream at home an average of 56 times a year.

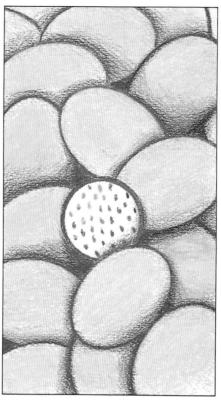

Tell Me Why At classy restaurants, it seems the management has decided that we are not to be trusted with a pepper mill and someone else must handle the decision-making about how much we want or are allowed—although they leave us alone with the salt. Do they think we will use too much of the pepper—or are they afraid we will walk off with one of those gigantic pepper mills sticking out of our back pocket?

What Makes Popcorn Pop?

According to Harold McGee, author of *On Food and Cooking: The Science and Lore of the Kitchen* (Scribner's): "...The protein is a very hard, shell-like layer just under the skin of the kernel. The center of the kernel is an area mostly taken up by starch granules. When water within the kernel gets to the boiling point, it vaporizes, expands in size and enters the starch granule. This causes the starch to soften and expand. Forces inside the center keep building, because the protein shell holds things back for a while. Eventually, the kernel is blown open by the force. The water vapor expands the starch granule and protein into the white stuff of the popped corn." Ah, so!

People Weekly

In One Day

Americans eat 75,000 pounds of pimiento, a small pepper used to make the pimiento tape that's stuffed into green olives. That much pimiento will make 3,500 miles of pimiento tape—enough to stretch from Griffin, Georgia, the pimiento capital of the United States, to Lindsay, California, the stuffed-olive capital, via Washington, D.C., the martini capital.

¶ Americans produce 110,000 tons of salt. That much table salt would fill a salt shaker 214 feet tall and 138 feet in diameter.

¶ Americans eat a quarter million pounds of lobster, a seafood dinner worth at least $2 million. The national surf-to-turf ratio? One pound of live lobster to 600 pounds of live beef.

¶ Americans eat 170 million eggs. That's enough unbroken eggs to completely cover a 100-acre golf course. Americans also eat 12 million chickens.

¶ Americans gnaw on 90,000 bushels of fresh carrots. That's equal to one 2,300-ton carrot, 26 feet wide at the top and 179 feet long.

¶ Americans eat 1.7 million pounds of canned tuna—enough to make 15.7 million tuna-salad sandwiches.

¶ Americans eat 815 billion calories of food—roughly 200 billion more than they need to maintain a moderate level of activity. That's enough extra calories to feed everyone in Mexico, a country of 80 million people.

Americans eat 2.8 million pounds of fresh cucumbers. That's equal to a cucumber 100 feet long and 28 feet thick.

¶ Americans eat 12.5 million pounds of cheese, including 85,000 pounds of blue cheese, 700,000 pounds of cream cheese, 650,000 pounds of Swiss, and 5.8 million pounds of cheddar. Cottage cheese alone makes up more than 2.5 million pounds, or 312,000 gallons, of the daily diet.

¶ Thirty-four million Americans pack more than 2 million bushels of lunch to work in lunch boxes and brown paper bags.

¶ Americans eat 8,500 tons of fresh lettuce. Measuring 90 feet in diameter, an 8,500-ton head of iceberg lettuce would in fact make a pretty respectable iceberg.

Tom Parker, In One Day

The Shortest Quote In This Book "Meals," says Barbara Kafka, contributing editor of *Vogue*, "are diminishing."

BIG BUSINESS OF FOOD

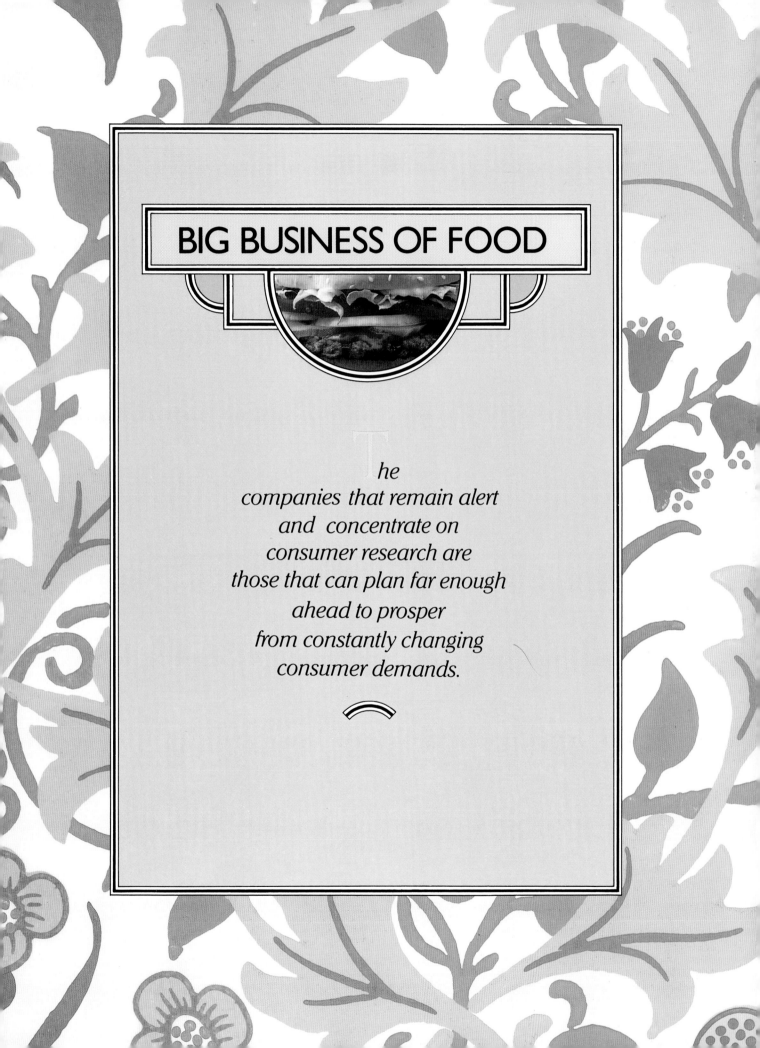

The
companies that remain alert
and concentrate on
consumer research are
those that can plan far enough
ahead to prosper
from constantly changing
consumer demands.

ABSORB-A-BUSINESS

President Eisenhower warned of the dangers of the military-industrial complex way back in the 50s, but now we have bigness in almost every aspect of our daily lives. Just as there are only a handful of large oil companies, major banks and huge investment companies, so too the advertising industry has regrouped into fewer firms, each wielding enormous influence. There are only three or four major television networks; newspapers are merging, as are publishing houses, real estate agencies and food companies. The recent acquisition of Beatrice by Kohlberg, Kravis, Roberts, and General Foods by Philip Morris are just part of a pattern that we can expect to see continuing into the future. As companies extend their markets into giant international conglomerates, the only way to fend off the competition is to absorb other companies, their distribution systems and other areas of specialized expertise.

Vertical integration is the goal because it is the way to achieve maximum efficiency and cost-effectiveness in the highly competitive food industry. The company that can grow its own products, control the price of all or most of the other commodities that go into the pro-

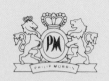

Philip Morris could, if they wished, offer us and their Marlboro Man a nice cold beer from their Miller Brewing Company or a crisp soda from The Seven-Up Company. They have also stepped into the kitchen with the acquisition of the General Foods Corporation, whose well-stocked pantry prefers Oscar Mayer and Louis Rich products, Claussen pickles, Post cereals, Log Cabin syrups, Entenmann's baked goods, Jell-O, Cool Whip, Baker's chocolate and coconut, Calumet baking powder, Certo and Sure-Jell, Birds Eye vegetables, Stove Top stuffing mix, Shake 'n Bake, Ronzoni pasta. And to drink: Kool-Aid, Crystal Light, Tang, Country Time lemonade, Maxwell House coffee, Yuban, Sanka and Brim.

cessing of its foods—while at the same time providing its own packaging and distribution system—clearly has a considerable economic edge over one that has to depend on others for its resources. Those companies that also concentrate on consumer research are those that can plan far enough ahead to prosper from awareness of changing consumer demands.

This last point is well illustrated by Heinz U.S.A. For years, competitors had watched enviously as the Heinz advertising lured the largest market share of tomato ketchup buyers by extolling the slowness with which the Heinz ketchup could be coaxed out of the bottle. The message was that the slower it poured, the better it tasted; thickness was achieved by using more and meatier tomatoes. Catching on to this idea, the research scientists at a rival company after not months, but literally years of dedicated experimentation and reformulation, thought they had figured out how Heinz had done it and got their ketchup to pour as slowly as Heinz's. Heinz, of course, watched all this scurrying around, but they didn't care. Just at the time it was thought that Heinz was

matched, Heinz announced the introduction of the new plastic squeeze bottle that gets that thick ketchup out onto the plate "quick as a whistle."

This is very serious business because a point or two of difference in the market share can add up to very big bucks. For some companies, however, another point is not worth the effect if they essentially own the market. Campbell's, for example, for all practical purposes owns the soup market, just as Hellman's has virtually got the mayonnaise market and Fleischmann's name is synonymous with yeast. When this situation occurs, and one corporation has close to 100 percent of the potential sales, it is not worth the millions of advertising dollars that it would take to reach the last point or half point. Instead, it is wiser to diversify into other areas. As you will see from the boxes on this page, the most successful companies are those that have absorbed other related businesses. Some of these function autonomously, while others share common services with the parent company, such as long-range planning, financial expertise, promotion and advertising. ●

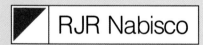

In case you don't recognize the name RJR Nabisco, Inc., it is the former R.J. Reynolds Industries and mightily has it grown with its acquisition of Nabisco. You don't have to even walk a mile from its Camel to stumble across its many and diverse properties including: Kentucky Fried Chicken, A.1. Steak Sauce, Del Monte canned fruits and vegetables, Ortega taco shells, Chun King canned foods, Shredded Wheat, Grey Poupon Dijon mustard, Regina Red Wine Vinegar, Life Savers, Care-free gum, Oh Henry and Butterfinger candy bars, Blue Bonnet and Fleischmann's margarine, Planters peanuts, Oreo cookies, Premium Saltines, Sunshine crackers, Ritz crackers, Triscuits, Canada Dry, Hawaiian Punch, Harveys Bristol Cream and Smirnoff Vodka.

There is much more going on at Pillsbury than the much-loved Bake-Off competitions. Among the many good things we can put into our grocery cart from Pillsbury are Van de Kamp's frozen seafood and ethnic entrees to be eaten along with all the Jolly Green Giant canned and frozen vegetables. Also microwave pizza, pancakes and popcorn, Poppin' Fresh biscuits and rolls, Soft Breadsticks, Pillsbury's BEST (TM) Apple Danish and Cinnamon Rolls, All Ready Pie Crust, Häagen-Dazs and Sedutto ice cream, Tofutti, LeSorbet, Jack Rabbit dry beans. And if we want to dine out, we may choose a Pillsbury restaurant: Steak and Ale, The Chart House, Luther's Godfather's Pizza, Moxie's Deluxe Grille or even Burger King.

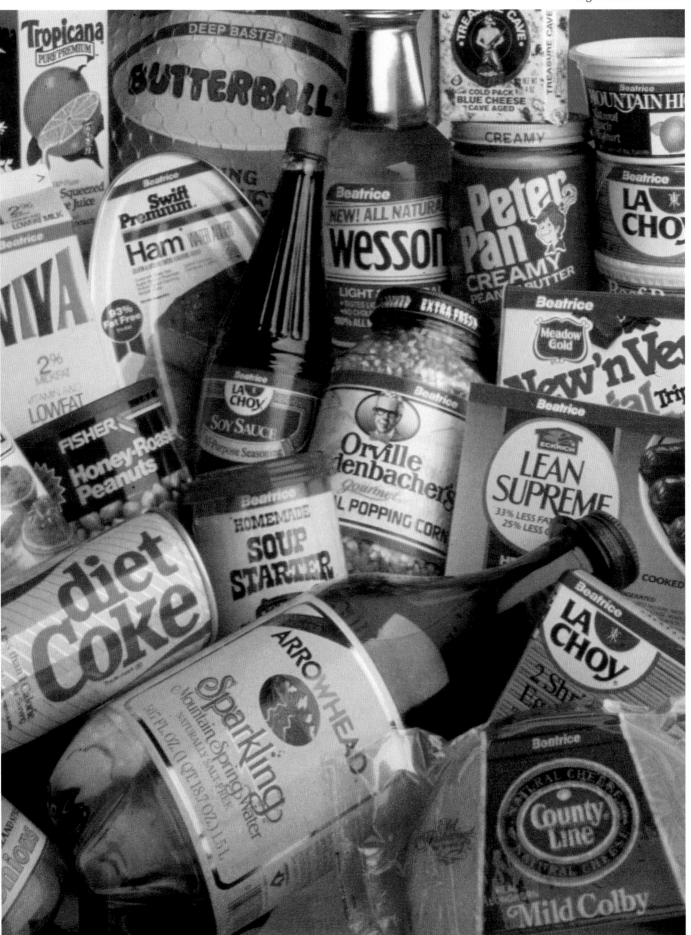

Beatrice can table everything you'd need for a three-meal day, and hasn't forgotten popcorn for the late show.

CAMPBELL'S: AIMED AT THE FUTURE AND LIGHT ON ITS FEET

Food is hot! Qualification: Food companies are hot.

You don't have to be a Wall Street gnome to know that. Stock quotations tell the story in plain numbers. The price of shares in the giant packaged food companies have played leapfrog over the last couple of years, climbing 60 percent in 1985 alone. The once-plodding dinosaurs are bounding ahead like gazelles, some of them racking up annual sales figures that stretch out hungrily toward the $10 billion mark.

Last year, old-line companies like General Foods and Nabisco Brands became the appetizing targets of successful takeovers by, in order, Philip Morris (for $5.75 billion) and R. J. Reynolds (for $4.9 billion). Very hot stuff indeed!

Savvy insiders find the reason for the transformation of these companies in the marketplace, which has turned topsy-turvy since the olden days when Mom would crank up the station wagon for her weekly assault on the local market and return home with 50 pounds or more of staid staples to feed her family.

Mom is still out there, but today she has lots of company. There are shoppers roaming the aisles with appetites that go beyond the basic meat-potato-vegetable-bread-dessert diet that for countless years has defined what food companies would produce for foodmarkets to put on their shelves.

Are you one of the 79 million?
Suppliers now have to reckon also with the appetites of the 21 million Americans—unmarried, separated, widowed or divorced—who live alone and love it. And add another 58 million singles who think like the loners but prefer life in tandem.

The individuals comprising this madding crowd increasingly are calling the food shots. They're self-pleasers, and they aim high. They demand good taste in top-of-the-line items—frozen meals, entrées and desserts, refrigerated salads and packaged breakfasts they can quickly heat and eat. Quality, above all quality, but with as little effort from the consumers as possible. They have too many other interests to spend time studying recipes and crafting a meal from scratch.

They're preoccupied with health, weight and fitness too. On any given day, 50 percent of the U.S. population is on a diet. Ob-

session with the narrow waist and agile step has elicited a torrent of "light" frozen foods, boosting this part of the food business, it's estimated, by one-third.

The food companies heard their message loud and clear, and are reaping the rewards for being good listeners.

Tracking the wild consumer
Remember the Campbell Kids—those plump, cheerful toddlers who started romping, skating, tumbling and dancing their way through Campbell Soup Company advertisements in 1905? They were rarely far from a can of Campbell's soup, and often sang its praises in naive couplets:

My, how Campbell's makes us grow!
Everybody tells us so.
We just beam with health and pride
With our Campbell's soup inside!

Your mother, if you're part of the right generation, would open the classic red and white can, add water and prepare a steaming bowl of, probably, chicken noodle soup, while you cut out the chubby, red-cheeked darlings and pasted them in your scrapbook.

If those playful innocents from 1905 were transported into the Campbell Soup Company of our day, they might well wonder if they hadn't taken a wrong turning along the way. Because the old homestead has

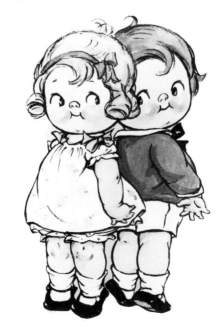

We just beam with health and pride.

changed. Oh, how it has changed from the company Joseph Campbell and one partner founded in 1869. And even from the time of the Kids' birth in 1905, when the company marketed exactly 21 varieties of condensed soup plus pork & beans in a can.

It's the Campbell product line that would probably first dazzle the Kids' popping eyes today—more than 1,000 items are sold worldwide, a bursting cornucopia of food products, with more than 400 created between 1980 and 1986. Frozen soup in plastic tubs you can heat in a microwave and crisp, sophisticated salads that come fresh as the morning in plastic bowls out of the refrigerator case.

The names go on forever
Then they'd ponder with amazement all the strange companies named on the labels, bags and boxes they see. What do Franco-American, Swanson, Pepperidge Farm, Vlasic, Mrs. Paul's, Recipe, Win Schuler, Prego, Casera, Le Menu and Godiva have to do with The Campbell Soup Company?

Or Pietro's Pizza Parlors and Annabelle's Restaurants?

Or Triangle Manufacturing Company, an outfit that makes physical fitness products?

And how about these tomatoes, mushrooms, avocados and salmon? They aren't in cans. They're fresh. It can't be!

Yes, it can. Read the small print, Kids. Never mind the names, product and place. They're all Campbell's, no less genuine Campbell's than the tomatoes, vegetables, jellies, condiments and mincemeat that Joe Campbell first put in cans a few years after the Civil War ended.

It really blows the Kids' minds, though, when they start to look below the surface and see what stands behind the old firm's staggering array of labels, names and products. They find plants that manufacture Campbell cans in such quantity that the company is the third largest producer of metal containers in the world. And they discover the Campbell Institute of Research and Technology (annual budget of more than $35 million) dedicated to new product development, and the Plastics Research Center, opened in 1984, where troops of people who aren't afraid to dream the impossible dream are searching for the elusive plastic compound that will do everything a metal

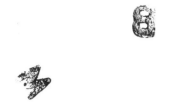

can does to protect its contents and more.

But one thing the Kids would find unchanged is the company's commitment to soup. The word is still an integral part of its name, The Campbell *Soup* Company, which was officially adopted in 1922.

Soup belongs to the people

There's one very good reason Campbell considers soup the centerpiece of its business and never stops adding to the line. Americans have a permanent love affair going with soup. We spoon down more than ten billion bowls of soup in the course of a year. Turning that figure around, 98 percent of all U.S. households purchase soup, with 93 percent of them buying Campbell's. No wonder Campbell has never given up on soup. It accounts for about one-fourth of the company's consolidated sales.

But—and it's a very big but—this is not The Campbell Soup Company of 1905.

The change is more than a matter of size, of growing from a company that peddled soup in a few U.S. locations to one with sales in 120 overseas markets. Growth is a given in the world of business, where the iron law of the marketplace is grow or perish; there is no standing still.

Spaghetti was the first

Like most consumer product companies, Campbell's growth over the decades was primarily nourished by acquisitions, beginning with Franco-American, its first, in 1915. The company's strategy still includes growth by acquisition, and in 1985 it acquired controlling interest in Continental Foods Company, a Belgian diversified food processor, and a 20 percent interest in Australia's premier biscuit maker, Arnott's Limited.

There are a couple of distinctive features to Campbell's acquisitions over the years. For one, they have all been food-related, and the company has never swerved from its dedication to the business of serving the health and nutritional needs of consumers. That allows even Triangle, the maker of physical fitness equipment acquired in 1983, a place in the Campbell family (second cousin, maybe?). The standard that the company now marches under bears the rubric "The Well-Being Company," which makes relatives out of any products that promote the real but indefinable quality of feeling fit and healthy.

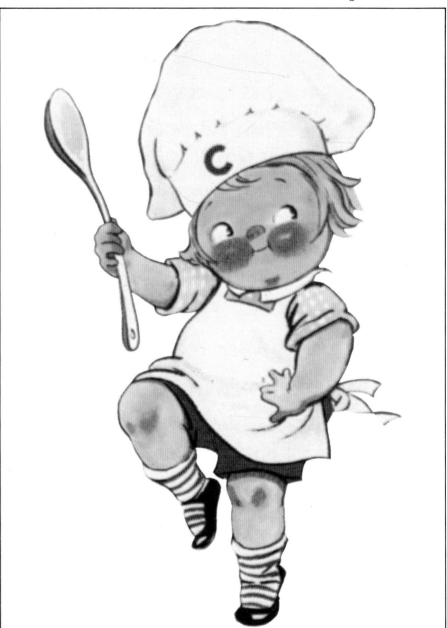

We blend the best with careful pains in skillful combination.

Up and down, Campbell does it all

Campbell's acquisition strategy has made it that rarity among the processed food leaders—in the jargon of the trade, a "vertically integrated" company. Translated, that means it's active at every stage of the business. Campbell produces much of the food it uses, including tomatoes, chicken and salmon; processes the ingredients; makes the cans for hundreds of its food items; and, finally, packages and distributes the products to the marketplace.

Truly a unique player in the $200-billion-plus food business.

And yet for many years Campbell was measured more by its size, dominance in the market and competitive staying power than by qualitative attributes such as innovation, leadership, vision. The word often heard was "stodgy"—a reliable performer but stodgy. One Wall Street analyst who keeps tabs on the food industry was heard to say, some years ago, "Following Campbell is like watching the grass grow."

It's generally agreed that the observed Campbell stodginess was a function of the company's playing off its traditional strengths: superb manufacturing technology, a lock on domestic and international raw materials and immense marketing and distribution muscle.

Booby traps

These great resources had evolved, as is typical with successful companies, in response to market demands. So, during its halcyon years, Campbell concentrated on producing and supplying a growing range of products with mass appeal. After all, that's the kind of market everyone saw out there—what ele-

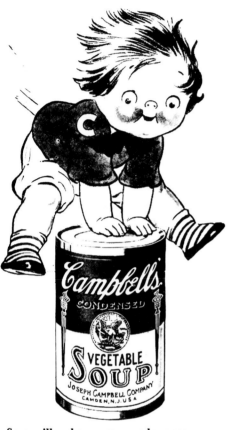

Soup will make you spry and prancey.

mentary economics textbooks call, logically enough, the "mass market."

Something the textbooks tend to obfuscate is that you run the risk of building future booby traps when your basic strategy is to throw your marketing loop around the whole of society.

Oversimplified, here's what happens. Mass appeal depends on the existence of look-alike tastes. So, what do you do? You pour products into the market that match those tastes, products you're able to manufacture economically and also have stored in abundance in distribution centers all around the globe. You expand the list by acquiring companies that make similar products. And you run such a mass business best through a highly centralized organizational structure.

If it isn't broken, don't fix it
For many years such a strategy worked, and worked well, for The Campbell Soup Company. It had iced its competitors in the condensed soup market and was a strong first or second player in other mass-market areas, like canned beans, vegetable juice, pickles and frozen dinners. Even if some of those categories showed signs of losing consumer appeal, why worry? It takes an awful lot of competition to halt a juggernaut.

But what if it's a change in the market, not tougher competition, that's eroding your business a little? What if there are simply fewer people buying the products you're selling?

That's a shocking, but pivotal, hypothesis, and it's one that Campbell was slow to consider. It was also slow to appreciate that the consumer market was slipping little by little out of sync with its awesome capabilities.

The splinter factor
A lot of factors were at work: rapidly changing lifestyles due to the huge increase of live-alones and singles; rising levels of education, affluence and sophistication; new definitions of the "good life"; a booming elderly population with money to spend. Taken together, they smashed the old stable mass market into lots of individual markets.

As R. Gordon McGovern, promoted in 1980 to Campbell president from the same position at Pepperidge Farm, a wholly-owned subsidiary, is fond of saying, "The market is no longer mass. It's micro."

It's almost impossible to say exactly when Campbell began to act on its sense that the consumer world was moving away from it. Somewhere about the close of the 70s is probably as close as it can be calculated.

That's close enough. Dating the moment is nowhere near as important as understanding the company's challenge as it faced off against an aggregation of consumers who displayed no uniform, consistent approach to food and eating. That challenge was nothing less than to retool totally its approach to serving those consumers.

What did you say your name was?
The biggest piece of that challenge was getting to know consumers all over again. You can't decide what to produce until you have a clear view of whom you're selling to, what they're buying, at what price and in what kind of package. That's another way of saying that marketing, getting yourself in tune with the markets, comes first and production follows.

This summary statement sketches the depth and range of the questions Campbell had to answer. The company, early in the 1980s, was starting at ground zero. The answers couldn't be found in its past experience, or in products already on its shelves, or in the rising, successful companies it might acquire.

The consumer had the answers, and there's no doubt that Gordon McGovern led the Campbell charge out into the world beyond corporate headquarters, to get as near to the source as possible. As he once put it, phrasing the objective as a question: "Who is this phantom, the consumer, and do we really know them?"

Try anything, maybe it will work
A lot of the effort took the form of orthodox market research. But McGovern isn't satisfied with orthodoxy—taste polls, focus group discussions and the like. He's an experimenter, and he'll try anything that might draw a face on that "phantom."

One of the most daring is called "Campbell's in the Kitchen." This puts Campbell executives into about 500 kitchens throughout the country, thoughout the year, observing ordinary people preparing their meals. The

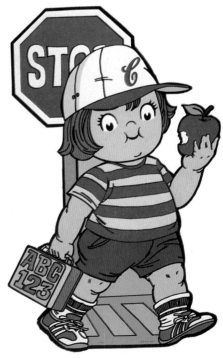

Campbell's takes us off to school.

exercise has added significantly to Campbell's store of consumer knowledge. Executives learn first-hand why their products sell or don't sell and how people actually use food products in the kitchen.

No absentee landlord, McGovern has put the program to the test by visiting kitchens himself—eating in them, too. He has also been known to scout grocery store aisles across the country, a shopping bag in one hand and his briefcase in the other.

Company employees pull a similar duty in Project Grassroots. They're stationed in supermarkets on weekends to canvass shoppers on why they select their purchases.

Freezer burn

Probably the most striking result of turning all this exhaustive market research into product strategy is Campbell's Le Menu dinners. A company study of consumer attitudes toward frozen dinners indicated there was a large untapped market for a more upscale product.

Consumers said they were willing to pay the price for higher quality, more interesting fare and greater variety. Campbell research and development people went to work and came up with Le Menu. It offered gourmet-style fare on a plastic plate, all of which you could microwave and put on the table without embarrassment.

Bullseye! Le Menu ended its first year in national distribution with almost $200 million in sales, advancing Campbell's frozen food business by 43 percent, and in 1985 topped $250 million. The wave of the future that Campbell has been riding ever since takes no consumer group for granted and offers products that are tailor-made to specific requirements. "We don't try to persuade consumers to buy what we have or can make," McGovern says. "We create what they tell us they want."

The Campbell creative drive goes beyond product development. Food products can only be as good as the container they're in allows them to be. It depends on what you want—convenience, freshness or garden-grown flavor. Choose any one of the above or, most difficult to attain, all three at once.

The future awaits

Product and package can't be divorced. That's the *raison d'être* of Campbell's new

Plastics Research Center. It's testing every imaginable plastics technology and layered combination to discover what role plastic may have in keeping foods at peak quality whether they're frozen, refrigerated or stored on an open shelf, no matter how they're to be prepared or eaten by the consumer—the ultimate end of the production line.

As in every aspect of its business, the company is keeping its options open. It's looking at metal, paper, glass as well as plastic—a searching and thorough look—to explore every possibility.

Food, Campbell has found in its long history, can be as fussy, as demanding, as unrelenting, as the consumer who buys it. The Campbell Soup Company is listening attentively and caringly to both, and its formula for success is a very simple equation: Product plus package equals quality. ●

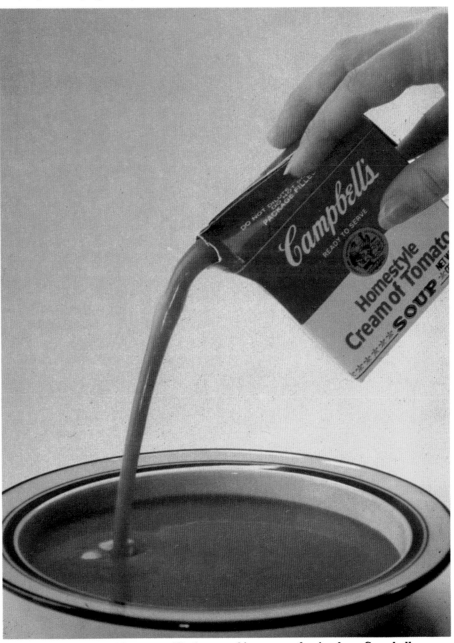

Squeeze and pour, nothing more. The last word in soup packaging from Campbell.

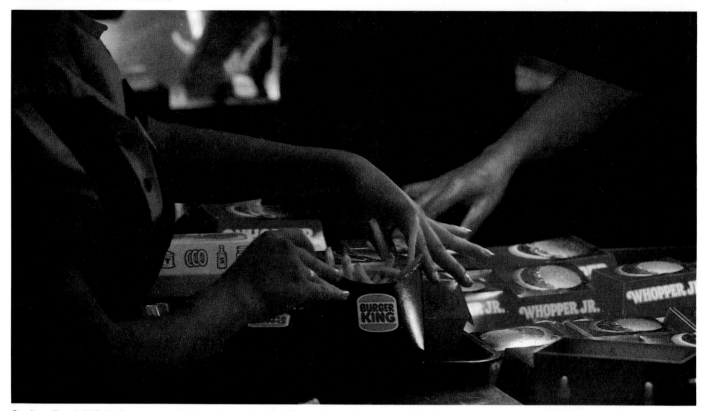

On Any-Road, U.S.A., burgers and fries change hands. The strip needs no name; it's just another hungry driver's street of dreams.

THE STRIP

Columbus, Ohio—Tooling down Route 161, cutting through the northern tip of this synthetic all-American city, you see them. Red roofed cubes. Wooden rectangles with glass-sheathed fronts. Orange neon signs. The kings of the road: McDonald's, Flakey Jake's, Burger King, Pizza Hut, Wendy's, G.D. Ritzy's, Sister's Chicken & Biscuits, Rax, White Castle, Showbiz Pizza Place, D'Lite's.

The hallowed names of fast-food America.

Route 161, with its neighboring roads, is Fast-Food Row in what is championed as the fast-food capital of the world. Some 450 fast-food eateries (67 McDonald's, 59 Wendy's, 35 Kentucky Fried Chickens, 27 Pizza Huts) crowd the Columbus metropolitan area. Because of its youthful population, mass-market tastes and central location, Columbus has long been a popular market testing ground for everything from detergents to bowling-shoe bags. Eight fast-food chains are based here, including Wendy's, the No. 3 empire after McDonald's and Burger King. Columbus is where the modern drive-thru window system was developed. Columbus is where the first Burger King on wheels was unveiled to the world. And, within Columbus, Route 161 is a strip that has become noteworthy as both a cradle for many fast-food infants and a graveyard for others.

"You want something for the stomach?" a

local resident remarked. "Drive that car down Route 161 and you'll see more eating than you ever saw in your life."

The fast-food industry was born 30 years ago. McDonald's Speedee Service Drive-in, the first outlet in the late Ray Kroc's fabled network of more than 8,000 McDonald's, opened its kitchen at 400 North Lee Street in Des Plaines, Ill., on April 15, 1955. And the rest, as any hamburger-eating schoolboy knows, is history.

Since that humble beginning, the selling of speedily made meals has ballooned to a $44.8 billion industry, almost four times what it was 10 years ago. Fast-foot establishments constitute the most lucrative, quickest-growing piece of the food-services pie. And thus there are more than 340 chains pushing superfast hamburgers and chicken and tacos at some 60,000 restaurants. Almost every week, it seems, another individual infected by the dream of, perhaps, instanteous pork chops opens up a kitchen and imagines himself Ray Kroc.

The whole face of fast food, however, has changed. Though the wafer-thin hamburger remains the core of the industry, a spate of new concepts is shaking things up. The hottest new subcategories are gourmet hamburgers, chicken products and "healthy" fast food. "Upscale" is the word on everyone's lips: The generation weaned on fast food is older now, and fussier, so every chain is being forced to overhaul its menus and ambiance.

The industry has had a trying recent past. Sales languished from the fall of 1979 to the fall of 1983, when the economy was soft, but revenues have been rebounding since.

But it is not an entirely merry 30th anniversary. The ominous news is, no matter how rapidly Americans demolish their meals, there are too many chains, too many similar dreams. "Everyone's jumping into new categories that are doomed to failure, because of the saturation," says Charles Bernstein, editor of *Nation's Restaurant News.* "How many gourmet hamburger chains are there room for? Probably one."

Michael Culp, a Prudential-Bache analyst who eats many fast-food meals in order to compute an edibility index, predicts unprecedented bloodletting in plastic America over the next two years. "There is a very serious long-term problem," he says. "It's called too much competition."

He and others envision slow, but solid growth for the survivors—something like 10 percent a year, compared to the 1970s when the industry regularly enjoyed sales increases of 20 percent and more. But they foresee a handful of powerhouses—the likes of McDonald's, Burger King, Wendy's, Kentucky Fried Chicken, Taco Bell, Pizza Hut—ruling America's roadsides, driving all but the sturdiest of the smaller combatants out of the game. Already, the ten biggest chains serve half of all superfast meals and their shadows are lengthening over the industry. ●

N.R. Kleinfield, reporter, The New York Times

On The Run Exponentially

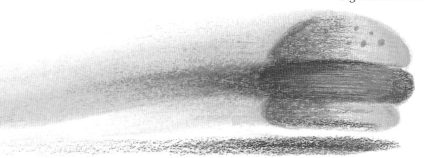

"Now here, you see, it takes all the running you can do, to keep in the same place. If you want to get somewhere else, you must run at least twice as fast as that!"

Lewis Carroll
Through the Looking-Glass

The cunning of the fast feeders lies in that simplest of all the market maxims: continuous, inexorable growth. Every fast-food chain in the country is adding new links as fast as it can, called units. Growth means profit, greater every year, providing investor confidence and rallying and supporting feeder suppliers—the smaller companies that do business with the giants.

If that's hard to follow, think of chain *letters*; they work similarly with less to go on, and they huff and puff and everybody makes some money until the proposition loses credibility, whereupon the scheme collapses. No enterprise in the free market is really any different. All work on the premise that there is

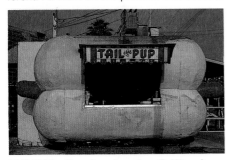

Tail O' The Pup, Los Angeles, California

no end to growth, to profitability. And to prove that, the fast-food companies are quite prepared to go to the ends of the earth—or at least, certainly, to Taiwan.

They'll get a warmer welcome there than they did recently in the affluent village of Great Neck, Long Island, where it came as a nasty jolt to residents that they were about to be joined by Burger King.

Burger King! some citizens exclaimed. You might as well have said Queens or The Bronx to them. "Tempers began to broil," quipped The *New York Times*, meaning a joke upon the Kingdom's open grills.

Petitions unscrolled all over town.

"We don't want it," said one burgher.

"Why? Because we're snobs. It's that sim-

ple. I tell it like it is."

Another protestor charged that the manifestation of Burger King "would change the character of the old village of Great Neck," which is a community of 9,000 simple, discerning people. He then went on to define a wave of the future that is as inevitable, in the global marketplace, as Noah's Flood.

"Next," he recited, "comes your McDonald's, your Roy Rogers, your Kentucky Fried Chicken and who knows what else."

The man was not speaking hyperbole. It may be that he reads the trades and understands the economic necessities which drive the fast feeders. It's all built right into each company structure to proliferate until they saturate—then (sigh) die. So here they come, like it or not, into every spot near *you* where enough fast food can be sold to produce a margin of profit. So far, that would be everywhere in this country where there's a vacant lot or a convertible dwelling that's zoned commercial.

The American fast-food industry now does $44.8 billion in business annually, according to *The New York Times*. In the past 10 years, this industry has quadrupled in size, and there are now 340 different chains sponsoring more than 60,000 outlets. Considering the next decade, if you multiply that by eight, you get 2,720 chains sponsoring 480,000 outlets. And if you wonder what your quality of life will be by then, think about whether you'd prefer Taco Bell for a neighbor or—if you're lucky—Wendy's in your livingroom. ●

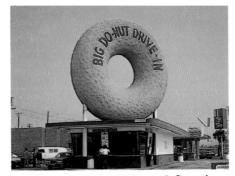

Big Do-Nut Drive-In, Inglewood, Georgia

The Miller Lite Analogy If you were going to start up a fast-food operation for health-conscious people, what would you offer them? Tofu Surprise? Mung bean loaf?

Not so Doug Sheley, a veteran entrepre-

neur who by the mid-70s had opened 18 outlets of Wendy's in eastern Tennessee. He wanted to create a menu that would be healthy and appealing at the same time.

His first D'Lites outlet opened on Peachtree Street in Atlanta in 1981. The menu featured lean burgers on high-fiber, multigrain buns; a vegetarian mulch shoved into a whole-wheat pita pocket with sprouts; and a frozen yogurt dessert with 40 percent fewer calories than ice cream.

"Lite" is the watchword. Even the mayonnaise is "lite." And so is the beer. *"L-i-t-e,"* says Sheley, "means a reduction of something bad for you, but not to the extent that it ends up being bland." D'Lites does not cut calories at the expense of taste or nutrition. They like to say they sell "reduced-calorie" foods, not "low-calorie" foods.

Sheley now has 38 restaurants in 11 states, and 22 more are in construction. If plans go according to schedule, there will be 600 D'Lites in America by 1991, and everything in them will be very "lite." ●

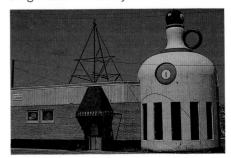

Sandy Jug Tavern, Portland, Oregon

No Cha-Cha At Chi Chi's Poor Chi-Chi's. A mere three years ago, analysts were predicting for it an annual earnings growth of 50 percent. This Mexican dinner house was the darling of the market, a leader among the young companies coming up fast in the wake of the giants. But its stock plummeted at the end of '84, losing half of its value, and the share price went even lower after that. Expansion problems took the rap, nor is that unusual with new, eager outfits.

Consider Mrs. Winner's Chicken & Biscuits, based in Nashville. Its earnings sank 50 percent in 1984. Says M.V. "Buck" Hussung, Jr., president of Winners Corp.: "We all suffer from trying to do too much too quickly. You can't grow beyond your ability to manage." ●

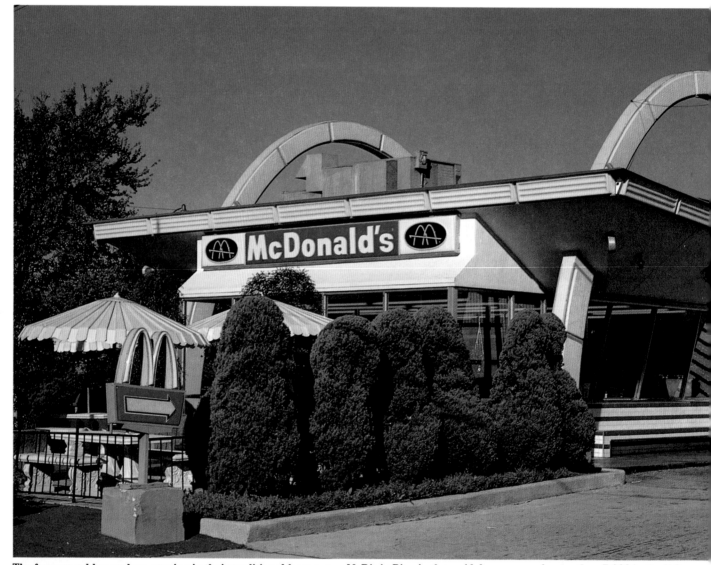

The famous golden arches, curving in their traditional form over a McD's in Birmingham, Alabama, one of more than 7,000 in the U.S.

McFacts

McDonald's McPublic Relations Department says that:

If you lined up all the 50 billion burgers they've sold, they'd circle the earth 19 times. And if you stacked them straight up, they'd reach the planet Pluto, 3,185,000 improbable miles away.

The late Ray Kroc, senior chairman of the McDonald's Corporation:

"We take the hamburger business more seriously than anyone else."

"We've worked out the precise formula for making a hamburger to the public's liking—down to the exact size of the bun, three and a quarter inches, and how much onions go on it, one-fourth of an ounce."

"It requires a certain kind of mind to see beauty in a hamburger bun."

AdWeek reports: "Despite ever increasing competition in the fast food field, McDonald's said last week that it anticipates opening 500 new stores worldwide, a rate of growth the company has maintained for over a decade. About 200 of the planned stores would be in the U.S., with the others spread through the other 40 countries McDonald's operates in. If expansion goes as anticipated, by the end of the year McDonald's will operate 9,401 stores worldwide."

By our calculations, this means that McDonald's is opening 1.37 stores every day, or one store every 17 hours. You wouldn't think there was that much McSauce in the world to go around.

Consider that in the last two minutes alone, McDonald's served 16,800 hamburgers.

And consider as well the observation of Michael Culp, of Prudential-Bache Securities Inc., that McDonald's "is the dominant factor in its field. . . . It's the chain with a restaurant on virtually every corner in the U.S." ●

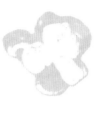

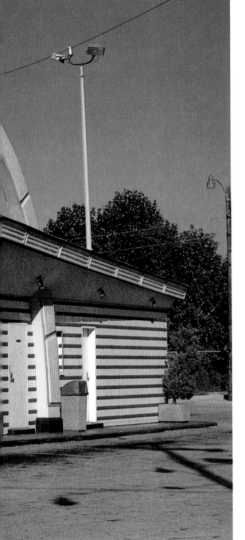

They're Just Trying To Get Our Attention Through the first nine months of 1985, McDonald's spent $226 million on network and spot TV, 20 percent more than it spent in the first three quarters of 1984 and 65 *percent* more than in '83.

Burger King's TV ad outlay, January to December 1985, was $110 million, up 10.4 percent over the previous year.

Wendy's spending, up 15 percent, was $63.2 million in the same period. Other third-quarter figures in '85: Kentucky Fried Chicken, $54.6 million; Pizza Hut, $48.6 million; Taco Bell, $30.1 million; Hardee's, $24.5 million; Long John Silver's, $19.4 million; Denny's, $17.4 million; Arby's, $11.6 million; Sizzler, $10.3 million; Jack in the Box, $9.3 million; Dairy Queen, $9.3 million.

According to *Advertising Age*, when the final computations are made, the fast food industry is expected to have spent $1.075 billion on TV ads in 1985. ●

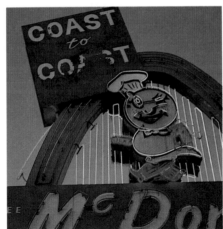

The way it's done in Azusa, California.

How Now Dow Chow? Rainbow Specialties of Riverside, California, knows a parody prospect when it sees one. And, oh, has it seen one.

It may be barking up the wrong tree, but the company has introduced Yuppie Chow.

"Your yuppie has the potential to build greater prestige and a healthier wallet by indulging in a new nutritional gourmet cuisine developed to ensure a hearty six-figure income," Rainbow says. "Yuppie Chow is recommended by four out of five financial analysts."

And what is Yuppie Chow? Why, packaged popcorn. We got the brie flavor, which comes at a yupscale price—$7.95. ●

ADWEEK

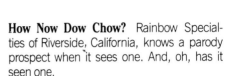

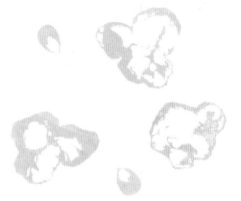

Every How Often? Along with breathtaking statistics that show a new McDonald's or Wendy's outlet opening while you blink your eyes, there's yet another that is troubling to the industry.

Every 27 minutes, some fast-food unit somewhere in the country is victimized by robbers. They threaten, brutalize and terrorize staff and customers and seize all the cash in the till, usually in a matter of two to three minutes, usually in the night hours (but also sometimes after the lunch rush, when robbers know they can expect a large haul). The cash loss, rarely more than $500, is usually covered by insurance. ●

Burger King Rolls Recently it struck the Burger King management that their units didn't have to just sit there, cemented to their bases, waiting for customers to come. Some units could be mobile, could ride on wheels and roam about the topography in search of customers.

The Burger King "Express" units were born—with every menu feature except the salad bar—and their targets will be college campuses, seasonal resorts, construction sites and military bases.

Meanwhile, the operation is a toe into the home-delivery business, which Burger King is contemplating. ●

Wendy's Goes To The Hospital The chain recently received its first on-site hospital lease. The setting is the Miami Valley Hospital in Dayton, Ohio. According to hospital spokesman Doug Paplaczyk, it would have cost Miami Valley $200,000 to renovate the tired old coffee shop they had on the premises. In this arrangement, Wendy's was willing to put up $500,000 to renovate the leased space. Wendy's also pays the hospital a percentage of the unit's gross sales.

But why did the hospital choose hospital-inexperienced Wendy's, when a certain larger chain is already in the field? According to Paplaczyk, Wendy's is considered to be the leader of the fast-food chains when it comes to developing foods that might be considered to have more nutritional value. This, he felt, had been demonstrated by the company's early implementation of salad bars and its recent unveiling of a "light" menu. ●

I CAN'T BELIEVE
I ATE THE WHOLE THING

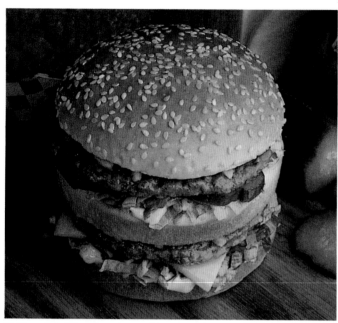

McDonald's Big Mac: meat with munchies, cheese and such.

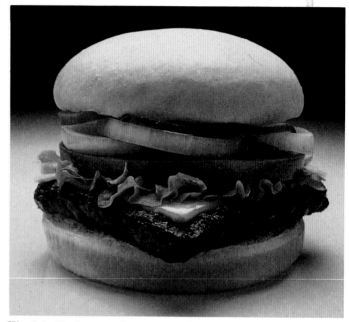

Wendy's Single: meat is square and onion is there.

Let's pretend you're a big-time corporate investor and you're very hungry for some fast food. According to current investment pundits, you could be onto a good thing. Fast-food outfits didn't look particularly delicious in yesterday's market—too soft, too uncertain for acquisition then. Takeover appetites are for red meat and baked potatoes, something very substantial.

But cash-rich companies have been looking at a wide-variety of consumer-oriented companies in recent times, and Wall Street has wondered aloud, through the columnists who write in its journals and newsletters, whether some of the fast-food outfits are not now ripe for the plucking, and whether what they term a "fever" is not hotting up in the direction of McDonald's, Wendy's and the like.

We know that somebody put the moves on McDonald's in 1985 in a suit that was not reciprocated, because the company announced that it was taking new anti-takeover measures, prompted by what it termed the "current abusive takeover environment." Wall Street analysts and speculators were intrigued, and Emanuel Goldman, of Montgomery Securities, told *The Wall Street Journal* at the time that "fast food may be the next large arena in terms of acquisitions."

Why should this be? To quote the *Journal:* "High-quality fast-food chains offer high-profile consumer franchises that are recession-resistant, produce consistent earnings, have healthy balance sheets and benefit from lower commodity prices.

"Unlike food processors, the best fast-food companies offer the additional promise of substantial unit growth and annual double-digit earnings gains, even during sluggish economic periods."

Investors are particularly attracted to "substantial unit growth," which is a built-in, do-or-die feature of the chains. So long as the company's units proliferate, the investor can expect appreciable annual earnings growth. And that is what the investor wants.

John Weiss, also of Montgomery, follows restaurant and food stocks. Companies he named with an annual earnings growth potential of 25 percent or more include Jerrico, Collins Foods, Shoney's, Church's Fried Chicken and International Kings Table. (In comparison, Weiss predicted that McDonald's earnings will grow at about 12 percent; Wendy's International, and Pillsbury's Burger King, he pegs at a 15 percent annual growth rate.)

Analysts say that McDonald's is the choicest target, but at $7.5 billion or so, the most prohibitively expensive hamburger in

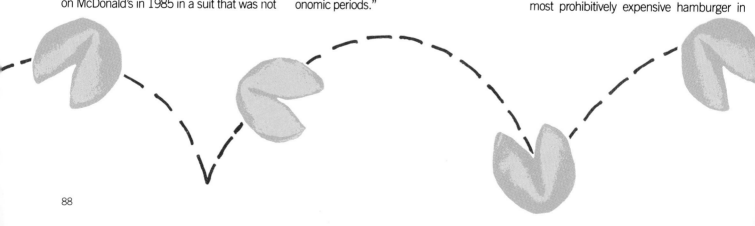

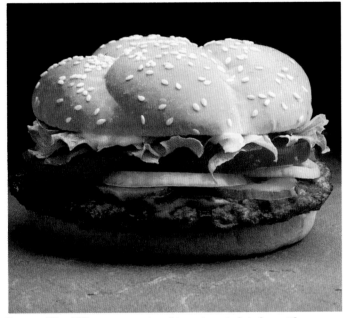

Burger King Whopper: meat and tomatoes twixt elegant bun.

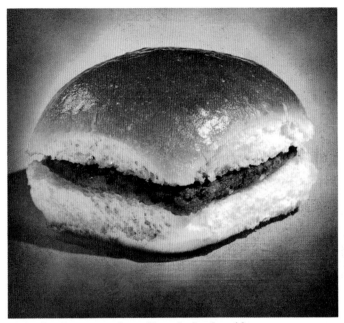

White Castle: meat and good bread, simply said.

town. Also, the company is not prone to receptivity and will use all its muscle to beat off an intrusion. One easier prospect named by analysts is Jerrico, which owns Long John Silver's Seafood Shoppes. They believe that Jerrico will be bought "sooner rather than later," and that this move will bring on market "fever" to go for other chains as well.

The talk is that PepsiCo might seek to embrace Jerrico. It already has Pizza Hut and Taco Bell in its tummy; with Italian and Mexican fast food already on its plate, it could have an appetite for the fast-rising seafood end of the business.

Wendy's also looks plump and comely; costly, to be sure, but ripe and alluring.

All Wall Street knows for certain is that when big fish get hungry, they go looking for little fish . . . or hamburgers . . . or chicken . . . or tacos . . . ●

Chinese Fast Food, Sweet & Sour

It used to be said by the fast food franchise folks that Chinese food was no good in that market. The cooking is so complex, so delicate, so time-consuming, that labor costs were bound to be high. Thus there was no chance of offering prices lower than those in regular Chinese restaurants.

Craig Schowalter, a food technician for Nankin Express, has changed all that, and declares that, by standardization, he can cut labor costs from 50 percent of total operating costs to 5 percent.

In a six-month study of a cuisine that is at least a thousand years old, Schowalter developed a four-step process of which he claims that 80 percent of all Chinese recipes can be readily adapted.

"All the magic can be taken out of it," he boldly states.

There are now several companies eyeing Chinese food franchises, or launching them. Quick Wok, China Rose and Eggroll Express have—as does Nankin Express—national ambitions.

A component of this brand of Chinese fast food is that the franchises can be run by non-Chinese entrepreneurs and served by non-Chinese employees.

The only question, of course, is whether the American public will want the magic taken out of the oldest and possibly most loved cuisine in the world. ●

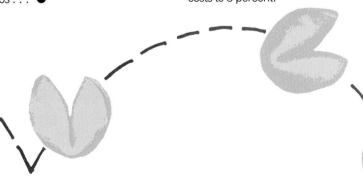

THE UNTAPPED DEMAND

Tom Monaghan insists on pepperoni when he's having a pizza. He wants sausage, onion, extra cheese and bacon too, but if it doesn't have pepperoni, he won't touch it.

Why do we care? Because Tom Monaghan is the founder and CEO of Domino's Pizza, Number Two after Pizza Hut in the usual competition, but front-runner in food service on wheels—a runaway craze that is going to revolutionize American eating habits and make a significant change in where the money goes.

Therefore, what Tom Monaghan likes on his pizza becomes automatically interesting; though more telling, perhaps, is the decisive way in which he lets you know about it.

Frank Lloyd Wright is one of Monaghan's major heroes. Knute Rockne is another. Ray Kroc (the guiding intelligence that built McDonald's) is also in the pantheon. All highly individualistic, driving men who had vision. It's not surprising that Monaghan's Law should be: "If there's an easy way and a hard way, take the hard way."

In 25 years, Monaghan has built Domino's Pizza from an Ann Arbor college kid outlet into a multinational organization. Domino's 1984 food and beverage sales totaled $626 million. On the way, he had hard times. He suffered near bankruptcy and lost control of the business for a time. Of that experience he says, "It tempers you. It's the best education in the world."

Today there are 2,472 Domino units, and the average unit volume is $450,000 annually. Monaghan's plans envision 10,000 units by 1990. "I think Domino's can get up to 10,000 stores in five years," Monaghan says. "The (home delivery) industry is at least that big again. It seems to me that we've just scratched the surface."

All this is based on Monaghan's carefully designed system for delivering piping hot pizza in less than 30 minutes of taking the order. Nothing less will do.

Monaghan, 48, grew up in orphanages and foster homes. He is an ex-seminarian and an ex-Marine. In 1960, he and his brother borrowed about $1,000 to start a pizzeria in Ypsilanti, Michigan. One year later, he and his brother made a deal: Tom's care for his brother's share in the business. Today he owns 94 percent of the enterprise.

The reason for Domino's success, says Monaghan, is going "the additional step of providing a service beyond what anyone else does and delivering it dependably. The secret of doing that is trying not to do everything else too. The system is very simple. Domino's people are pizza people, period. They try to do one thing and do it well."

As for himself, Monaghan says, "Being stupid is a blessing. I believe, because I'm not too bright, that I want to have everything going for me. I want everybody on the team pulling for me. And the only way everybody on the team can be pulling for me is if I really treat them well. Try never to talk down to anyone. People work for me, but I really work for them. Give everybody autonomy. Let them make mistakes. Just sit back and watch them go. Have no secrets, share my dreams and ambitions. Be as open as you can be."

It seems to work. Domino's employees operate with split-second timing. Every step is plotted in a process which begins well before the customer calls. In optimum conditions, Domino can turn out a pizza in six minutes. Then the race is on to deliver insulated, hot pizza to the customer. More often than not, Domino meets its commitment.

So far, there is no fast food out there on wheels that can beat Domino, and Domino means to keep it that way. ●

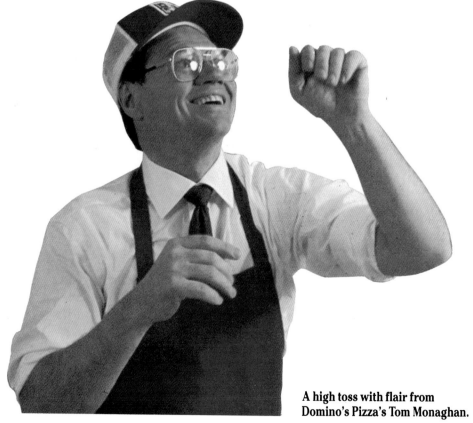

A high toss with flair from Domino's Pizza's Tom Monaghan.

One With Anchovies, Hold The .38

When Daniel and Monika Crotta decided to spice up their San Diego pizza business in 1983, they settled on a police motif. They decorated the store to look like a precinct house and called it the New York Pizza Department, or NYPD, since Monika got her recipes from an uncle in Manhattan. For orders to go, the Crottas hit on the notion of delivering in two white "squad cars." Daniel cleared the idea with the San Diego police. Says he: "They didn't endorse us, but they didn't discourage us."

But that was before the police started getting complaints from people who confused the NYPD cars with real SDPD vehicles. One citizen tried to flag down an NYPD car after seeing a burglary and was outraged when the pizza man kept right on going. To prevent such mix-ups, the state legislature is considering a bill that would bar vendors from using vehicles that look like police cars. To avoid a showdown, the Crottas have made some changes. The word pizza now appears in seven places on their cars, and the NYPD logo has been enlarged. But the confusion may just be starting. Business is so good that the Crottas hope to open pizza precincts in Arizona, Colorado, Texas and Utah. ●

Time

Itza Good Idea Anybody who has ever trudged regularly into a college dining hall will remember such delicacies as "mystery meat" and "the green death." It's mostly in the eye of the beholder, but when you are the possessor of a meal plan, everything served looks pretty dreary after a while.

The Campus Dining Division of ARA Services feeds students on 240 American campuses and, while they have never consciously served "the green death," they would sometimes notice a sullen expression on the faces of their young clients, and a vast number of empty cardboard pizza cartons in the dorm trash barrels.

In the summer of 1984, ARA introduced Itza Pizza, a campus outlet designed to resemble a chain pizzeria. The chain did $3 million in its first year; in 1986, with outlets operating on 100 campuses, they expect to make over $7 million.

ARA bustles. Local ads are emphatic. "Itza great! Itza authentic!" And Itza Pizza "hotline" numbers are posted near telephones. Students who skip dinner in the dining hall are entitled to vouchers worth $2.50 a time at Itza Pizza.

Not everybody is so crazy about Itza Pizza, however. In Potsdam, New York, local merchants have been trying to shut down the outlet on the Clarkson University campus. Local pizzerias said their delivery business was down 30 percent. Merchants have filed a complaint charging that the campus is not zoned for commercial restaurants like Itza Pizza.

Itza crying shame. ●

We Were Just Kidding, Folks! Early in 1985, Pizza Hut was running a comic commercial down in South Carolina which portrayed a condemned man eating a pizza as his last meal. That was fine, until a condemned man in a South Carolina prison ordered a pizza for his last meal before going to the electric chair. His choice was duly reported in the press, and this instance of life imitating art offended four South Carolinians sufficiently that they complained to Pizza Hut headquarters in Wichita, Kansas. Pizza Hut immediately withdrew their convict commercial from South Carolina TV.

Unkindest cut of all: The real-life condemned man ate a hearty meal of pizza . . . but it wasn't from Pizza Hut. ●

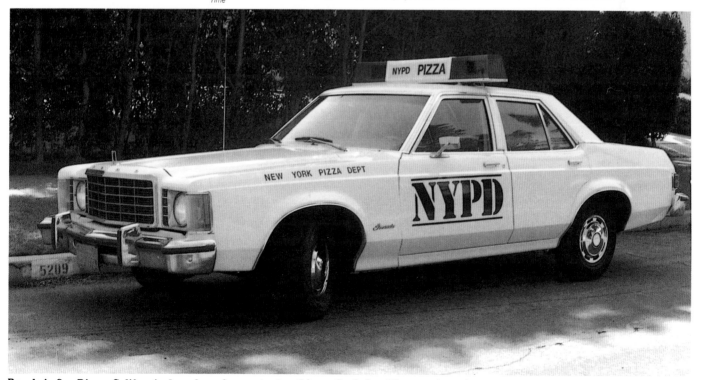

People in San Diego, California, have been known to stop this car for help with more than pizza.

IS WHAT YOU EAT REALLY WHO YOU ARE?

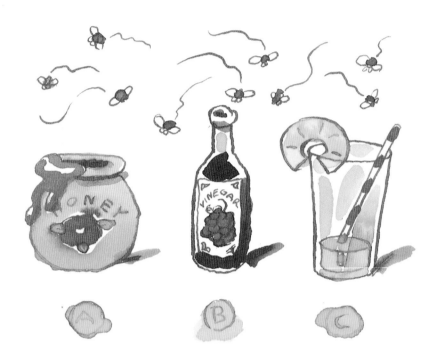

Mother Hubbard's Multiflavored Personality Inventory Test

Section I: Theory

In each category pick the statement that most closely corresponds to your cherished beliefs.

1. Aesthetics:
   a. Nothing becomes a lobster like boiling sea water.
   b. The wilder the cherry, the sweeter the juice.
   c. It's never a mistake to order a plain grilled chop in a fancy French restaurant.

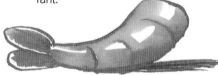

2. Tradition:
   a. Serving chive cheese with lox is the compromise of a timid soul unable to face up to a slab of onion.
   b. I always butter my bagel before adding cream cheese.
   c. Sweetened cheeses aren't so bad.

3. Individual Talent:
   a. I always shell my own shrimp.
   b. I always use heavy cream on my corn flakes.
   c. I never eat at a place called Ma's.

4. Morality:
   a. Thai food that doesn't bring tears to the eyes is inauthentic.
   b. Cocoa skins are probably good for you.
   c. Most people, when offered a fruit salad with miniature marshmallows and a sour-cream-mayonnaise-maraschino dressing, will eat it if they are sure no one is watching.

5. Philosophy:
   a. Brown foods are better for you than white ones.
   b. The above statement is truer for sugar and chocolate than for rice.
   c. And applied to eggs and mushrooms it's a distinction that exists only in a brainwashed consumer's imagination.

6. Value Systems:
   a. Too many cooks spoil the broth.
   b. Toast crusts make your hair curly.
   c. Kind words butter no parsnips.

Section II: Practice

Complete the following statements with the answer that best describes your preferences.

1. Pizza crust should be
   a. thin and staunch.
   b. thick and crunchy.
   c. easy to fold.

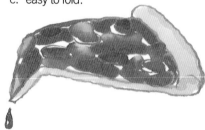

2. Beans in chili are
   a. an abomination.
   b. yummy, but then, I'm not from Texas.
   c. OK, but what I really like is the spaghetti.

3. Ice cream on Indian Pudding is
   a. a barbarism, as the *Joy of Cooking* so rightly recognizes.
   b. a problem, in that the exact proportions of cold Häagen-Dazs to hot pudding are impossible to determine until the second helping, and sometimes not even then.
   c. good.

4. More flies are caught with
   a. honey.
   b. vinegar.
   c. last night's unfinished piña colada.

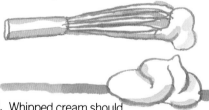

5. Whipped cream should
   a. hold its shape.
   b. melt over the sides of a slice of cake and sweep the surrounding plate like an incautious curtsy.
   c. be sweetened.

6. When scrambling eggs
   a. slow cooking is imperative, in order to

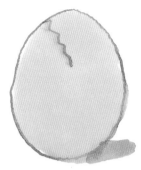

achieve the proper tapioca-like consistency.

   b. a few crusty brown patches actually make a nice textural addition.

   c. it is not necessary to mix yolk and white before the egg hits the pan.

7. Chocolate cheesecake is

   a. a crime against nature.

   b. the best of two worlds.

   c. seldom transcendent but worth pursuing.

8. The best coffee is made

   a. with spring water and home-roasted, freshly ground beans.

   b. in a shiny espresso machine in a little café that has marble-topped tables and pictures of Italian soccer stars on the walls.

   c. in a machine capable of turning itself on just before the alarm goes off in the morning.

Section III: Essay Questions
Answer only one.

   A. Comment on the following statement by a young urban professional: "I'd rather eat mediocre food in a great room than a wonderful meal in a place no one goes." (Hint: Explore the relationship between moral fiber and bran fiber.)

   B. "You are what you eat." Comment, drawing on historic example. (Hint: Trace the literary and sociopolitical development of this idea from Eve to John Belushi in *Animal House*.)

   C. Explain the simultaneous recent rise in popularity of sushi and cocaine. (Hint: Expound on the known sinus-clearing properties of green horseradish.)

Scoring: If you find yourself drawn mostly to A answers you're a Purist, confident·that there is a best in this uncertain world and that you're just the soul to recognize it when you see it. Speaking of souls, whether their incorruptibility takes the form of sophisticated gourmet dining or a rigorous health food regimen, purists have no doubt that their gastronomic lifestyles are based on sound moral judgement.

   B boys and girls (I'm speaking of answers, natch)—you're the Romantics in the crowd. You let your emotions get tangled up in your dinners. Although you suspect the purists

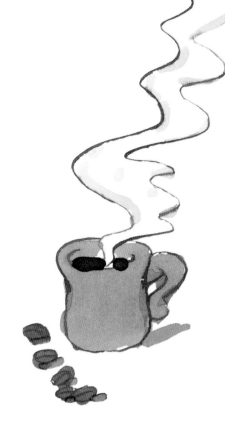

may be right about the connection between eating and morality, you keep letting your taste buds sweep you away.

   Mostly Cs? Practical you. You know what you like and what you're not going to waste time on. Other people think you have the palate of a Neanderthal, and sometimes you do. But you're too hard-headed to be blinded by fads that can fool a Purist and too hard-hearted to be troubled by Romantic guilt.

   The months ahead: As Libra's balanced dietary influence begins to wane, beware of stepping off your scales. The advent of Scorpio, ruler of food additives and hidden calories, will make Purists glower, while feeding Practicals' and Romantics' worst impulses.

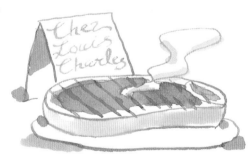

But the Purists will have their revenge under Sagittarius, who always shoots his own game. Not until Capricorn, that goatish omnivore, takes charge (just in time for the holiday season) will Romantics, Practicals and Purists be able to share the same table in any sort of harmony. ●

Ariel Swartley, freelance writer. The Boston Phoenix

CHRISTOPHER IDONE'S GRILLED MINIATURE VEGETABLES
Baby vegetables are for the true grown-ups.

Serves 6

Ingredients:
3 long Japanese eggplants
3 red bell peppers
3 yellow bell peppers
3 "chocolate" bell peppers
3 heads garlic
6 ears fresh baby corn, unhusked
3 white baby eggplants
6 miniature zucchini with blossoms
6 miniature yellow squash with blossoms
6 miniature pattypan squash with blossoms
1 cup fruity olive oil
Salt and freshly ground pepper
$1/4$ cup chopped fresh thyme, sage, rosemary or chives, optional

Method:
1. Prepare an outdoor grill, preferably with grapevine cuttings as kindling.

2. Slice the Japanese eggplants into thirds lengthwise, leaving them attached at the stem ends. Fan the slices out from the stems.

3. Halve the peppers lengthwise and remove the stems, seeds and veins.

4. Cut a small slice off the stem and root ends of the garlic leaving the skin on. Cut each bulb in half crosswise.

5. Remove the corn silks, but leave the husks on.

6. Leave the baby eggplant, zucchini and squashes whole.

7. Brush the vegetables with the olive oil and season to taste with salt and pepper.

8. When the coals have a dusty red glow, grill the vegetables for about 7 minutes, turning to cook evenly, until they are charred.

9. If you have grilled over grapevine cuttings, the vegetables will need no further seasoning; otherwise, sprinkle them with the chopped fresh herbs before serving.

THE OUTER LIMITS

For those of you whose memory may have gone astray in a time warp or who simply weren't there then, fifty years ago a package was something you received in the mail, often from Grandma. And a label—well, you stuck a label on the package *you* were mailing to Grandma or, if you were one of the contrary people who trusted no cooking but your own, carefully fixed one on the Mason jar—after retrieving it, steaming, from its boiling bath—so you wouldn't serve the kids tomatoes instead of strawberry preserves to spread on their bread.

For "good old days" read BS—before supermarkets. Not before food chains, you understand, but supermarkets, because in that distant time you could find an A&P (represented on the marquee as The Great Atlantic & Pacific Tea Company) that today, of course, would be swallowed up in the greeting card section of one of our giant, super-duper drug emporiums.

As for shopping carts! You might as well have tried to drive your car down the aisle. You asked your genial proprietor to snatch any item out of reach with an extending mechanical hand.

Way back, when grandma was there

And Grandma, or her surrogate, was there, too, smiling out at you from jelly jar and cookie tin. A can shaped like a log cabin sent the comforting message that the syrup therein had been gathered right out of the trees. Messrs. Post and Kellogg offered their basic cereal in boxes that were as dry and colorless as their contents: Add milk and hope for the best. The cook displayed on the Cream of Wheat box held a bowl of pale mush wreathed in steam, wore a chef's hat, and flashed a toothy smile that clearly implied you were in for a lipsmacking treat when you tasted *his* cereal.

A different scene. No arrogant cat defying you to tell *him* what to eat. No psychedelic designs in day-glo colors to trumpet a shampoo you can use to seduce Don Johnson or a box of dried soup that suggests it has been lovingly prepared in the kitchens of Lutèce. No packages that grab you by the throat, shake you silly and make you buy, buy, buy.

And no mind-boggling array of 12,000 different products—from herb teas to pâtés to gourmet specialties with a ravishing Cordon Bleu taste—that greets the numbed eyes of 1980s shoppers when they enter their temple of blatant consumerism to replenish empty larders.

No, none of these. Just a simple choice among the staples you needed to keep life and the family going.

Farewell, Grandma. You don't live here anymore.

Dispatch from the packaging front

It's rarely talked about in public, but there's a secret war going on under the surface of the glitzy world of contemporary packaging. Well, maybe "war" is putting it a bit strong. Let's call it "tension," as between two disagreeing states, where neither side takes any overtly hostile action but each side, although occasionally teaming up with the other out of self-interest and in the cause of mutual survival, represents in essence an opposing ideology.

On one side of this unacknowledged contest stand the package designers, the masters of optical illusion, driven by an ambition to stop shoppers dead in their tracks and persuade them to drop the "sizzle" into the cart before checking on the "steak" inside. In the trade, this is sometimes called the "first strike." Its thesis? The product that hits quickest puts the enemy (the competing products) at a severe disadvantage.

For package designers, packaging is marketing, a device, like advertising, to capture the attention of consumers so winningly that they won't take the time to put their brains in gear. Packaging in design terms is decoration, adornment, seduction, if you like.

The outside story.

You sense a bias here, an animus against talented pros who only play around with the surface of things?

More like a divided mind. Anybody who's

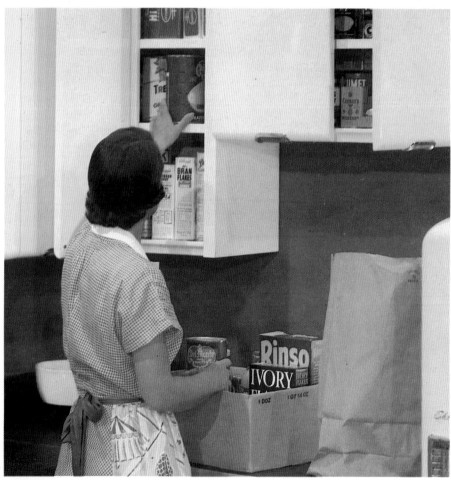

Back in the old days, life was simpler . . . and so were the labels.

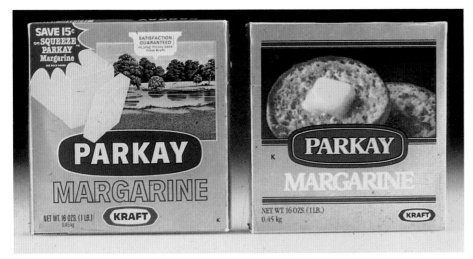

It's still an oleaginous paste, but with its new cover Parkay is irresistible.

dedicated to improving the appearance of our ugly urban/industrial/commercial environment gets my vote. And Alvin Schechter, one of the most successful package designers, is working off a cogent insight when he calls the package a "continuing billboard" and says packages are (almost) forever. So true. A TV spot lasts 30 seconds, you throw away the magazine after a couple of days, but the package stares you in the face week in and out, on the supermarket shelf or in your pantry.

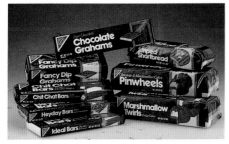

A face lift turned strangers into family.

But . . . oh, I have quite a few buts.

Like, but hey, fellows, do you have to take yourselves so seriously? Reading interviews with package designers in the trade press (they will talk, and talk, and talk, at the drop of a microphone), you have the impression that a lot of them think their peers are Picasso and Modigliani, when they're really more like copycat Andy Warhols looking for those 15 minutes of celebrity that the aging con artist said everyone in the world would one day experience.

The sugar-coated phrase

And the language they use to describe their work and inspiration is, pure and simple, confectionery, landing about as much punch as a bowl of Jell-O. I, for one, could take the designers' genuine successes a lot more seriously if they deleted from their vocabulary mandarin phrases like "strategic package design," "vital signs" (of a product), "visual bonding" and "creative flashes."

But (a "but" on their side) despite all the hype and the hip chatter, we do owe this fancy breed a debt of gratitude for the way they're cleaning up the visual pollution that clogs supermarket shelves. They're coordinating, simplifying and clarifying the packaging design of product lines that occupy huge swaths of shelf space, such as pet foods, dairy products, detergents, soft drinks and cookies.

John Lister, an executive and co-founder of the respected ListerButler design firm in Manhattan, gave focus and appeal to the Parkay Margarine pack when he deleted what he calls "the swamp" from its background, and his design for the various Nabisco cocoa-coated cookies cooled down the glaring, conflicting colors of the different brands to a soothing, discreet chocolate brown with gold trim.

If your eye is pleased by the new look on some baby food, soup mix, soda, cigarette and detergent packages, thank Alvin Schechter. New Coke, Coke Classic and the new cigarette emblazoned with Yves Saint Laurent's elegant logo, all arrest the eye with-

out blinding it. No mean feat.

These designers, too, are not above sticking their neck out and taking a stand. A couple of bright, funky ladies named Millie Falcaro and Mary Tiegreen are a good case in point. One of their clients, a manufacturer of Italian condiments, wanted to splash bright colors all over its toothpaste-like tubes (a neat idea in itself) of garlic, onion and tomato pastes.

Falcaro and Tiegreen held out for a black box and a black tube as the ground for crisp, bright photographs of the vegetables pureed within. And they won.

The dignified sound of silence

Can you imagine anything more subdued and understated than basic black, which may well become the reigning chic supermarket color? It's just possible we're on the threshold of a new era, where dignity and originality rather than visual "noise" are seen

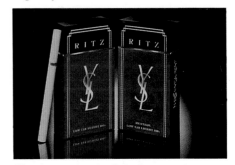

"Putting on the ritz," designer style

as the high road to the shopper's heart. Hope springs eternal!

This hope gets a lot of support from a raft of energetic and inventive entrepreneurs scattered throughout the United States, unknown except to their customers, but just the same a constant leaven working on the lumpy loaf of commercial, manufactured packaging. Their specialty is the made-to-

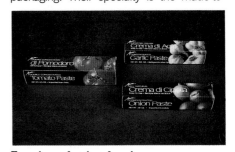

Even in packaging, less is more.

order package, exquisitely tailored, like a Savile Row suit, according to the precise requirements of the individual customer.

It's happening, for example, in specialty food shops and departments, where "we aim to please" is the first rule of marketing.

Surprises downstairs

Expression Unltd., in Warren, New Jersey, is one of these. Descend a corner staircase from its ground floor chock-a-block with domestic and imported palate-tingling treasures and you'll find yourself in a spacious room where clever artisans are eager to work instant miracles on your purchase. With elementary ingredients such as paper, ribbons, baskets and the like, they will transform your tins of tea, pâté and caviar into a surprise package you'll be reluctant to open, it so artfully makes *your* personal statement.

On a slightly more grand scale, but glowing with the same inspiration, The El Paso Chile Company, in (where else?) El Paso, Texas, proceeds on the principle that the product itself is the package. Confronted with this creative company's panoply of handmade Chile (their spelling) wreaths, ristras and Indian corn wreaths, all infinitely edible, you will hesitate to break the spell they cast. Surely, they are too good to eat!

How do we exit from such a dilemma? Well, we buy two of everything, and keep one for the wall, where its beauty can daily refresh our eyes.

End of the outside story. . . .

But (my final, and basic, "but"), this is only half the packaging story. If you end the tale here you've broken the narrative at the point where it really starts to build interest and excitement, where the serious drama is going on—within the container.

The "inside" story

The chief actors in this drama are scientists, technicians, researchers and chefs, and their first concern is the product inside the package. Call them masters of fact. Their stages are in laboratories, on manufacturing production lines, in test kitchens, and without cease they test, measure, question—always question—the way the food products that line this country's commercial and private shelves are processed, packaged and presented to consumers.

For them, packaging is technology, and in

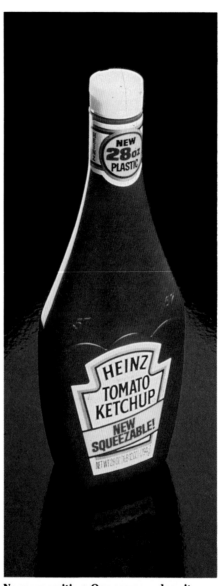

No more waiting. One squeeze does it.

researching new ways to process and package food, they take their lead from the food itself. It's the food that sets the specifications for the package. Here, the eye of the beholder is irrelevant. The proof is in the eating.

Despite the bad-mouthing packaged, processed foods continue to suffer, these point men on the research and development front have one objective: to improve the quality of the convenience foods that in our congested, rush-and-gather days are becoming ever more indispensable to us—the quality of their nutrition, ingredients, flavor, texture and appearance.

Quality versus convenience

The operative word is convenience of preparation, but at the lowest possible cost of losing the intrinsic attributes of food as it comes straight from Mother Nature. To deliver convenience *with* quality, that's the challenge faced by the teams of research scientists and their assorted professional allies at the giant food companies—General Foods, Beatrice, Campbell Soup, Nabisco, General Mills, Pillsbury, Kraft and Stouffer's, to name some of the biggest players—and at dozens of other food processors out there scrabbling for the consumer dollar.

To those of us outside the business, the challenge of convenience foods—items that can be opened and served with the least hassle—is obstinately arcane, a struggle against shadows. Perhaps a quick review of the subject will help set the stage.

Basically, convenience food is the end product of two related activities: processing and packaging. Sometimes the food is processed after it's sealed in a container (called "retorting"), as in the traditional cans of soup, or baked beans, or calamari, or mixed veg or Spanish rice, in fact, just about anything the palate fancies. All you have to do at home, then, is open the container, heat the contents (assuming the item is to be eaten hot) and serve.

In the other traditional approach, the food is processed first, then packaged and either refrigerated or frozen. The variety is virtually unlimited—from full meals, entrées, side dishes and desserts to the juice, milk, yogurt and cheese in the dairy case ready to be poured, spooned and sliced at your need.

The spoiler lies in wait

While the technology for processing food and the containers for keeping it have evolved over the years, the basic challenge on both sides of the processing/packaging equation remains the same: how to keep the food from spoiling, keep it eatable.

The great enemy here is oxygen. Ironic, isn't it? We can't live very long *without* oxygen. Food can't live very long *with* it—with oxygen, food will decompose.

Even retorted food is at risk; oxygen is in the food as well as in the space not filled by the contents. That's why additives for preservation are included among the ingredients. They're unnecessary in frozen foods, where freezing prevents organic deterioration.

Trouble is, as food processors have long known, retorting and freezing aren't perfect processes. Freezing breaks down the basic food cells, altering texture and, to a modest degree, taste. In retorting a canned product, the long cooking time—up to 70 minutes for some foods—isn't very kind to the ingredients. In consequence, the flavor of canned food doesn't compare to that of food prepared from scratch in your own kitchen.

Testing the equation

In recent years, researchers have focused on both sides of the convenience food equation: process and package. On the process side, they're studying, for example, fermentation, curing, drying and freezing, and testing various sources of energy, such as irradiation, heat, microwave and extremely low temperatures.

They've made the greatest, or at least most conspicuous, progress in packaging, leading to the appearance on supermarket shelves of containers that are stunning in their versatility, convenience and quality—and seem to break every traditional packaging rule.

The container that really fits that bill bears probably the most unbeautiful, unappealing name you could tie on a food package—aseptic. Makes you think of medicine and of things hygienic, colorless and therefore without taste, doesn't it?

Hygienic the aseptic package may be, but its contents are anything but tasteless. You'll know this packaging best in those squatty little boxes and flat foil envelopes filled with fruit juices that have now debuted and are beginning to push canned juices to the wall in many supermarkets.

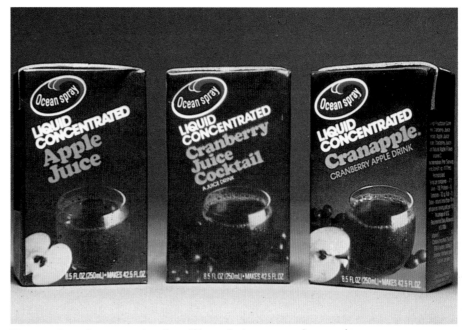

The aseptic package promises long life, enduring taste and convenience.

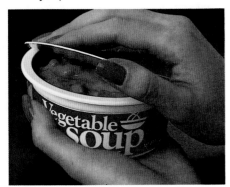

Lift the lid, heat and eat. Perfect.

But juices are only the beginning. Wine, tomato products and various fruits are being carried in these multi layered, laminated paper-and-foil containers. The most startling addition to the line is milk; though not yet widely available in this form, it is possible, as improbable as it may sound now, to store milk safely without refrigeration for up to six months.

The future has no horizon. Packaged food companies are testing aseptic packaging of foods they would otherwise retort in cans. The advantage is all on the side of taste, because retorting only takes a few minutes in an aseptic package, and delicate ingredients like wine and herbs can be added to the mix. Today, fruit juices. Tomorrow, beef stew, clam chowder, veal piccata, chow mein; you name it, it's yours.

But the magic stuff that has really launched packaging toward a future no one dares prefigure is plastic. Plastic, food processers are convinced, is the fast lane toward creating packages that are as safe and convenient as cans but deliver foods that have the pristine taste of frozen.

Some of these products are already on the shelf. Early and elementary are the ubiquitous plastic soda bottles, towering monsters that would strain your back to lift if made of glass.

Aim . . . squeeze . . . bullseye!

Next came the squeeze bottles loaded with salad dressing, mustard, ketchup, jelly, marmalade, margarine and barbecue sauce, with no end in sight. This particular innovation has not always been greeted by unadulterated praise. The squeeze bottle has also become the high-tech water pistol that has sent mothers scurrying for their high-tech detergents and bleaches to remove the stains administered during a shoot-out at some neighborhood OK Corral. An item, regrettably, with multiple uses!

The plastic bottle is strictly a convenience; it does nothing to enhance the product inside. But, like the aseptic container, plastic also assures an indefinite shelf life—without refrigeration—to pre cooked foods. All that's needed is a plastic that provides an effective barrier against the oxygen trying to get into the container.

It's here. You may already have seen plastic cans topped with easily removable metal lids: Just peel, pour and heat the contents. On the other hand, if you just want to open and eat, you can now buy applesauce in containers just the right size for an individual serving. Some food companies are test marketing soups lodged in plastic bowls that you take off the shelf, microwave and eat right out of the container.

The pouch wants a second chance

The *wunderkind* (somewhat aging now) of this family is the retortable pouch. Developed in the 1960s, the pouch went commercial in the 1970s but never really caught on with American consumers otherwise addicted to convenience. The procedure is simplicity itself. Food is sealed in the flexible pouch, retorted (not long), then put on the open shelf in a paperboard carton.

Cousin to the pouch is a retortable plastic tray, which requires about 30 percent less cooking time than a can. The flat cartons stack easily on your pantry shelf, and when you're ready to eat one you peel off the lid, pop it in the microwave, and sit down to eat in less than two minutes.

It's anybody's guess if the pouch will make it on reruns or the tray will get star billing when it goes national. For one thing, we don't desperately need these products; we have plenty of freezer and refrigerator space. And then there's the matter of anxiety. Ask yourself: How do you feel about veal parmesan sitting on the shelf at room temperature?

The old reliable

Uncertainty about the answer probably explains why some companies are hedging their bets and sticking with that old reliable, cold, and working to improve the containers for refrigerated products. Food companies are using thin plastic material (Cryovac is a prominent brand name) that strengthens the barrier to oxygen. Inside this wrap, broccoli florets enjoy an extra week of life in the cooler, and lemons are expected to last nine months instead of one.

More plastic packaging wonders are on the way, of course, including the breakthrough every food company is hoping it will have first: a single layer sheet that will be an impregnable barrier to all invaders and comfortably contain any food product.

From where I sit, the most fitting end to the current packaging story (which will have already left me behind as you read, so rapidly is plastic technology evolving) is with the dazzling achievements of a small Vermont firm, Gerard's Haute Cuisine.

M. Gerard Rubaud had the audacity to think he could successfully offer cuisine at its most *haute*, precooked and delivered to customers in plastic bags.

Sacre bleu! The mind curdles and the pal-ate retreats in horror at such an enormity. Salmon Rillette, Lobster Terrine, Chocolate Marquise—and in plastic! *Impossible!*

Not so, whatever language you speak.

With a little help from friends

M. Rubaud has done it. He had some help, of course. A couple of chefs with three-star experience and the highest quality ingredients available . . . state-of-the-art vacuum packing technology . . . and plastic sheet that comes as close to being the perfect barrier as one can hope for today.

The items are prepared, sealed in a pouch, then refrigerated on ice—absolutely critical for home storage, too. Even the most delicate items, like scallops in *beurre blanc*, will remain at their peak for ten days.

Cuisine en plastique, as it's called in France, is accepted without question in Europe, and in this country, where dining out is becoming the rule rather than the exception, restaurants are turning to gourmet fare in a bag because there aren't enough chefs around who can go it on their own.

Miracles are yours to make

As for you, in the privacy of your home, imagine this scene. Dinner guests you must impress, and you're behind the closed kitchen door. Out come the precious chilled envelopes. You drop them in boiling water and a few moments later what darling culinary treasures you carefully arrange, on a nicely preheated plate.

You first present, like an overture, tiny zucchini, their tender, delicate yellow-and-orange blossoms filled with lobster and graced by a lobster sauce scented with tarragon. You follow with a fillet of poached salmon, accompanied by tiny young carrots, wearing a cap of green for color, and thin *haricots verts* girdled with strips of sweet red pepper. And over all a lemon-butter sauce delicately laced with basil, chives and chervil. You conclude with chocolate mousse cake and a passion fruit *entremets*.

With some embarrassment (well concealed) at the deception, you accept the kudos. Technology and art have triumphed. *Quelle miracle!* ●

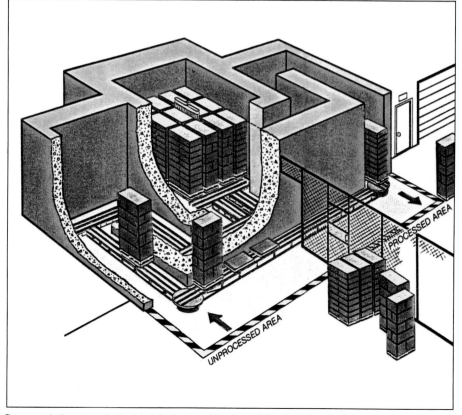

Conveyed along tracks behind fortress walls, food is bathed in a radioactive shower.

Nuke Your Food

There's been a lot of talk lately about irradiating food—zapping it with the equivalent of your dentist's x-ray machine. The food industry claims irradiation disinfects and preserves food harmlessly; critics aren't so sure it's so harmless. But let's get one thing straight: Irradiating an apple will not make the fruit—or you—glow in the dark.

Irradiating food first come into use in this country by the military during World War II and the process has remained essentially the same: Food is carried on a conveyor belt into a shielded chamber, where it is exposed to radiation from a machine or from a chunk of radioactive mineral. The radioactivity—usually x rays or gamma rays—breaks apart molecules in the food and in the bugs and bacteria that have taken up residence inside it.

Proponents claim that irradiation represents an improvement over using pesticides and other methods of preservation. Irradiated strawberries, for example, can remain free of mold for as long as two weeks, and meat and fish may last three weeks instead of three days in the refrigerator. Irradiation can slow down the ripening of fruit, keep onions from sprouting, increase loaf volume of bread, and break down some of the oligosaccharides in beans—the main reason the legumes are so flatulent. Irradiation enthusiasts also argue that the process is as harmless as passing luggage under an airport scanner.

Critics, on the other hand, charge that the process may make food less palatable. It can turn fruits such as grapes and cherries mushy and it breaks sulfur bonds in dairy products, producing a revolting taste. There is mounting evidence, also, that irradiation destroys some vitamins and other nutrients.

But more important, irradiation may make food dangerous to eat. It's not that it renders food radioactive. But the chemicals that are produced as a result of the radiation—the so-called radiolytic products—may be toxic or carcinogenic, according to some studies, including ones conducted by the Department of Agriculture.

So far, about 30 countries market irradiated food and in the U.S. the Food and Drug Administration recently approved the process for use in killing trichinosis-causing parasites in pork as well as destroying insects in fruits and vegetables. ●

HALLIE DONNELLY'S CALIFORNIA ROLL SUSHI
One roll makes one complete package.

Makes 4 rolls or 30 to 35 pieces

Ingredients:
4 1/4 cups water
3 1/2 cups Japanese short-grained rice
5 teaspoons salt
6 tablespoons sugar
2 tablespoons rice wine vinegar
1 ripe avocado, preferably the dark, bumpy-skinned type
Juice of 1 lemon
4 sheets nori (dried seaweed)
2 tablespoons wasabi (Japanese green horseradish paste)
1 cup cooked crabmeat
Soy sauce and additional wasabi, for serving

(Note: Short-grained rice, rice wine vinegar, nori, wasabi and bamboo mat for rolling sushi are available at Japanese and some specialty food stores.)

Method:
1. Preheat the broiler.
2. Put the water, rice a pinch of the salt and a pinch of the sugar in a 2-quart saucepan and bring to a boil. Cover the pan and cook over moderate heat for about 10 minutes until the water has been absorbed. Reduce the heat to very low and cook for 5 minutes longer. Remove the pan from the heat and let the rice stand, covered, for 5 minutes.
3. While the rice cooks, combine the vinegar with the remaining sugar and the remaining salt in a small saucepan. Mix thoroughly. Cook over moderate heat just until the sugar dissolves. Remove from the heat and cool to room temperature.
4. While the rice is still very hot, transfer it to a wooden bowl. Add about half of the dressing and gently toss the rice with a rice paddle or wooden spoon. Fold the rice by using a downward cutting stroke, being careful not to mash it. When the first addition of dressing has been absorbed, add more gradually, taking care that the rice does not become mushy. Fan the rice as you toss it, until it has cooled to room temperature.
5. Cut the avocado in half lengthwise and remove the pit and the peel. Cut the flesh into long strips, 1/4-inch wide. Put the strips in a bowl and gently toss them with the lemon juice.
6. Toast one side of each piece of nori by running it under the broiler for 3 to 5 seconds, until crisp.
7. Place one sheet of nori, shiny side down, on a bamboo sushi mat. Cover it with 1 cup of sushi rice in an even layer, leaving a 1-inch border at the top and a 1/4-inch border at the bottom.
8. Spread 1/2 tablespoon of the wasabi in a line down the center of the rice. Place 1/4 cup of the crabmeat in a thin line over the wasabi. Arrange a quarter of the avocado strips in a thin line over the crabmeat.
9. To roll the sushi, hold the lines of the fillings with your fingertips, flip the edge of the mat over the filling, and roll the mat into a long cylinder. The two ends of the nori will be brought together. Press firmly and remove the mat. You should now have one long roll.
10. Cut the roll into 1-inch slices with a sharp knife. Wipe the knife with a damp cloth after each slice to prevent sticking. Repeat the filling, rolling, and cutting procedures with the remaining ingredients.
11. Serve the sushi with little bowls of soy sauce and dabs of wasabi, to be mixed by each diner.

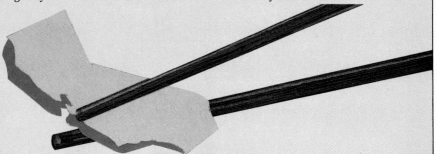

It All "Ads" Up — To Billions

Is the food industry trying to get your attention? You bet it is. The amount of U.S. advertising dollars spent annually— $2,760,816,000—sounds like the gross national product of a middling-size country.

Food and food products lead the advertising field, ahead of the automotive industry. To break the billions down into somewhat more digestible sums: It's not surprising that television gobbles the major share of the cake. Last year, $1,404,590,000 in ad bucks went to the mighty networks, with $872,704,000 spent on "spot," or local, commercials. Moving right up there is cable TV, weighing in with a healthy $58,360,000. Billboards just aren't significant in the food world—ads total a mere $9,595,000.

By far the biggest spender is McDonald's, which put up $100 million to hoopla the McDLT, its hot burger-with-cold-lettuce-and-tomato. Hard on McDonald's heels is Burger King, which spent $40 million on their mystery man Herb. Herb, disappointingly, did not build sales. We won't see him again. According to a bigwig from the ad agency that created the campaign, it was an error to make Herb a "lovable nerd." Instead, "He should have been a surprisingly attractive individual."

Radio accounts for about 723 million of food advertising dollars. "We get people at the point of decision making," says the vice-president of marketing information for The Radio Advertising Bureau, a trade association. "We get them in the car going to the supermarket—95 percent of the cars in America have a radio—and we get them in the act of food preparation. We know that half the kitchens in the country have a radio." Supermarket commercials now are heard on sports shows because surveys show that 40 percent of all food shoppers are men.

"Most advertisers try to go after what is called the 'heavy user'," says Kim Rotzoll, head of the prestigious Department of Advertising at the University of Illinois. "That's the proportion of the population that uses the largest amount of the product." To use beer as an example, 20 percent of our citizens drink 80 percent of the suds, and beer ads are targeted to that audience.

Similarly, there is a great deal of data available on viewers who watch specific shows and their food preferences: who watches what game show, who uses what mustard and how old the mustard eaters and game show watchers are. "Matching media with target market is pretty much computerized," says Mr. Rotzoll, "but the creative ad is anything but scientific. So much of it is a matter of intuition." ●

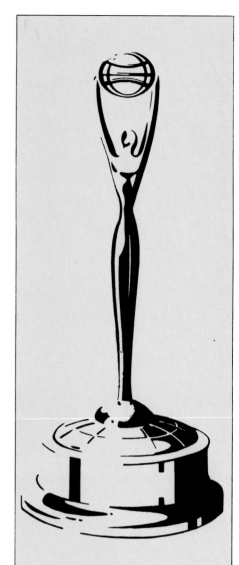

The Clio Awards

The annual Clio Awards, now in their 27th year, are to the advertising business what Oscars are to the film industry. Emphasizing creativity in selecting the winners, the Clio organization, a private company, invites only advertising "creatives" such as creative directors, art directors, copy writers, producers, commercial directors, editors, animators and cinematographers to serve as judges. Marketing and account executives do not have a vote.

Although ads for print, radio and other media are now honored by Clio, TV awards are considered the highlight of the event. This year, over 1,000 judges considered more than 21,000 entries from 53 countries. It took them over three months to select the 1986 winners.

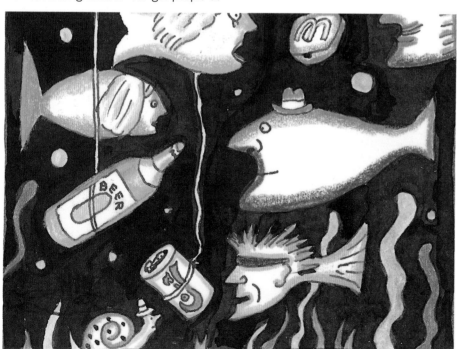

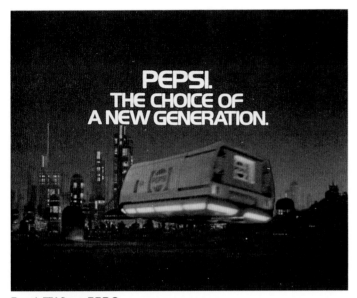

Pepsi, TV Spot, BBDO

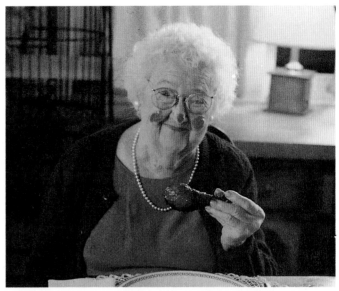

General Foods Shake 'n Bake, TV Spot, Ogilvy & Mather

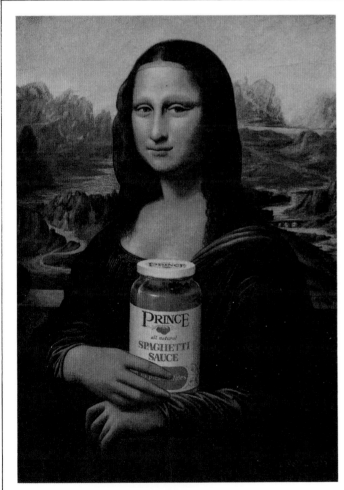

Original.

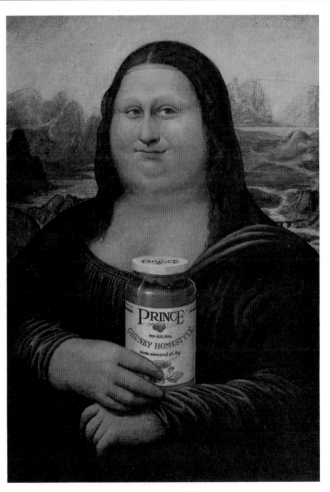

Chunky.

Prince Spaghetti Sauce, Outdoor Poster, Fallon McElligott

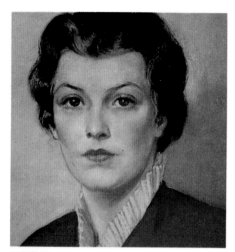

1936

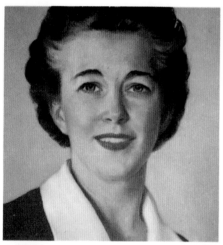

1955

Betty Crocker: Looking Good At Any Age

She was born in 1921, first showed her face to the public in 1936 and just had her portrait painted again—she's Betty Crocker, General Mills' durable homemaker. At her debut, her image featured plucked eyebrows, marcel-waved hair and pleated white collar; she was the epitome of the modern, stylish homemaker of her day. In her present incarnation, still looking an impeccable 32, she is now clearly also a career person, complete with floppy go-to-business ties.

Betty saw us through the Great Depression, World War II, the Korean conflict, Watergate, the space race and all the years between. She first appeared in the Swing Era and has weathered Progressive Jazz, Bebop, Rock 'n Roll and Punk Rock.

As times changed, so did Betty. Her hairstyle, makeup and clothing reflected each new era but the essential serene countenance remained the same, reassuring us that no matter what turbulence reigned outside the kitchen, all was well—Betty Crocker was in charge. Fittingly, therefore, her 1955 portrait coincided with her first frosting mix and the 1968 version brought us Pineapple Upside Down Cake.

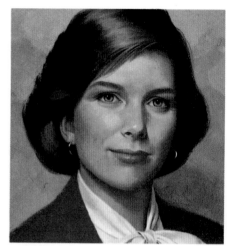

1986

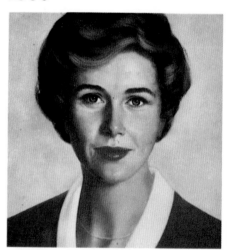

1980

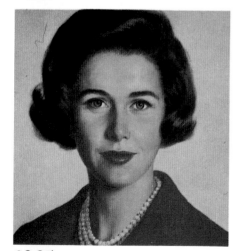

1965

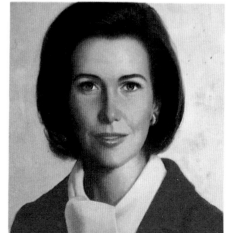

1968

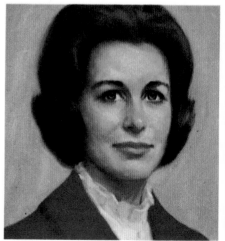

1972

Food Public Relations Associations

Every year, The American Lamb Council organizes an educational seminar for a few fortunate food writers and other food professionals. The purpose is to get the message of the lamb "industry" to the public and it does so most effectively by taking a small group directly into the field to observe, to ask questions and to learn. Having seen and tasted, it can then be stated with absolute confidence that American lamb is the best in the world when it is eaten in its native land.

There are similar trade associations for almost every commodity—grapes, for example, catfish and strawberries. These groups frequently supply the recipes and photographs that are seen in magazines and newspaper food pages. They are bonded together under the banner of the International Food Service Editorial Council (IFEC) and can be reached by writing to 82 Osborne Lane, East Hampton, New York 11937.

Alaska Seafood Marketing Institute
(206) 285-7082

American Catfish Marketing Association
(601) 887-5401

American Egg Board
(312) 296-7044

American Lamb Council
(303) 399-8130

American Sheep Producers Council
(303) 399-8130

American Soybean Association
(314) 432-1600

American Spice Trade Association
(212) 420-8808

Beans of the West
(206) 285-7082

The Beef Industry Council
(415) 984-6193

California Apricot Advisory Board
(415) 949-3100

California Artichoke Advisory Board
(408) 633-4411

California Cling Peach Advisory Board
(415) 541-0100

California Dry Bean Advisory Board
(209) 591-4866

California Iceberg Lettuce Commission
(408) 625-2944

California Kiwifruit Commission
(206) 285-7082

California Olive Industry
(415) 949-3100

California Pistachio Association
(415) 861-4949

California Prune Board
(415) 984-6193

California Raisin Advisory Board
(415) 984-6193

California Strawberry Advisory Board
(408) 724-1301

California Table Grape Commission
(206) 285-7082

California Fresh Market Tomato Advisory Board
(209) 591-0437

California Tree Fruit Agreement
(209) 252-9150

Canned Food Information Council
(312) 836-7142

Chocolate Manufacturers of America
(212) 977-9400

Florida Celery Committee
(212) 420-8808

Florida Department of Citrus
(212) 977-9400

Florida Fruit & Vegetable Association
(212) 420-8808

Florida Tomato Exchange
(212) 420-8808

Halibut Association of North America
(206) 285-7082

Idaho Frozen Foods
(415) 891-9034

Idaho Potato Commission
(212) 977-9400

International Apple Institute
(703) 442-8850

Leafy Greens Council
(312) 524-0398

Maraschino Cherry & Glace Fruit Processors
(206) 285-7082

Michigan Cherry Committee
(517) 321-1231

National Capon Council
(312) 524-0398

National Cherry Growers & Industries Foundation
(206) 285-7082

National Dairy Council
(312) 696-1020

National Duckling Council
(312) 524-0398

National Fisheries Institute
(202) 296-3428

National Kraut Packers Association
(212) 752-8610

National Pork Producers Council
(417) 882-5050

National Red Cherry Institute
(616) 774-0831

National Turkey Federation
(703) 435-7206

North American Blueberry Council
(206) 285-7082

North Atlantic Seafood Association
(216) 781-6400

Ocean Spray Cranberries, Inc.
(212) 887-8032

Pacific Coast Canned Pears
(415) 541-0451

Peanut Advisory Board
(912) 386-3470

Pickle Packers International
(212) 752-8610

Pineapple Growers Association of Hawaii
(415) 956-7470

The Potato Board
(415) 984-6193

Rice Council
(713) 270-6699

Walnut Marketing Board
(415) 984-6193

Washington Apple Commission
(209) 252-9150

Washington Asparagus Growers Association
(206) 383-2223

Washington State Fruit Commission
(206) 285-2222

Washington State Potato Commission
(206) 285-2222

Western New York Apple Growers/New York Cherry Growers
(716) 924-2171

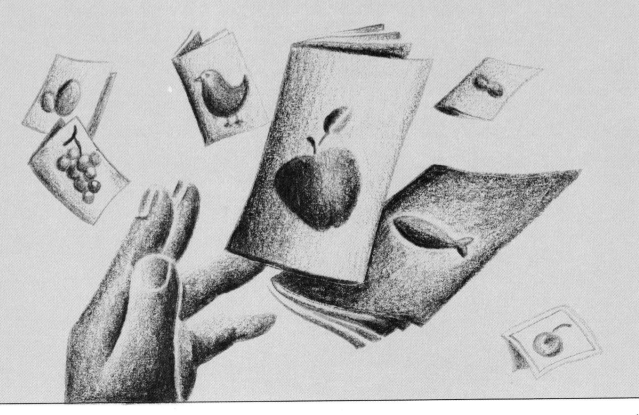

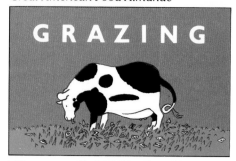

GRAZING

Bagel With Lox, Hold The Mayo

The Bagel Capital of the World is a title claimed not, as one might expect, by New York City, but by Mattoon, Illinois (population 19,800).

Mattoon is the Midwest home of Lender's Bagels, which recently opened a 150-yard-long bagel bakery on State Route 121. The Mattoon plant produces a million bagels daily, which are then frozen, packaged and shipped to stores in the West and Midwest.

Until recently, bagels were primarily an East Coast phenomenon, with a few bagel outposts scattered in places like Los Angeles and San Francisco. In 1984, six million bagels a day were sold in the U.S., but in 1985, that figure shot up to eight million.

One reason for the bagel boom—and for Lender's brand-new Mattoon plant—is the so-called bagel war currently raging between Lender's and Sara Lee. Lender's started producing frozen bagels in 1962, in New Haven, and had pretty much cornered the national frozen bagel market. But in August 1985 Sara Lee (as in cheesecake) got into the act, introducing its line of frozen bagels and launching a national ad campaign to promote them.

The effect of the advertising has been to help sell not only Sara Lee's bagels, but Lender's as well, with frozen bagel sales up by 30 percent since the "war" began. Stores specializing in freshly baked bagels are benefiting, too—even in places as unlikely as Tulsa, Oklahoma. There, one store owner reported in a recent *New York Times* article that cowboys wander in asking for "bangles" or "bockles."

Did They Ask Someone To Do Them A Flavor? Pigs and cows that are raised to become food for our tables are being fed flavored food—or rather, feed. (For some reason, food that is fed to future-food is not called food, it is called feed.) This may be dark-rum flavored (which cows like) or root-beer flavored, orange-flavored or even butterscotch-flavored. (Eaten any funny tasting steaks lately?)

Regional Preferences

There may be no longer such a thing as "American taste" in food and drink; a CREST Household Report recently cited by *Advertising Age* indicates that there are at least nine district regional variations. As shown below, the preferred top three foods and beverages, chosen from a given list, differ markedly in the following regions of the continental U.S.:

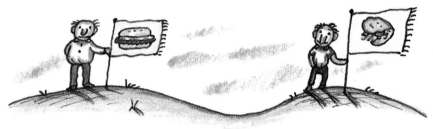

Region	Foods	Beverages
New England:	1. Heroes/subs 2. Fish (not fried) 3. Salad sandwiches	1. Diet non-colas 2. Wine 3. Regular coffee
Mid-Atlantic:	1. Heroes/subs 2. Salad sandwiches 3. Veal	1. Hot tea 2. Uncarbonated soft drink 3. Decaffeinated coffee
East North Central:	1. Chili 2. French toast 3. Cheese	1. Decaffeinated coffee 2. Regular coffee 3. Diet non-colas
West North Central:	1. Mashed potatoes 2. Pan pizza 3. Soft-serve ice cream	1. Hot chocolate 2. Colas 3. Milk
South Atlantic:	1. Breakfast sandwiches 2. Fried shellfish 3. Non-fried shellfish	1. Iced tea 2. Colas 3. Diet colas
East South Central:	1. Vegetable platters 2. Breakfast sandwiches 3. Fried fish	1. Iced tea 2. Colas 3. Diet colas
West South Central:	1. Enchiladas 2. Nachos 3. Fried vegetables	1. Iced tea 2. Colas 3. Beer
Mountain:	1. Tacos 2. Burritos 3. Enchiladas	1. Uncarbonated soft drink 2. Hot chocolate 3. Non-cola drinks
Pacific:	1. Burritos 2. Enchiladas 3. Taco salads	1. Wine 2. Hot chocolate 3. Hot tea

EATING OUT

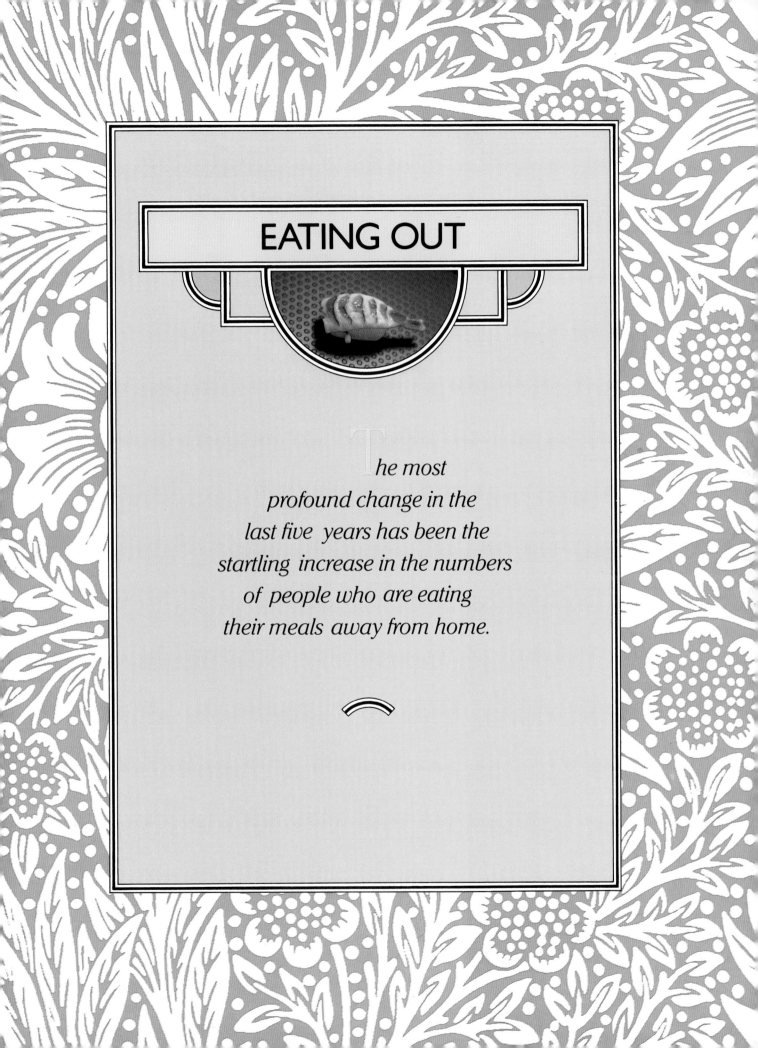

The most profound change in the last five years has been the startling increase in the numbers of people who are eating their meals away from home.

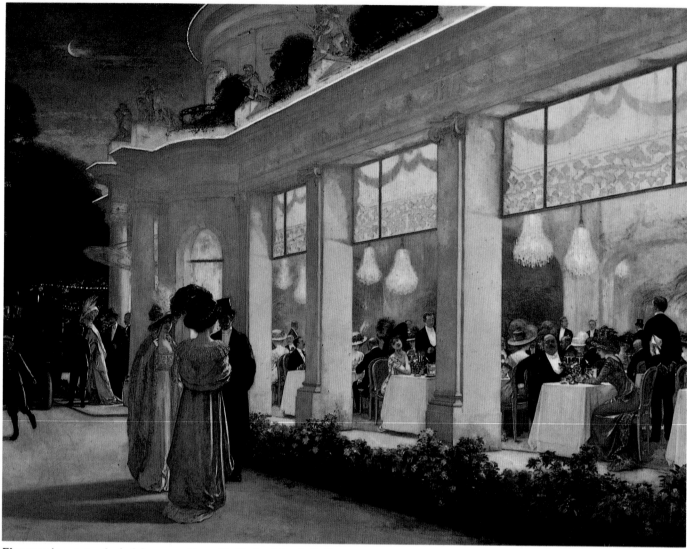

Elegance is a state of mind, borrowed from the Paris of the Belle Epoque . . .

THE RESURGENCE OF HOTEL DINING

Several years ago, restaurant developer and consultant Joe Baum addressed a group of hotel executives in New York. "Thank you," he said, "for bringing all those people into our city and sending them out to dine at our restaurants."

Typically, the hotel dining room has fed and fed off a captive audience. Travelers ate where they slept because it was convenient, and because they didn't know where else to go. Hotel guests still do that, but their on-premise choices today range from elegant continental dining to cafeteria food and often what the hotel offers is as good as or better than what's outside.

The aggressive food and beverage director today has to be as market-wise as the best independent operator in town, not only to satisfy hotel guests but also to attract the local trade, and convert them to customers of the hotel's far more lucrative banquet and

conference facilities. As Fred Rufe of *Hilton International* puts it: "The locals are your product and the guests are dessert."

So, in a startling reversal of their once-complacent attitude, hotels have transformed dull, moribund dining rooms into gloriously attractive, trend-setting, competitive dining palaces. Indeed, in many cities today, the hotel restaurant is *the* place to eat, *the* destination restaurant. True, it is not happening everywhere and the attempt does not always work. There is a great polarization, but those that succeed are very successful.

Perhaps the best example of this trend is Dallas where seven of *The Ten Best* on restaurant critic Michael Bauer's (of the *Dallas Times-Herald*) list are hotel dining rooms. But it is also happening in every major city and at times seems like a duel of the giants, with a few independents caught in the battle. In Seattle, the headquarters hotel of the

Westin chain goes head-to-head with the Four Seasons Olympic and a surprisingly fine Sheraton.

In Boston, the same high level rivalry goes on among the Parker House, the Meridien, Seasons at the Bostonian, the Westin and, in its home city, the Sheraton Boston Hotel and Towers. In New York, the Maurice stands out in a crowded field which includes the ever-dependable Pierre, La Récolte at the Intercontinental, the Barbizon and a whole phalanx of elegant hotel dining rooms. Each has poured thousands upon thousands of dollars into equipping, decorating and staffing its restaurants, and each offers extraordinarily fine dining in luxurious settings.

In many cases, one restaurant alone is not enough, and a hotel will often provide a gourmet restaurant, a specialty restaurant, i.e. a seafood room, a less expensive dining room and a coffee shop, as well as a lounge, each ranking very high within its respective category.

In the best hotels today, nothing is spared in the search for a competitive edge, whether it's a world famous chef, a celebrity maître d', or art and furnishings that dazzle the eye. Whatever it may take, the hoteliers and their food and beverage directors aren't hesitant to spend the money needed to build a clientele.

"Great hotel dining rooms," says Joe Baum, "represent a mini-trend within a larger trend. The majority of hotels still don't want to be in the restaurant business. Hotels make their food and beverage dollar from their banquet rooms, not from restaurants. They grudgingly produce restaurants because they have to have them, not because they really want them. Those hotels that are producing strong restaurants are doing so for marketing reasons.

"It has little to do with the profit and loss statement, it has to do with creating attractions. The business is becoming overcrowded. Too much capacity has been built in too many cities and one way of distinguishing a hotel is the quality of its restaurants."

In the cold eyes of the controller, the food and beverage operation is not a great profit center. In 1984, Laventhol & Horwath, consultants to the lodging industry, report an average 74.3 percent return on room sales, against 16.9 percent for food and beverage revenues. The full-time employee in food and beverage was worth $25,000 in dollar productivity, while room workers brought in nearly $60,000 each. In dollars and cents, even telephone operators, with a median productivity of $50,000, according to Laventhol & Horwath, made a greater contribution to hotel revenues.

But, as Rufe of Hilton International likes to tell his associates, "A hotel without a restaurant is a motel." Dennis Lombardi, a principal of Laventhol & Horwath, furthers the motion. "Hotel companies realize that to have a good average return on investment, they need a profitable food and beverage operation. And while the return on rooms is so much larger, a good food and beverage operation will itself generate a reasonable profit and will also help the hotel's occupancy rate. Hotels, like any other business, bank dollars, not percentages."

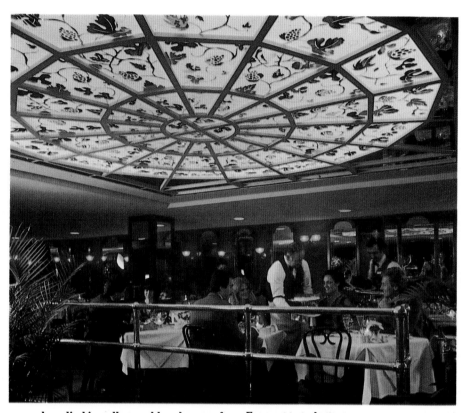

. . . and applied in yellow, gold and green; from Fouquet to today.

Producing those bankable dollars is what keeps executives like Rufe and Walter Staib of Omni/Dunfey up late at night. Concept is their buzz word. Rufe harkens back to the creation of The Four Seasons in Manhattan.

"Joe Baum, who was then running Restaurant Associates, said we had to innovate, we had to build a restaurant with no basis for comparison, something that would be fresh even 20 years later. And if you go into the Four Seasons today, it still looks new and never gets old.

"When we built the Vista Hotel in lower Manhattan, where practically nobody ever went in those days, we wanted a restaurant that would be unique. So we built the American Harvest, the first restaurant in New York to specialize in American food. You have to offer the public something they can't find anywhere else and you have to show the customers you're thinking of them."

Doyle Wayman of Laventhol & Horwath's design unit, INDEX, explains, it is all a matter of satisfying the hotel traveler. "We are designing hotels that have upscale restaurants and at the same time offer a service for the guest who arrives on that late-night plane and wants something simple, maybe just a sandwich, something that he might eat with a beer in the lobby or carry upstairs in a brown bag.

"In the not too distant future, you may see retail delicatessens dropped into some hotels to eliminate the problems of running a full-scale restaurant. But there will always be fine hotels with fine restaurants. It is a matter of serving the public, in all of its requirements." ●

Mort Hochstein, food reporter, *Market Watch*

The Brightest Spots	
Maurice	Parker Meridien New York
Jean-Louis	Watergate Hotel Washington, D.C.
The Dining Room	Ritz Carlton Chicago
La Tour	Park Hyatt Chicago
Squire Room	Fairmont San Francisco

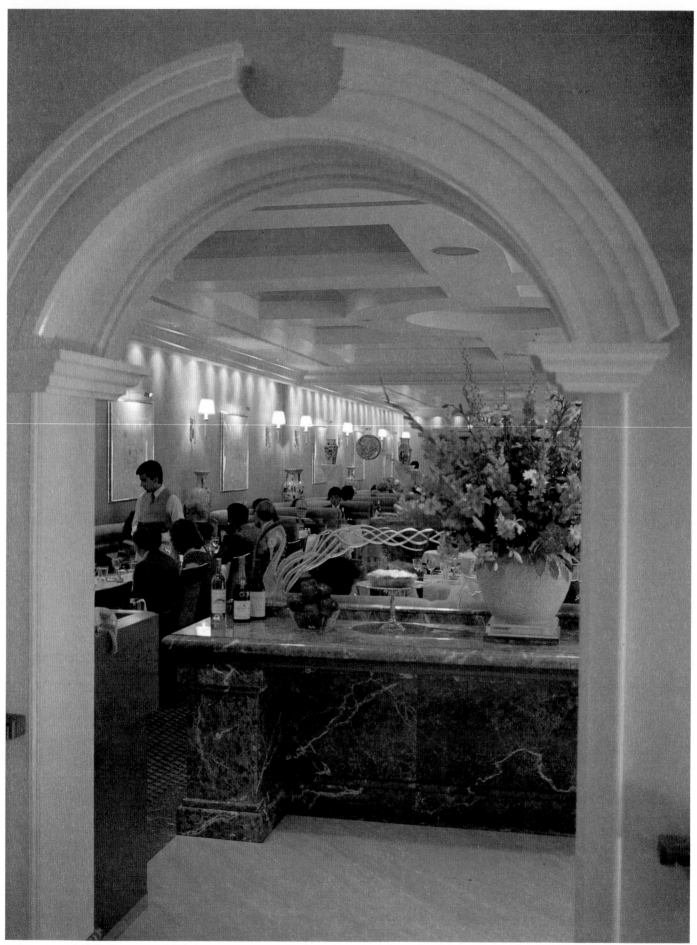

Light, space, and air fragrant with flowers are yours at Campton Place restaurant, San Francisco.

The New Restaurants

In case you hadn't noticed, restaurants are not what they were. In former times, restaurants sat there quietly, waiting patiently for customers. Today, so many people are clamoring to eat away from home that, in the most popular of big city restaurants, reservations are required weeks in advance. Further, with some elite establishments it is necessary for the would-be patron to reconfirm the date and time of the reservations, as if making a commitment to the Concorde.

Restaurants have a problem with giddy people who reserve a table and then fail to show. Costs of operation these days are so great that an empty table can cause grief to the management. In the wind is the notion of demanding a penalty from no-shows. How would it work? The restaurants would take your credit card number at the time you called to reserve; in the event that you failed to appear, you would be billed for your dereliction.

The long, leisurely dinner is also doing a vanishing act, and the tables truly are turned. Forget prime time; everybody else gets there first. You have a choice of dining too early—at 6:30—or too late—at 9 or 9:30. Consider the plight of the restaurant owner who is faced with the dilemma of a couple who gaze rapturously at each other, on and on and on, while the couple next in line, collapsing with hunger and steaming with impatience, wait at the bar for a table they booked weeks before.

Gone now is the clutter that used to be the hallmark of excellence. Gone are the silk dresses and the corsages, gone are the rolling silver service trolleys that held their barons of beef in a sultry sauna. Gone are the haughty headwaiters who may have greeted you a hundred times but never recognized you once. Gone are the ponderous, brocaded wallpapers, the crystal chandeliers and the prevailing gloom.

Here comes the sun

In place of all that, we get open kitchens, right in front of everybody. We get light, bright space, embowered in fresh flowers. We get generous, commodious bars where people alone are welcomed to dine. And a few of the bolder, more forward places even offer single diners the option of being seated at a communal table. This is not too surprising in light of the fact that 21 million Americans now live

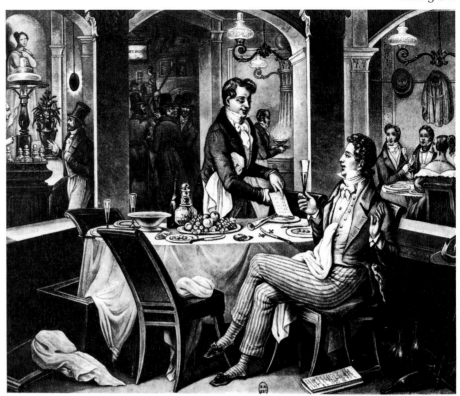

An American in Paris: This young Yankee doesn't know he has been stuck with the tab.

alone, and their numbers are increasing three times as fast as any other category of household. When a restaurant policy makes a single person feel welcome and well-looked-after, then that single person, who might well have friends, may come again with some of those.

Drinking is not what it was, and thus bars are more than they were. Today, the bar is a place where one can choose privacy or companionship, a drink or none at all. Menus there offer everything available in the dining room and then some—finger-foods and "littlemeals" for grazers.

Today, dining out is theater, and there are several reasons for this. One of them is that the theater itself is moribund; there's not much going on and what there is costs the earth. People don't go to the movies as much as they did because most movies are made for 14-year-olds; those that are meant for grown-ups can be seen on the VCR. So where else are we to go for spectacle? Where else are we to go for that sense of uplift that cathedrals provided in an earlier time? We go to a big, bright restaurant, and observe our fellow man, and bow our heads over our plates, and leave an offering behind. We spend 40 to 60 cents of every food dollar eating away from home, and we find it's worth it.

They want us

Restaurants strive to accommodate our needs for food and satisfaction. They serve lunch, stay open for bar meals during the afternoon, and then sponsor two seatings for

dinner. To further maximize their investment, they open for breakfast too, and even afternoon tea.

Twenty years ago, going out to dinner, more often than not meant that we ordered a steak large enough to feed a family of eight in Tibet, and accompanied it with a baked potato slathered in butter and sour cream. Prime ribs and roast beef were regarded with a reverential awe shared only by Old Glory and the Constitution of the United States of America. People still go to steak houses . . . but guess what the Steak & Ale folks have lately added in all the restaurants in their chain: fresh fish!

Menus can no longer be mistaken for graduation diplomas from obscure Balkan universities, with illegible calligraphy and bedecked with silken tassels. We still have our excesses—Nebraska Mesquite Grilled Ear of Wild Boar with Wild Michigan Morels, Garnished with California Carambola, for example—but at least we can read the words. And the special of the day has taken, now, a back seat to the wood of the day. Will our grilled, range-fed chicken be cooked over oak, ash, grapevine or some other exotic wood on hand? Each is claimed to impart a particular fragrance to the chicken. It is a whole new area in which to become a member of the cognoscenti. The *new* cognoscenti, to be sure.

The pieties of the past have faded, replaced by surprises and the fresh pleasures of innovation and risk—and we find that restaurants today are more fun than they have ever been. ●

COURSE DESCRIPTION: A PENETRATING EXAMINATION OF THE CURRENT EATING HABITS AND POPULAR HAUNTS OF AMERICAN YOUNG ADULTS (UNDER 30 OR PURPORTING TO BE AND PASSING).
UNIT HOURS: 6 MINUTES.
PREREQUISITES: MINIMAL APPETITE.
COURSE REQUIREMENTS: 3 CARROT STICKS, 4 PIECES OF SMOKED TOFU, A SINGLE LEAF OF ARUGULA FOR GARNISH, AND ONE PUBLIC BAR TO LEAN AGAINST.

Grazing 101

Once, in recent memory, we thought of restaurants simply as places to go when we wanted to eat out. Today, attitudes of that sort are too simplistic to apply. Rather, the vastly increased frequency of dining anywhere but at home must be carefully examined in terms of the psychographic composite of the typical teenager raised on fast food, together with the implications of Trivia games upon Western civilization—with particular reference to the recently observed phenomenon of "grazing" among upwardly mobile American young adults.

Let's begin by talking about games. From the beginning of time, mankind has played games. However, in the 1960s our games changed radically, mainly because, in the era of the Haight-Ashbury, nobody liked rules any more. They still don't. The Trivia games were designed to entertain us, not to educate, and they became hugely successful because they conform to the American Way, the Democratic Ideal, which is that Everyone Wins. If it turns out that others think you lost, you can always maintain a tone of lofty moral superiority simply by declaring the entire exercise *trivial*.

Lists are very popular among Trivia players. People like lists a lot, and this is why the Wallechinsky *Book of Lists* was so successful. We can even argue that a love of lists is why people go to restaurants, for what is a menu, after all, but a very long list? (And getting longer every day.)

Other games we play now are much more meaningful than Trivia. Take the TV game shows, for example, many of which are, for many people, becoming a way of life (fueled, like the lotteries, by that most fundamental of motives, greed). "Wheel of Fortune," with its giant wheel of fortune, is seen every day by more than 43 million viewers.

The connection between Trivia games and game shows is that both test a contestant's knowledge of trivial facts; however, the TV version does so against a backdrop of dazzling lights, with a lot of people dashing about and very loud music.

You will see that, when people become comfortable with this fantasy setting, they also begin to feel at home in large, noisy, upscale versions of the school cafeteria, where the food is only marginally edible and such morsels as are eaten are picked up in the hand. Like children, we are eating "on demand" and, instead of having three "proper" meals, we linger over "littlemeals" all the time. And this is why we are never *really hungry* any more at what was once called, quaintly, dinner time.

New restaurant managements have understood this extended adolescence of ours very well, and they cater to it. They have also grasped the fact that, as we live in smaller and smaller apartments with scarcely any room to turn around in, we want to escape into vast spaces that are brilliantly lighted, brilliantly decorated and are brilliant backdrops for our meetings with our friends. They also know that, often, it matters little what is on the plates or, as in the school cafeteria, who is seated next to whom.

Bars in these restaurants are gigantic, accommodating the transient candidate who can drop in, view the scene, have a drink, stay or leave, depending on the mood of the moment. The humanscape is constantly in motion, like the illuminated crystals in a kaleidoscope.

Because we no longer know what to say to each other, loud music is provided as our excuse for having no conversation. So there we sit, inundated by sound and light, eating very little or—often—nothing at all, all good little statistics in the exploding population of the culture of Lean Cuisine.

Other needs are being met, too. Not so very long ago, to be seated next to the kitchen was the very, very worst thing that could happen. Now it has become *quite* the thing to *want* to sit next to the kitchen. This may be because many young people grew up with mothers who were district attorneys or heart surgeons, and who were never at home peeling the carrots and potatoes. So to watch the activity in the kitchen fills a deep psychic need, in that you feel nurtured in seeing a meal being prepared just for you. In this instance, of course, you pay for it in dollars rather than in guilt. Small wonder that personal nutritionists are replacing psychiatrists in the young adult's budget.

We must redefine ourselves, then, not by what we eat but by what we do when we are *working*. Here lies a problem, because our language, once perfectly adequate for conveying such simple notions as "I love you" or "Please pass the salt," no longer serves our need to communicate with our peers: Each of us speaks in tongues that have been developed to deal strictly with specific professional needs.

Thus, the words, symbols and terminology of the theoretical astrophysicist cannot be understood by the astrologer, who thinks about Gemini and Taurus and circling planets in a way incomprehensible to the astrophysicist. Nor, in similar fashion, can a chef understand the menu of a computer programmer.

So, if we cannot communicate, what shall we do? It won't be long before we'll be seeing a toaster-like device on every restaurant table, in which His and Hers video cassettes pop up. Adjoining screens will enable her to watch "Places in the Heart" while he watches "Rambo" and both eat their *crème brûlée* (recently rediscovered after decades of neglect). The same device may well double as a means of ordering from the pantry—and as the order is entered there, the funds

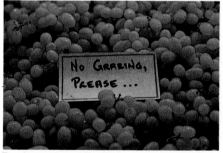

Don't touch me! I'm little, round and juicy.

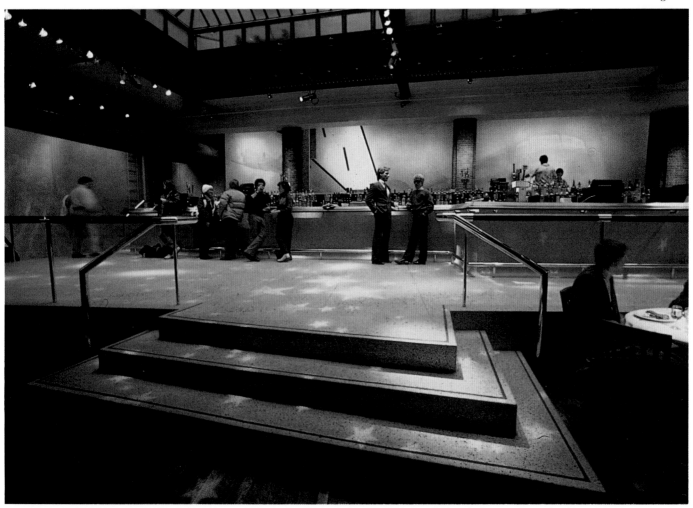

It's show-yourself time at New York's America restaurant, where you go, maybe to eat, but chiefly to admire and be admired.

to pay for it will be deducted automatically from the personal bank account.

The proposition of eating as entertainment has caught on greatly in recent times. This explains why it is that when you invite a friend to choose a restaurant for dinner, the response will hinge not on whether the place serves decent food at a decent price, but on whether your friend has already *seen* it.

Simply knowing which restaurant to choose proves you to be one evolutionary notch above your fellow man. And it is not always easy to exercise the skill of knowing. Increasingly, the chic new places do not have names on the doors. What's worse, they have unlisted phone numbers and, like the smart nightclubs of the 1940s, admit only those who are wearing garments that match the drinks and the decor.

If we do penetrate the new sanctum, we won't eat much. But we will be awed and humbled by the sheer artistry of it all, exemplified by the geometric placement of five pâtés, topped by four different kinds of caviar, nestled in a pool of three sauces, counterpointed by a lone crawfish pirouetting on a single, sublime pea.

You may have noticed, also, that the earnest young folk seem to favor very large, very

sweet drinks that come in all manner of interesting colors, none of which appear in nature. The latest craze is for Mexican and Italian food, and we may soon be seeing margaritas and pasta being merged into a balloon-shaped glass containing tequila and a single strand of spaghetti. You will recognize this item on the menu as a Conquistador Carbonara.

Where will it all end, you ask? The answer is at hand; we just have to cast our nets wide enough to see the whole picture. Clearly, our future leaders will not be the traditional gray-bearded tutors, but Jolly Young American Chefs who take lessons in public speaking while they study sauce- and pastry-making. Their mission is not so much to cook for us as to amuse us, and long gone is the notion that Real Chefs do not give interviews or appear on talk shows.

The diners of yesteryear have evolved into the chic American bistros of today, filled with flowers and with lithe, spare waitpersons—unisex beings of great charm and attraction. The waitperson is, in reality, an actperson out of work or—to be more accurate—out of the *preferred* line of work. In order to experience personal satisfaction, waitpersons compete each evening for the Escoffier Oscar, which is

given for the best soliloquy in the form of a dramatic reading of the evening's specials.

Nothing is as it was. And it's puzzling to discover that the mousse has been taken off the menu and instead has become something to be combed through our hair. The once familiar chips, formerly companion to the fish, have turned to silicon, and the special of the day has been replaced by the wood of the day. Now we have to agonize over whether the ubiquitous redfish is to be blackened over mesquite, ash or oak chips.

Is it possible to relate our current eating habits in this country to the international banking system, to the United Nations, to the EEC, to any organization that seeks union out of diversity, that promotes equality, harmony and righteousness? Are we eating all these ethnic tidbits, are we providing ourselves with bistros, brasseries and teahouses so that we may become, symbolically, at least, part of the global family of man? It would be nice to think so, but who knows?

Only one thing seems absolutely certain at the moment: that each one of us should go and contemplate a frozen chocolate-cranberry-bran-calcium-enriched-tofutti truffle . . . and let the cookies go crumble where they may. ●

Conversation With A Waitperson

Sam Cagnina has a long day. He has acting class from 9:30 to 1. He has dance class from 2 to 4. On Tuesdays and Thursdays he fits in a voice class. And on Wednesdays, Thursdays and Fridays, from 5 to midnight, Sam is a waitperson at the Zona Rosa, a chic Tex-Mex emporium, cooly Art Deco, on East 59th Street in Manhattan.

The owners of the Zona Rosa encourage their waitpersons to be individuals, and they all oblige. Sam's presentation includes a sleeveless black tee shirt, extremely baggy pants with big pockets (for putting money in) and black-rimmed spectacles. The spectacles are a prop, he confides.

"The glasses are for Sam the waiter," he says. "They're a mask that makes me into a new person. I can arrive here sad or depressed but I put my glasses on and I'm somebody else. Every night is a fresh performance."

For our conversation, in the late afternoon at the Zona Rosa, Sam took his glasses off.

How old are you, Sam, and where are you from?

I'm 25, but I'll be any age they want me to be. I was born in Key West, raised in Miami. And from the time I heard there was a New York, I wanted to come here. I tried it first when I was 18, and the city chewed me up.

So this is my second try. I've been here a year and I've defied all the laws of New York. I got an apartment in two days, I got a job in two weeks. Hated the job, though.

What was it?

Waiter, in a place on the East Side. They make you stand around polishing the silver when there's nothing to do; I was miserable. So I called on my higher powers and I went out looking and I found the Zona Rosa. I'm really happy here. I can be whoever I want to be.

Who is that?

I don't know. Whatever's necessary. I'm an actor acting a waiter, and it's fun. It's fun for the customers. After all, they pay money to come here and I want them to get their money's worth. We've got 14 flavors of Margarita and I can recite them in about five seconds; it makes them laugh.

We've seen you moving around here like greased lightning, yet your customers are always amused and happy. You seem to find personal time at every table. How do you do that?

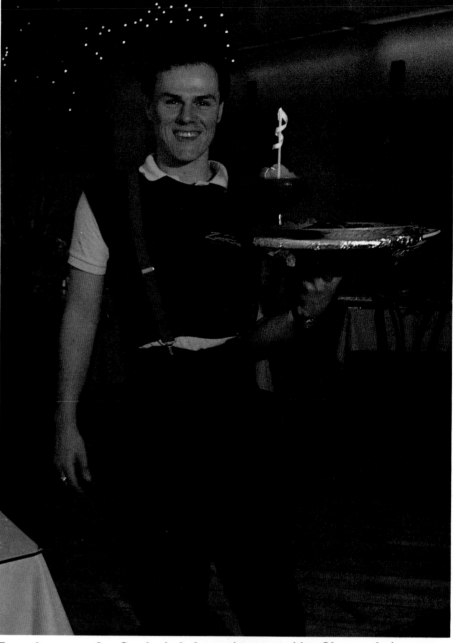

By random survey, Sam Cagnina is the best waitperson waiting. Of course, he is an actor.

Concentration. I have a seven-table station, and sometimes I have to take more tables than that, and serve drinks up in the lounge too. (I take the steps three at a time.) I just . . . pay attention.

What are your plans?

Well, I don't expect to be a waiter all my life. Some people are, and they're very happy with it. But I've been in ballet since I was a kid—I was with Harkness House here, and the New York City Ballet—and now I feel that, more than anything, I want to be an actor.

I know I could get a Broadway show this year, but it's a question of timing. I'm not ready yet. My philosophy is that you can be anything you want in life, if you just keep taking the smaller steps. Why be negative? I believe there's plenty of work out there. People

have this precognition that they want to be superstars. I just want to be as good as I can be at what I'm doing. It may be 20 years before I reach my dreams and can consider myself a skilled actor. But like a dancer, I must spend my time at the barre before I go on stage.

People say to me, "You're already 25 years old. What have you done?" They never ask me, "How have you lived?"

How have you lived?

For my family. I love my whole family. My father had a third-grade education, but he's a self-taught man. He reads philosophy. My mother is running a boarding house. She's like Charro. You think *I* have energy, you should see her. I have a brother, too, and two sisters. My dreams don't focus on me, you see. They focus on them.

Sam, what is the worst thing about being a waitperson?

Getting stiffed. It's only happened to me twice, and it's so perplexing. You give good service, the customer is all smiles—in one case, this woman was even giving me her phone number—and you come back to the table and there's no tip, or maybe a little change.

But the worst thing that ever happened to me was on New Year's Day. They didn't expect anybody to come in, and I was the only waiter for this whole restaurant, and more than 200 people came in for lunch! And I was down by the cash register, waiting to run a charge, and I reached in my pocket and all my money was gone. More than $800. We're our own bankers, you know, we account for everything later.

So you don't know my feeling when there was nothing in my pocket. I'm responsible, you see. The owners were very nice about it. They're letting me pay it back on a weekly basis. I'm still paying it back.

Sam laughed then, and turned to notice that customers were starting to come in. The adrenalin flow was almost visible as he made his farewells, stood, put on his glasses, and embarked on yet another great performance. ●

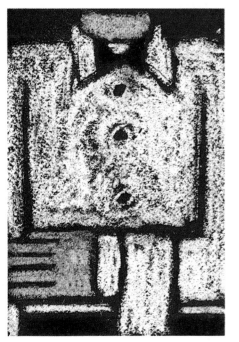

GEORGE LANG'S SURE-FIRE RECIPE FOR AN AMERICAN BISTRO

Serves one good-sized bistro

The Cooking Utensils:
About 4,000 square feet of space near a paved road. One very long lease, which is like the girdle on a fat lady: Maybe it's tight but it still lets her breathe.

Ingredients:
For the dough:
Several sackfuls of money, preferably not yours and without strings attached

For flavoring:
1 well-seasoned chef, male or female (between 120 and 200 pounds), preferably one whose ego has to be fed only once a day
1 bouquet garni of assorted cooks and key personnel (average age should be 30 years old with a minimum of 20 years experience)
1 head bartender with 4 hands and no pockets
A medium-sized, all-purpose kitchen planner

Yeast:
1 fully-grown manager who will make the *bistro* rise without too much kneading

Making the sauce:
1 fully-ripened interior designer (do not remove the backbone)
1 fine-grained graphic designer and 1 uniform designer (optional)

Additional ingredients:
5 billion kilowatts of energy combined with the firmness of Bo Derek
The combined leadership qualities of de Gaulle and Genghis Khan
The optimism of a person who is getting married for the seventh time
1000 gallons of tact and resourcefulness (or more as needed)
A sprinkling of well-sifted originality

For the topping:
1 public relations person, whipped until a froth has formed

Method:
Before combining ingredients:
Conduct market study to match the taste of your market and the planned restaurant with your location, considering dozens of changeable and unchangeable conditions. After completing it, read it carefully and go with your instincts.

1. Consider the total interlocking picture before beginning the cooking process.

2. Mixing the dough: You must control budget and scheduling, otherwise you'll end up with a disaster.

3. You must define each segment of the preparation and cooking process; then divide it into individual tasks giving them out to different specialists, and at the end—if you did your job properly—the recipe will add up to a living *bistro*.

4. You must be sure to train everybody as a true professional, remembering at all times that the American *bistro* is a democratic and egalitarian institution where everyone should be treated with equal hospitality.

5. What was called *Art de Cuisine* in the near past must be transformed into Good Food with a point of view served to a non-captive audience within a dining (not eating) ambience.

Serving directions:
1. In order to lower the failure factor you must consider the American *bistro* as a social institution, a place for recreation and entertainment.

2. You must learn how to produce quality in the age of short cuts, serving food which is not of the blow-dried variety.

3. This recipe will be considered a success by others as well if the *bistro* offers flavor, freshness and friendliness and contributes happily towards the guests' hedonism.

Note: If you have carefully followed the above steps, you are ready to cast your jalapeño-cornbread upon the waters and let the good times roll . . .

George Lang is an international restaurant consultant, journalist and owner of Café des Artistes in New York City.

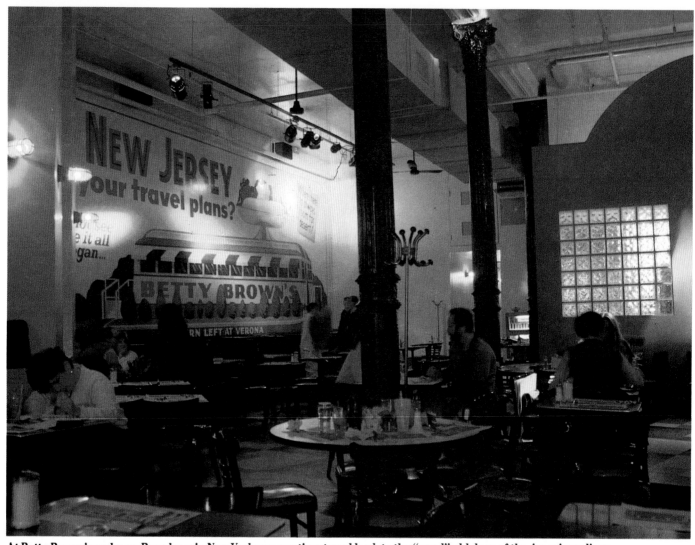

At Betty Brown's on lower Broadway in New York you can time-travel back to the "good" old days of the American diner.

A Bowl Of Bossy

If restaurant tycoon Michael Weinstein—of America, Ernie's, Metropolitan Café and Albuquerque Eats fame—is to be believed, the much-heralded new American cuisine is dying. "It's been killed in a year and a half," he says. "It's been overdone."

But Weinstein figured there was still some *old* American cuisine that hadn't been fully explored. So, in December, he and his Ark Restaurants partners opened Betty Brown's Broadway Dining on lower Broadway, between Bleecker and Houston. This, then, is Weinstein's uncharted territory—the New American Diner.

The food at Betty's might best be described as retro, with Sloppy Joes, "sliders" (yes, hamburgers à la White Castle), fruit-Jello-O molds and macaroni-and-cheese casseroles as menu mainstays. Stools are covered in candy-apple-red flecked vinyl, and prices dip almost to fifties levels (chicken à la king costs $5.95).

Many dishes are described in a bizarre diner slang, unearthed at Radcliffe's Schle-singer Library by William Lalor, the Ark partner in charge of "food concepts." A Bowl of Bossy is hobo talk for beef stew, and a Brace of Beagles is a side order of sausages. The Frito Pie is actually a ripped-open bag of Fritos topped with chili and cheese—"junk food from New Mexico," Lalor says. And Betty Brown's has a 138-item ice cream menu.

Already the place is attracting the young-and-restless NYU crowd, ready to move on from Bar Lui across the street. But don't haul out your poodle skirt or your buckskin bag just yet. Know first that the place is about as cozy as an airplane hangar, that earplugs are needed to muffle the whine of "He's So Fine" and that the food—well, let's be kind and call it "fun."

Betty Brown's does not stand alone. The New American Diner is a national trend. In Chicago, a fifties-style diner called Ed Debevic's is such a success that creator Richard Melman's group is branching out. And New Jersey, where real diners are still manufactured, will be home to the Ark group's next ventures—possibly a Betty Brown's in Paramus and an America's Diner in Verona.

The Fonz would love dinner at the New American Diner. Laverne and Shirley would, too. Even residents of the 1980s might occasionally yearn for the low-down taste of a South Philly cheese-steak hoagie, home-style meat loaf, or an ice-cream sundae studded with cinnamon hearts—or even a slice of Betty Brown's Brown Betty. ●

Jane Freiman, cookbook author and restaurant reviewer, New York

If I Can Make It There I'll Make It Anywhere Manhattan is an irresistible magnet for venturesome restaurateurs. Despite the fact that 80 out of 100 restaurants fail every five years, about 15,000 new ones are opened every year, according to the number of permits issued by the health department for all of New York City. Although most of the population lives in the outer boroughs, the majority of these new restaurants are in the heart of Manhattan—where one restaurant exists for every 200 inhabitants.

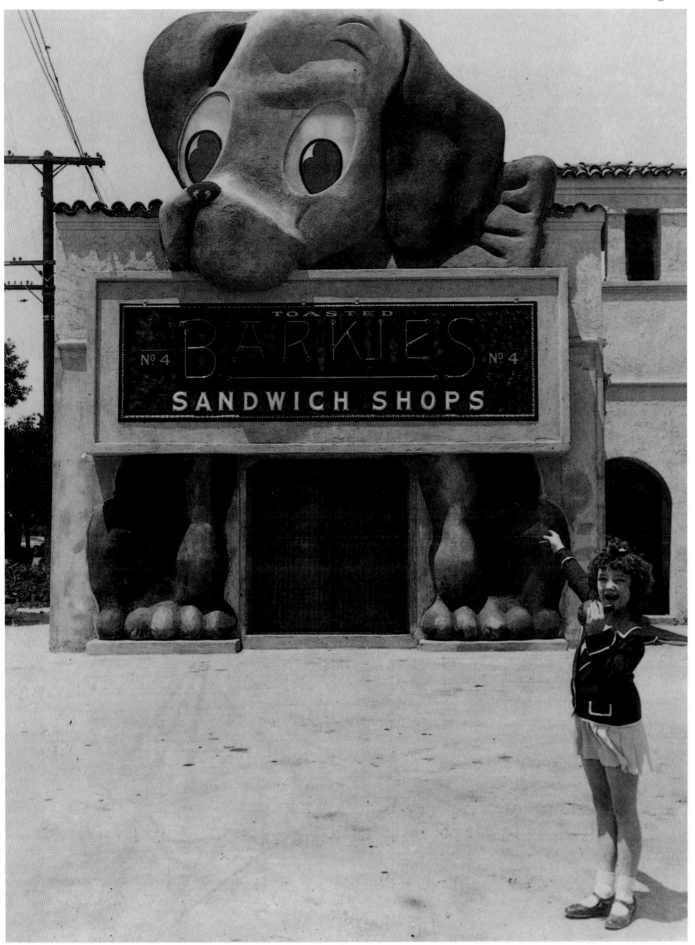

If you like being ogled by an outsized puppy as you sneak in for a snack, then Barkies, outside Los Angeles, is your house.

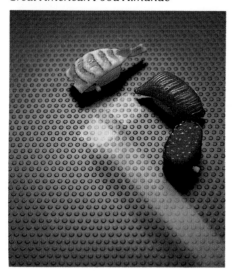
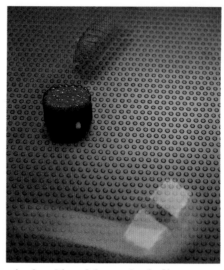
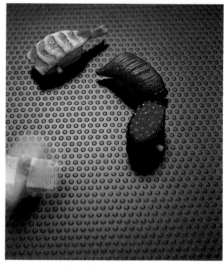

The latest thing for sushi lovers, any age—motorized sushi models on wheels. Now you can have your sushi and eat it, too.

I Hate Sushi

Irene Sax

I am not a picky eater. I'm game for kidney and sweetbreads; I actually like octopus and eel, and although I'd rather not eat squirrel, I can't say I wouldn't taste it if someone cooked up a pot of traditional Brunswick stew. But I just can't stomach sushi.

I know I'm the only person in America who feels this way. I know that 90 percent of the thin and stylish people in Manhattan can't wait to get to the nearest sushi bar so they can tell the guy in the headband to wrap them up another piece of flying fish roe and raw fluke. I even know an 18-month-old who says only 15 words, but one of them is "sushi."

At first I thought they were all pretending. But not the kid: He can hardly talk, much less lie. I still have a hard time believing them when it's time to go to lunch and everyone gets excited about eating Japanese. I want to say, "O.K. guys. Let's be honest. Low fat, sure. Chic, too. But good?" Of course, I don't say anything. I go to the restaurant, order tempura and put up with the sight of them all smacking their lips and enjoying themselves.

I hate everything about sushi. I don't like the texture of raw fish. I don't like the taste of seaweed. I don't even like the sticky rice, and I've heard some sushi lovers admit that the only thing they do like about it is the rice. I sink so low as to dislike the soy sauce and horseradish, which causes the kind of ecstasy these days that used to be reserved for pesto and orange-flavored Hollandaise.

Why, you ask, (and a sensible question it is) do I feel so strongly? I feel about sushi the way I used to feel about opera. It bored me. I couldn't sit through an opera without wishing I was at the movies. But I knew there had to be something there. I mean, Lincoln Center didn't have two opera companies, tickets didn't sell for over $50, the critics didn't write all those vicious reviews for a hoax. I was just jealous that everyone else was getting pleasure from something that left me cold. And that's how I feel about raw fish! ●

Irene Sax is a food writer.

Panache!

Charles Morris Mount

My most memorable restaurant experience was a lunch with Mr. Baum when that famous restaurateur was still operating Windows on the World. With me were several clients who were a bit nervous about meeting "the legend." One of the jittery clients knocked over a bottle of wine, much to his embarrassment.

Seeing the man's mortification and trying to ease it, Mr. Baum took the bottle of wine and poured the rest of it over the tablecloth. He then just snapped his fingers and waiters lifted up the whole table and took it away. Then they brought back a new table already set. To me that's style. That's Joe Baum. ●

Charles Morris Mount is an interior designer.

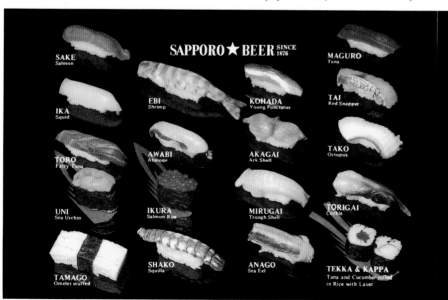

For those who don't hate sushi, a wide selection.

Nouvelle Hell
Mindy Heiferling

MENU

APPETIZERS

Sea Urchin Roe with Goat Cheese, Served on Blue Cornmeal Crepes	$8.00
Individual Pizza with Starfruit and Toasted Pine Nuts	$6.50
Baked Elephant Garlic with Three Peppers and Three Caviars	$10.00
Grilled American Buffalo Sausage with Tamarillo-Cherimoya Coulis	$8.00
Venison Carpaccio with Hazelnut Oil and Nasturtium Blossoms	$9.00
New York State Macoun Apple Soup with Pesto Cream	$4.50

ENTRÉES

Fresh Mint Fettuccine with Sun-Dried Tomatoes and Maytag Blue Cheese	$10.00
Buckwheat Ravioli with Blueberry-Pumpkin Filling and Lemon Thyme Butter	$10.00
Grilled Rare Duck Breast with Poblano Chile Confit, Grilled White Eggplant and Purple Potatoes	$14.00
Roasted Free-Range Chicken with Ollalieberry Salsa and Baby Vegetable Ragout	$14.00
Sauté of Muscovy Duck Livers with Kiwi Flan	$12.00
Chianina Beef Filet En Papillote with Blood Orange Beurre Blanc	$18.00
Poached Monkfish Cheeks with Fresh Ginger Mayonnaise	$16.00,

SALADS

Arugula, Radicchio, and Chicory Frisée with Duck Cracklings and Warm Sorrel Vinaigrette	$5.00
Belgian Endive, Walla Walla Onions and Lemon Cucumbers with Balsamic Vinaigrette	$4.50

DESSERTS

Cilantro Sorbet	$5.00
Mesquite-Broiled Crème Brûlée	$6.00
Ancho Chile Mousse with White Chocolate Sauce	$6.50
Rye Bread Pudding with Caraway Crème Anglaise	$5.00

Mindy Heiferling is a free-lance food writer and recipe developer living in New York.
She avoids restaurants serving tamarillo-cherimoya coulis.

TREND FOOD LUNCHEON

TALAPIA SALAD
AVOCADO

SEBASTIAN'S TRIO:
Yellowfin Tuna Charbroiled
Shark Brochette
Shovelnose Lobster Tail in Zucchini Boat

Mondavi Fumé Blanc, 1984

Luncheon menu created by: Chef Johnny Rivers for News Seminar Disney World Contemporary Hotel Saturday, February 22, 1986

Breadfruit
Baby Wing Beans

Carambola Dessert

Coffee   Tea

Fastest Gaining Food And Beverages In The Restaurants

Rank & Item	Two Year Growth Rate
1. Decaffeinated coffee	57%
2. Fruit	48%
3. Breakfast sandwiches	39%
4. Diet colas	39%
5. Mexican foods	36%
6. Main dish salads	31%
7. Rice	29%
8. Pizza	21%
9. French toast	17%
10. Cheeseburgers	17%
11. Chinese/Oriental foods	15%
12. Juices	15%
13. Large french fries	14%
14. Omelettes	14%
15. Cold cereals	14%
16. Large colas	13%
17. Chicken (non-sandwich)	11%
18. Tuna/chicken/ham salads	11%
19. Soups	10%
20. Other egg dishes	10%

National Restaurant Association

The Top Restaurants

Restaurant	Sales
1. The Hilltop Steak House Saugus MA	$24.2MM
2. Tavern on the Green New York NY	23.0
3. Phillips Harborplace Baltimore MD	14.7
4. Anthony's Pier 4 Boston MA	14.5
5. Smith & Wollensky New York NY	13.0
6. The Four Seasons New York NY	12.6
7. Spenger's Fish Grotto Berkeley CA	12.5
8. Old San Francisco Steakhouse Dallas TX	12.3
9. The Manor West Orange NJ	12.0
10. The Hard Rock Cafe New York NY	12.0

© 1986 Restaurants & Institutions, *a Cahners publication.*

High On The Hog

Russell Baker

I had never eaten where the truck drivers eat. All my life I had meant to. "Eat where the truck drivers eat" is one of the first maxims every American learns when he first takes to the road, but I had never done it.

Maybe I was scared. Truck drivers are mythic he-men in American lore. Maybe I was a little uneasy about pulling into a place where the truck drivers eat. They might not like having their restaurants invaded by the kind of man who wears a watermelon-colored sport shirt and drives a six-cylinder sedan with an automatic transmission.

Yes, that was it. In my mental picture file, truck drivers looked very much like a character named Bluto in the old Popeye comic strip, and Bluto looked as if he could play the entire offensive line for the Chicago Bears. Subconsciously, I probably feared having one of these Blutos challenge my right to eat where the truck drivers eat.

"Any man driving an automatic transmission," he would say, "has to beat me at arm-wrestling before he can eat where the truck drivers eat."

Well, not to make too much of my cowardice, I have eaten some incredibly bad food at franchised highway restaurants, solely because they seemed hospitable to the kind of people who wear watermelon-colored shirts, which is to say, the kind of people who don't make a fuss when their veal scaloppine arrives looking as if it could be either beef stew under water or—well, never mind, I am struggling to describe my dinner last Saturday at a franchised restaurant near Scranton, Pennsylvania, and thinking about it is making me queasy.

Sunday morning, with Scranton far behind, I resolved to eat breakfast in a place where the truck drivers eat. I had recently discovered a cousin who was a truck driver. He looked no more like Bluto than I do. The average place where the truck drivers eat, I figured, probably had a lot of truck drivers inside who are no better at arm wrestling than I am.

Besides, I had recently seen something on television suggesting that truck drivers

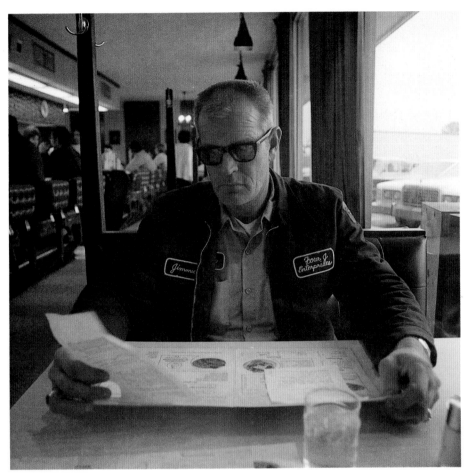

Truck Stop Stops Trucker: It's not easy to enchant a Texan on the road.

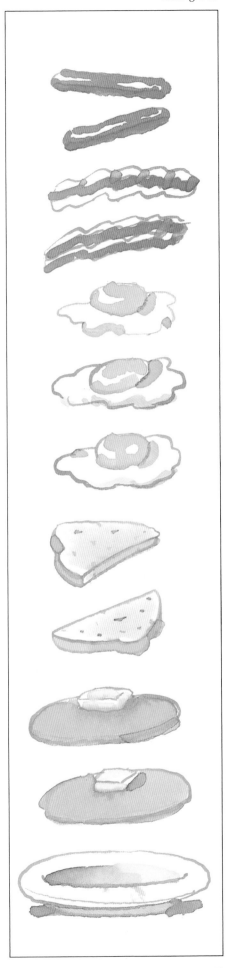

are devout church-going people. Though it was hard squaring this information with tales I'd heard about the Teamsters Union, Sunday morning seemed like the most propitious time to try eating where the truck drivers eat.

Sure enough, pretty soon, over the mountain rises this huge sign telling of the easy availability of diesel fuel and home-cooked food.

"We're going to eat where the truck drivers eat," I told my wife.

"If it's as bad as last night's dinner," she said, "I'm going to bring mine outside and pour it in their gas tanks."

Inside was full of big men. Big, big men. Several ran well over 300 pounds and caught your attention right away because of the intensity with which they were taking aboard eggs, mingled with slabs of ham, bacon and sausage, and the heroism with which the chairs supporting them refused to collapse.

There were a few women, too. Although all were in the heavyweight class, 190 pounds and up, since they were not tattooed I assumed they weren't truck drivers. There were a few men, pretty obviously drivers who were lean, but packing down breakfast like men who didn't expect to eat again in the present lifetime.

Not a soul among them showed any

interest in a stranger wearing a watermelon-colored sport shirt. Menus arrived. I hadn't seen menus like that ever, at any time, at any place, on any road, in all the years I have passed up chances to eat where the truck drivers eat.

Here were people who had never heard of cholesterol, or who, if they had, had said, "Life is too short to spend eating lettuce when you can get two biscuits covered with sausage, gravy, topped by two farm-fresh eggs sunny side up, and flanked by a quarter-pound of homefried potatoes."

"Even the home fries taste real," said my wife.

I was deep in a stack of pancakes with butter and maple syrup, topped by three eggs, over easy, and four slices of bacon with four pieces of toast drenched in real butter, so hadn't the energy for conversation.

That's all there is to say. I finally ate where the truck drivers eat, and eat, and eat. I have probably eaten several hours right off my life, but it was worth it, and I'd like to do it again some time if my appetite returns. Since Sunday's breakfast I haven't felt the need to eat a bit. ●

Russell Baker is a columnist for *The New York Times.*

A RESTAURANT WATCHER'S FIELD GUIDE

How to spot a good eatery

- Check whether the parking lot is crowded, then check again to see that it is crowded with local cars.
- Don't ask your hotel concierge or taxi driver for a recommendation; ask a policeman, an antique dealer or the proprietor of a bookshop. Or find a reputable restaurant that is closed or booked up, and ask there what other restaurant you should try.
- Some people trust a restaurant named after a person—be sure that person really exists and is still connected with the restaurant. A restaurant named after two people is a better bet, particularly if one of them is a woman.
- An even more promising choice is a restaurant named for a location, either its own (Florida Avenue Grill, Second Avenue Deli) or another place (Gulf Coast, New Orleans Emporium, Santa Fe Bar & Grill).
- If a steakhouse is your desire and you don't have a reliable lead, choose one outside of town in a near suburb. Before you commit yourself to dinner, ask if they make their own french fries.
- Similarly, if you're looking for a good café, ask if they make their own mashed potatoes or if their pie crusts are homemade.
- If either the waitresses or the customers are wearing housedresses, you can expect good home cooking.
- When there are children sitting around doing homework, your chances of a good meal are improved.
- When choosing between two unknown restaurants, try the one with the smaller menu, particularly one with a one-dish menu.
- A restaurant connected to a bowling alley or housed in a former gas station is a safer choice than conventionally housed equivalents.
- To choose a Chinese restaurant in an unfamiliar place, look for the one with the lowest proportion of chow meins.
- Never opt for a restaurant where there are reviews of the restaurant on the wall and the newest one is more than three years old.
- To get authentic local food, look for church suppers, outdoor food festivals and firehouse breakfasts; they are often advertised in the classified ads of the smallest local newspaper or on posters tacked to trees and telephone poles.
- In cities of less than two million people, never dine in a restaurant where waiters wear ruffled shirts.
- In a bar, cafe or roadhouse, look for hand-lettered signs of recent vintage that announce specials; somebody is likely to be actually cooking in the kitchens.

What to order

- Try dishes named for somebody, particularly for a child of the chef.
- Don't miss rare seasonal local specialties such as fiddleheads, melons, corn, fish from nearby waters.
- It's a good sign to find an unexpected ethnic dish, such as Korean Bulgogi on a Greek menu (as a chef explained in that case, the previous Korean owners had taught him the dish because customers had loved it).
- Appetizers are often better than main dishes, so if in doubt order multiple appetizers instead of a conventional meal.
- Opt for salads instead of cooked vegetables unless there are at least three green vegetables on the list.
- Sample anything the restaurant displays for carryout sales: its own salad dressing,

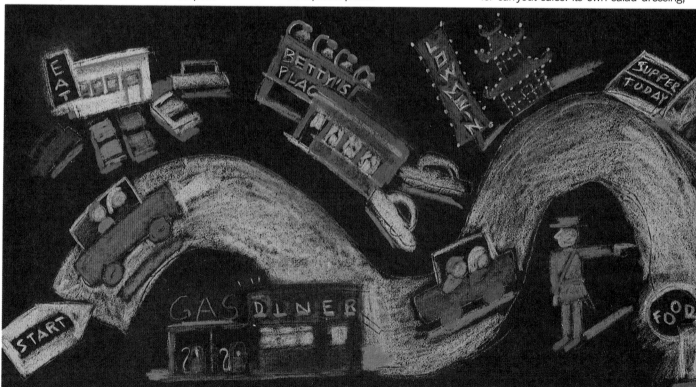

hams, breads.

- If the waiter tells you what he thinks is good, ask whether he has actually tasted it.
- Seriously consider any dish that is unexpectedly expensive (at Joe's Restaurant in Reading, Pennsylvania, the Polish creamed mushrooms were priced like steak and tasted like heaven).
- Chicken is safest in a small unknown café.
- Meatloaf is invariably at least decent.
- Nowadays, liver is a good bet.
- If there is a choice of soup or salad, opt for soup.

What not to order

- Avoid complex dishes on an otherwise simple menu; the Chicken Kiev, Veal Cordon Bleu and Beef Wellington are likely to be frozen.
- Lobster dishes, if there is no indication of whole lobsters in the kitchen, are likely to be made from frozen lobster tails or, in the case of lobster bisque, from a powdered mix.
- Potato skins, if there are no other potato dishes on the menu, are probably frozen; ditto fried clams, if there are no clams on

the half shell (except in Maine, where they don't know you can freeze clams), oyster dishes, if there are no oysters on the half shell, and fish fillets stuffed with crab, if there are no other crab dishes on the menu.

- Be wary of ordering steak in a restaurant that doesn't specialize in steak (but never pass up a chicken fried steak if you appreciate Southern cooking).
- Never order beef in sight of an ocean, or seafood more than three states away from the water unless you are in a major city.

Color code to ordering

- Southern states—white foods such as grits, corn puddings, spoonbreads or corn muffins (the best are made of white corn), hominy, cream pies.
- New England—brown foods such as brown bread, baked beans, Indian pudding.
- California—anything green.
- South Dakota—sepia foods.
- New Jersey—red foods such as beefsteak tomatoes, cranberries, strawberries, which are locally and deliciously grown. ●

Phyllis C. Richman, restaurant critic,
The Washington Post

What's Hot In '86? Garrison Keillor, host and chief writer of American Public Radio's *Prairie Home Companion*, gleaned from the new menu at Dorothy's Chatterbox Café and adapted for *Chicago Tribune* readers by cousin Flo, who took over when Dorothy left for Tucson: Six-can casserole with 40-day cabbage salad, Dorothy's "hidden treasure" meat loaf, liver o'gratin, Tuna ting-a-ling on chow mein noodles, eggs in baloney cups with liver sausage salad, Ritz cracker pie. ●

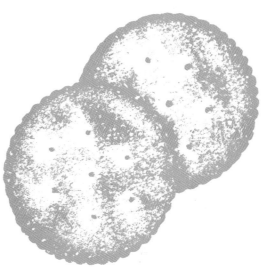

Watson! Come At Once! I Need You!
"I was once in a restaurant with my husband and a host. We had ordered lunch and it didn't come and didn't come. We inquired, but it still didn't come.

"Our host asked the waiter, 'Could you bring me a telephone?' 'But of course,' came the reply. 'I would like the number of the kitchen,' continued our host, 'to call and see about our order. Or failing that, I need the number of a good carry-out.'

"It was all done politely, and we did get our lunch and the point was made." ●

Peggy Katalinich, quoting Miss Manners (Judith Martin) in *Newsday*

Back To The Basics
"For my money, there's far too much originality in food these days. Sorry, but such New American fare as ravioli stuffed with chili, sauced with goat cheese and basil, is just not something I go around craving—or wanting to throw $16 at." ●

Arthur Schwartz, food editor, New York *Daily News*

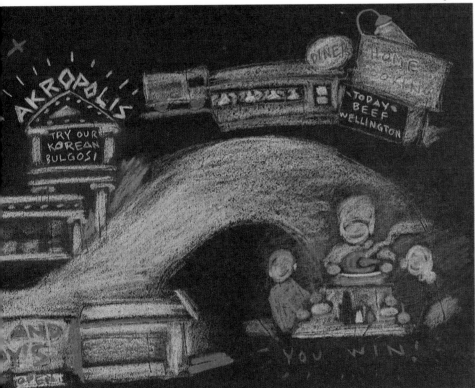

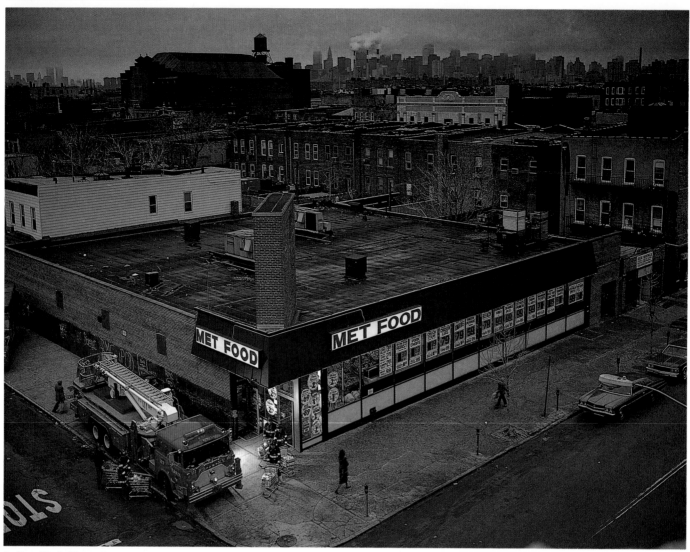

In New York City, a firefighting crew must never be separated; thus, when a firehouse cook forgets the pasta, everybody goes shopping.

THE FIREHOUSE COOKS

Some of the hottest restaurants in town do not charge more than $3 or $4 a person for dinner. They also do not accept checks, credit cards, reservations or, alas, customers, except for those who work on the premises. And all of the chefs are volunteers. Firehouse food, a simple, hearty cuisine with a long and distinguished history in many American cities, is going like a house afire. Working with recipes that are usually unwritten, and often passed down from hand to hand through the years, firemen-chefs are blazing new trails of culinary improvisation—and under rather difficult and unusual circumstances. As might be expected, the flavor of firehouse fare varies dramatically from city to city, from firehouse to firehouse and even from chef to chef within each station.

San Francisco, a city known almost as much for its food as for its fires and earthquakes, has almost as many firemen-cooks

as firemen. The fare at the city's forty-two firehouses does not much resemble the elegant new American cuisine for which the Bay Area is becoming famous, but it does reflect the fire department's ethnic makeup: mostly Italian and Irish, with a sprinkling of German. Thus, plenty of chicken and veal sautés; calamari in a fiery tomato sauce with pasta; a locally famous shellfish stew called cioppino; and roasts, stews and meat loaves.

The evening meal is the main event, and often the only time the entire house gathers at one time. Some firehouse cooks still favor what are known in the profession as "door slammers," simple dishes, like a roast and potatoes, that can be put in the oven and the door slammed after them. Increasingly, however, they are being replaced by more exotic offerings, such as homemade pastas, paella (often with crabmeat instead of lobster), chiles rellenos, and, on special occasions,

traditional beef Wellington.

Perhaps the best-known fireman-chef in San Francisco is Jim Neil, a 16-year veteran of the force. For the past three years Neil has been preparing a meal before the cameras every week for KPIX-TV's morning show, "People Are Talking." He tests some of his recipes on his colleagues at Fire Station 2. "These guys are really tough," he says of his firehouse critics. "I know that if they like what I make, it will be a success on the show and with the viewers."

In Houston, a city better known for oil and cattle than for elegant dining, firehouse cooking has a decidedly down-home flavor: chili, barbecue, more chili, flounder and jumbo shrimp from the nearby Gulf of Mexico, still more chili. Though the men are responsible for their own meals, the department's dedication to good eating begins at the top. Before he became Houston's fire chief, V.E. Rogers was an accomplished chef. "I cooked everywhere I was stationed," he recalls. "Corned beef and cabbage was my specialty."

In Boston, fireman Jack Corcoran's baked

beans and fireman Dan McHugh's codfish cakes rival those from better-known eateries in a city known as the home of the bean and the cod. Corcoran, who cooks for Engine Company 37 near the Museum of Fine Arts on the edge of Back Bay, soaks two pounds of beans overnight, drains them the next morning, and mixes in a generous handful of brown sugar, some molasses, and a few pieces of salt pork. (Measurements are casual at Boston firehouses.) He simmers the dish for just under an hour in a pressure cooker and eventually reheats it on top of the firehouse stove. "I'm a great believer in letting things sit overnight," says the robust rosy-cheeked Corcoran. " It helps the flavor."

McHugh, the cod-loving chef at Engine Company 33 in Back Bay, arranges two and a half pounds of codfish in a baking dish, puts it in a 300-degree oven for about 20 minutes, cools and then flakes the fish. He mashes six boiled medium potatoes, mixes them with the cod, along with a chopped onion, a cup of evaporated milk, salt and pepper. He shapes the mixture into cakes and bakes them at 400 degrees for thirty minutes. The result, in both cases, is the kind of simple, hearty dish that the men of Boston's 35 firehouses generally prefer over more ambitious offerings. Says McHugh, who trained as a chef at Boston's Copley Plaza hotel before joining the department, "They never like any of that fancy stuff."

In New York, which has 10,000 fire fighters, more than any other American city, at least 3,000 of them are of Italian descent. That has given New York's firehouse cuisine a heavy Mediterranean accent: Tortellini soup, chicken or veal rollatini, pasta and sausage bread are common offerings. The city also has a system of staffing its 220 firehouses that ensures a multitude of cooks.

Emilio Longo of Engine Company 263/Ladder Company 117 in Astoria, Queens (where kitchens have been fashioned out of what were once feed stalls for the horses), is typical of New York's firehouse chefs. Longo, who learned to cook from his mother, does the day's shopping in the station's predominantly Greek neighborhood before he arrives at work. If he forgets something, the entire company has to fire up an engine and accompany him: Department policy requires fire fighters to leave the station only in complete crews ready to speed to a fire and with the radio tuned to a boroughwide network.

As in San Francisco and Houston, meals are paid for on a cash-on-the-barrel basis, with an average dinner running about $3 per person. Longo once exceeded that informal limit to produce one of his tours de force, an elaborate chicken rollatini. When he presented the $4.50 per person bill, the diners nearly roasted him in his own juices before finally anteing up. Longo, however, insists that "camrady" is thicker than water. Realizing that complaints usually mean that he has scored a culinary triumph, he shrugs off all criticism: "For them, it's never good enough or cheap enough." ●

Donald Morrison, *Time* senior editor. *Cuisine*

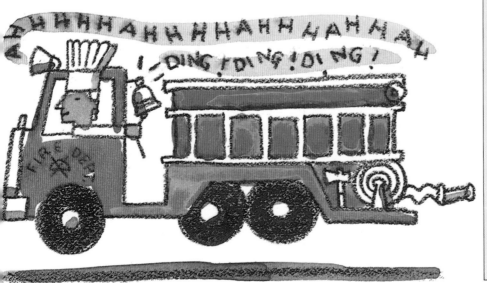

JACK CZARNECKI'S HOMINY GRITS WITH MUSHROOMS
A recipe to fire the imagination

Serves 4

Ingredients:
3 tablespoons butter
1/3 cup finely chopped shallots or onions
1 pound fresh wild or cultivated mushrooms, chopped
1 teaspoon salt
1 teaspoon sugar
1 tablespoon soy sauce
3/4 cup uncooked hominy grits

Method:
1. Heat the butter to foaming in a 1½-quart Dutch oven or heavy saucepan over moderate heat. Add the shallots and cook, stirring frequently, for about 5 minutes, until they are translucent.

2. Add the mushrooms, reduce the heat to low, and cook, covered, for 20 minutes, stirring occasionally.

3. Stir in the salt, sugar and soy sauce. Add enough water to bring the amount of liquid to 3 cups. Bring to a boil over high heat.

4. Reduce the heat to low and add the grits in a thin stream, stirring, to prevent lumps from forming.

5. Cover the pot and cook for about 50 minutes, stirring occasionally, until the grits are tender.

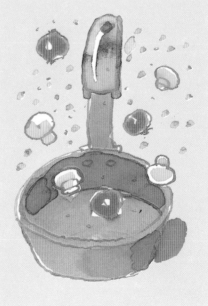

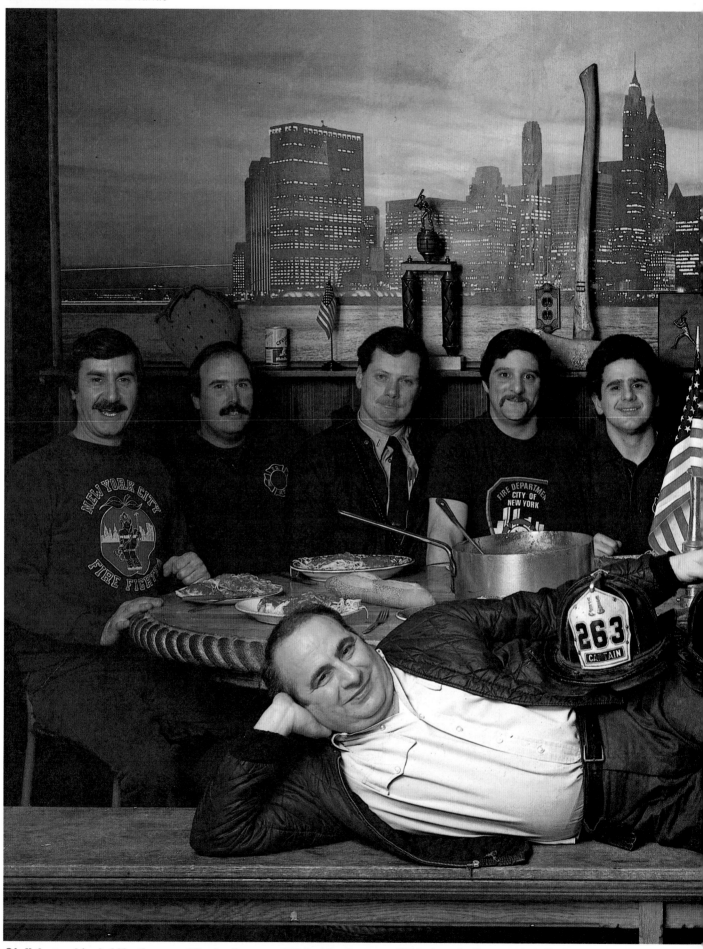

Of all the trophies held by the men of Engine Company 263/Ladder Company 117 in Astoria, Queens, their firehouse cook, Emilo Long—

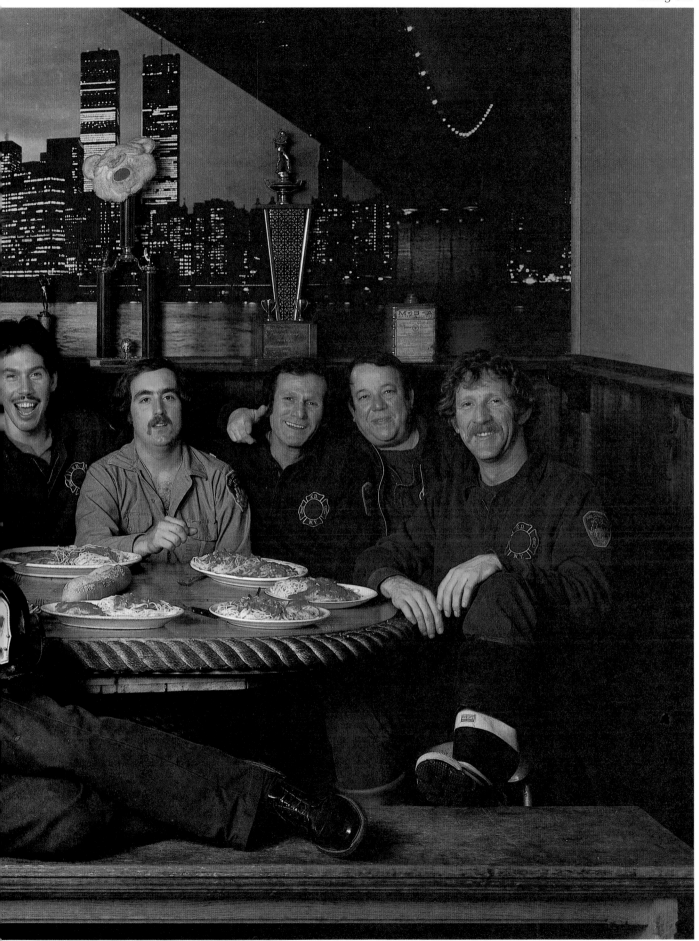

seen here supine before a groaning board and food fans—is by far the most cherished and appreciated.

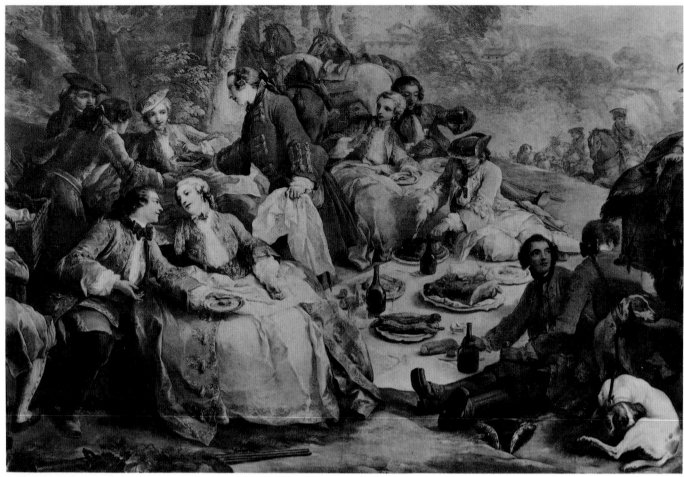

A cold bird and a bottle . . . or four or five . . . and a cool spot in the shade of a fine old tree; our European forebears showed us the way.

PICNICS

Eating outdoors is not everyone's idea of a picnic, but there are certainly plenty of people who think that nothing is finer than to eat sandwiches in the sand, bake a clam on the beach, barbecue in the backyard or carry a boxed lunch to the bleachers. Churches go in a lot for outdoor suppers and campfires burn as brightly as ever they did. There are millions who picnic in the park, backpack along country trails and toy with tidbits at the intermission of charming outdoor chamber music concerts in courtyards of museums. There are the fortunate who feast alfresco at music festivals, families who bring food on board boats and yet more who spend their summers having supper seated around swimming pools or perched on patios. Dining out is the *in* thing to do.

It seems that most of us like pretty much the same kind of food when we eat outdoors. We don't bother much with the kind of ditsy dinners we eat in the smart restaurants. We don't go in much, either, for all this low-calorie stuff. We kind of let ourselves go when we move outside. What we like a lot is hot dogs and hamburgers, coleslaw and po-

tato salad, watermelon and plenty of ice cold beer. Some folks like to have iced tea too. Advertising agencies tried to get us to drink lemonade a year or two back, promoting nostalgia. But for as long as we can remember, our elders just drank Dr. Pepper and Coca-Cola and root beer and plain beer, so we weren't fooled. Hardly anybody brings lemonade to a picnic.

On a hot summer evening, no one much cares about anything. We don't even mind if the barbecue grill smokes a bit and the smoke gets in our eyes. We even like it. Out of doors, people get along with each other a lot better than when they are cooped up inside. It has a lot to do with feeling like pioneers—cooking and eating outdoors. There is a bit of an adventure about it all. We never quite know if the meat will be overcooked or undercooked. Usually it is a bit of both at the same time.

In America, we have overcome a lot of the unpleasantness that people in other countries have to deal with. We don't, for instance, have to worry about the ants and the flies and the mosquitoes that are almost certainly there, though you can't see them in those pastoral paintings of picnics that Manet did so well. We like to spray the hell out of the area where we plan to eat—and a

radius of about half a mile around the picnic site too. Then just to be sure, we hang up those blue electronic flyswatters that zap anything that gets too close.

We are good at keeping cold food cold too. In Europe and in Great Britain, picnickers go in for all manner of fancy picnic baskets that have built-in leather loops for holding a service of fine tableware for eight and special places for the wine and the corkscrew and I don't know what all—except there is never much room for the food. And, curiously, no one outside the U.S. bothers with napkins. Fancy tablecloths yes, but no napkins. We Americans know to bring paper napkins to every occasion. Even if it's a picnic of a buttered roll or a doughnut and regular coffee to go—they always give us more napkins than we could possibly use.

No matter where we decide to have our picnic, we carry along a sensible styrofoam box crammed with food. We usually have enough for at least two extra meals, and fill up the corners with pickles, macaroni salad, potato chips and carrot sticks, though hardly anyone eats the carrot sticks.

Having a picnic is a great way to have a party—and there are no dishes to wash. Paper plates and plastic forks are the way to go when we commune with nature. ●

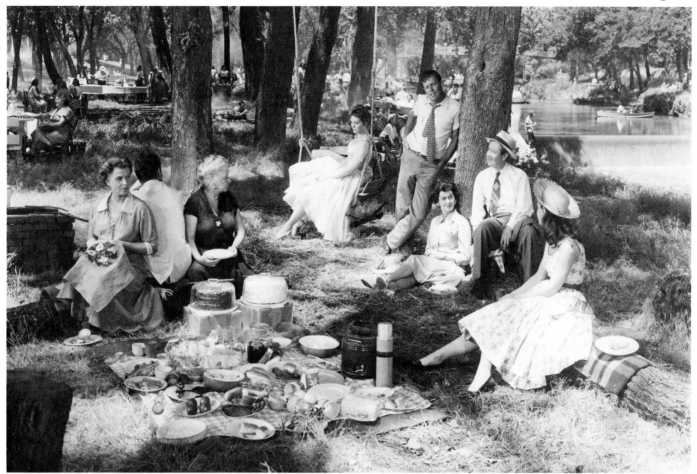

In "Picnic," Kim Novak sulks prettily, Bill Holden broods handsomely, and as for Roz Russell, she has no taste for eating out . . .

Hearts Remain Aflame For Our Beloved Bar-B-Q

High society calls it grilling, but most everyone knows it as "barbecue," that cooking technique in which food is prepared over charcoal or wood fire or electric heat.

By whatever name, barbecuing is fast becoming *the* way to cook, and the outdoor rotisserie is taking the place of the wok in trendy American homes.

The concept also is catching on in supermarkets. Sales of rotisserie-type barbecues in institutional foodservice and supermarkets is growing astronomically, says Steve Maroti, president of Hickory Industries.

Mr. Maroti would not disclose Hickory sales, but he says the rotisserie manufacturing company increased sales more than 300 percent since 1982.

While home barbecuing is popular, he says, those city dwellers who don't barbecue are relying on fast-food outlets, carry out places and even grocery stores to provide them with barbecued food.

As a new grocery product, barbecued food is a good profit-maker. While it does take some juggling of deli space, a chicken

bought by the store at 60 cents a pound can sell for up to $1.99 a pound barbecued, according to supermarket sources.

Because barbecuing isn't labor intensive, most of that is pure profit, Mr. Maroti says. The idea has caught on. More than 44 percent of grocery stores served barbecued products in 1984, compared with 36 percent in 1981, *Modern Grocer*, an industry trade magazine, reports.

Barbecued foods also have some appeal for health-conscious consumers. Grilling on a rotisserie means fat and excess oils drip off the food rather than being sealed in as in frying, says Robert Brown, a doctor at Boston's Massachusetts General Hospital. Nutrients are lost in frying, but barbecuing seals nutrients into the food.

There is one drawback to barbecuing, though. Chefs should be careful to keep meat rotating rather than just lying on the grill, Dr. Brown warns. There is some indication that charcoal or mesquite burnt meat may be cancer-causing.

However, the Food and Drug Administra-

tion reports that incidents of cancer are lower with rotisserie cooked foods than fried foods because carcinogens are cooked out of barbecued foods.

The most popular barbecued foods remain whole chicken, beef and pork ribs, chicken parts, sausages and specialty birds, Mr. Maroti says. ●

Julie Franz, columnist , *Advertising Age*

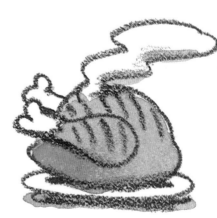

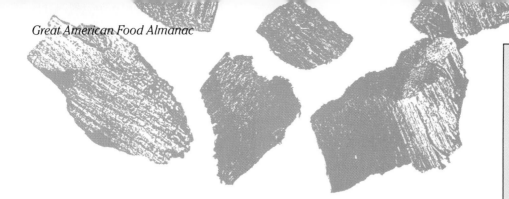

The Mesquite Mystique

It is lunch time here at the Williams home in north Dallas, and it is clear from the start that we aren't in for a light meal. The hors d'oeuvre of mesquite-smoked frozen pizza sets the tone. The rest of lunch is out back, smoking away on Ray (R.J.) Williams's latest invention, the Du-All 8-In-One Food Preparation Appliance, one of eight barbecue grills stuck all over the yard.

Spread around the mesquite-chunk canister in the middle of the Du-All, which looks like a Weber Kettle grill atop a wok with legs, are lobster tails, pork tenderloin, little quiches, asparagus with mushrooms, croissants and, for dessert, mesquite-smoked apple turnovers.

Above the jet-roar of the gas burner, R.J.—whose daddy, J.R., is also an inventor who helped him design an automatic tamale maker and an electric car—provides a little history. "Several million years ago, the first barbecue occurred when a forest fire cooked some animals," he yells, "but until about three years ago, this mesquite deal wasn't zip."

Today, mesquite is life itself for R.J. and Rozan, his wife. Behold Rozan bejeweled in her mesquite-wood earrings, pendant and bracelet, writing with her mesquite ball-point pen. Her family portrait includes a typically squat and bushy mesquite tree, and a friend walks on mesquite crutches. When she isn't helping R.J. run the family wood-chunk business, she performs presidential duties for a group called Los Amigos de Mesquite.

"I guess you could say we're fanatics," Mrs. Williams says.

She is right, of course. The Williamses are pretty extreme examples of what's going on with this mesquite deal.

Still, in this, Texas' sesquicentennial year—when the oil patch has dried up, and the Dallas Cowboys are again resigned to watching the Super Bowl on TV, and the prairie is dotted with acres of new unrented office space—the tree bears watching. The trendy fumes that recently seasoned dishes only at rarefied temples of gastronomy like Berkeley, California's Chez Panisse have quickly wafted into every Red Lobster restaurant and con-

vention hotel grill in America. And in a state that sold the world the cowboy boot and hat, not to mention the mechanical bull, when backyard entrepreneurs smell smoke, they figure money can't be far behind.

The economics of the mesquite business are mysterious, and the competitive spirit high (the Williamses believe their phone is tapped by competitors). But it is clear that most mesquite cutters and chunkers don't pay much for raw material.

In Bryson, Texas, R.B. Parkinson, a retired airline pilot, explains the dynamics of his MissKeet-brand wood-chunks business fairly succinctly: "People give me the wood, then we chop it up into little hockey pucks and ship it to New England and Hilton Head, South Carolina, for about $1 a (three-and-a-half-pound) bag," he says.

Times may be changing, though. "It used to be anybody would let you take it off their land for free," says Pat Morrison, who does business in Dallas as the Cowboy Cutter, shipping wood to distributors calling themselves things like "Coyote Pete" in places like New York's Long Island. Nowadays, he says, "you might have to pay somebody 50 cents to a dollar a cord to let you haul if off."

By the time the wood reaches places such as New York's Bloomingdale's or Zabar's in little bags, it can cost between $1.50 and $3 a pound—and it is often hard to find.

But if mesquite owes its recent good fortune to the fickle tastes of New York and California gourmets, trouble could be just around the corner.

Reached while loading a truck of mesquite logs headed for Tampa's Busch Gardens, Frank Kainer, the owner of B&B Charcoal Co. and C&C Wood Co. in Weimar, Texas, makes a startling revelation. "Some fellows from a big chain of restaurants in California just called on us," he says. "They want to know if we can supply them with a bunch of pecan wood, which we can. They're gonna start smoking all their stuff with pecan instead of mesquite."

Is it good? "Oh yeah," says Mr. Kainer, "All the old-timers down here cook with pecan." And it is, after all, the Texas state tree. ●

John Huey, reporter, *The Wall Street Journal*

JANICE OKUN'S BUFFALO CHICKEN WINGS

These wings fly off the plate.

Serves 4 to 6

Ingredients:
Blue cheese dressing:
1 cup mayonnaise, preferably homemade
2 tablespoons finely chopped onions
1 teaspoon finely chopped garlic
1/4 cup finely chopped parsley
1/2 cup sour cream
2 teaspoons fresh lemon juice
2 teaspoons white vinegar
1/4–1/3 cup crumbled blue cheese
Salt and freshly ground pepper
Cayenne pepper

Chicken wings:
24 chicken wings (about 4 pounds)
Salt and freshly ground pepper
4 cups peanut, corn or vegetable oil
12 tablespoons unsalted butter
3 tablespoons hot pepper sauce, or more to taste
Celery sticks

Method:
1. Combine the ingredients for the blue cheese dressing in a bowl. Beat until thoroughly blended.
2. Cover the dressing and refrigerate for at least an hour.
3. Cut off and discard the small bony tip of each wing. Cut through the joint to separate the two remaining wing sections.
4. Rinse the wings and pat dry with paper towels. Season to taste with salt and pepper.
5. Heat the oil to 375 degrees in a deep-fryer or heavy pot.
6. Cook the wings in the hot fat in several batches, until crisp and golden. Each batch will take about 10 minutes.
7. Drain the wings on paper towels.
8. Melt the butter in a saucepan and stir in the hot pepper sauce.
9. Arrange the wings on a warm serving platter and pour the butter sauce over them. Toss to coat the wings with the sauce
10. Serve with celery sticks and pass the blue cheese dressing separately for dipping.

The Catered Affair

Sean Driscoll, a founder of Glorious Food—Manhattan's caterer of choice to kings, potentates and mere multimillionaires—is the most articulate of men. But when asked who his major competitors and imitators might be, and there are plenty of both, his eyes glaze over and his mouth just cannot form the words.

"I imagine there *are* some," he concedes, "but I don't really take any notice. "We haven't the time to bother with that sort of thing."

When Driscoll has to bid on a job, he is aware of others in the field, but he rarely has to bid. "Mostly, it comes in over the telephone," he explains. "Word of mouth. Manhattan jungle telegraph." And what comes in are challenges to create and deliver brilliant evenings—from cocktails to sit-down dinners, for hundreds and sometimes thousands of people—in such settings as the Metropolitan Museum of Art, the New York Public Library, even in a parking lot.

When Driscoll started Glorious Food 15 years ago, it was thought that such feats could not be accomplished. But Glorious Food has proved not only that such things can be done, but that they can be done splendidly. The absence of kitchens in so many of these grand public halls has never been a drawback. The caterers bring their kitchens with them—in a fleet of vans and station wagons; and they cook where space can be found—in back corridors, in elevators and cloakrooms. They can convert the draftiest, most forbidding cavern of carved marble into a charming backdrop for an intimate dinner for 2,000 people—which would sound like a joke if they were not so good at it. Equally, they can cater a christening party for 20 people with the unobtrusive style that they bring to the National Gallery of Art, the Rotunda of the Capitol building in Washington, D.C. (they catered the inaugural luncheon there in 1984) or the bloated country cottages in Greenwich and Southampton.

"I have 15 full-time people," says Driscoll, "in administration and cooking, and I have 500 freelancers—butlers, chefs and all the waiters. Seventy-five of the waiters work exclusively for us. We find them by word of mouth, or they call us; we put them through a security check with the FBI, train them in seminars and give them a try.

"We don't have a waiter with us who isn't a

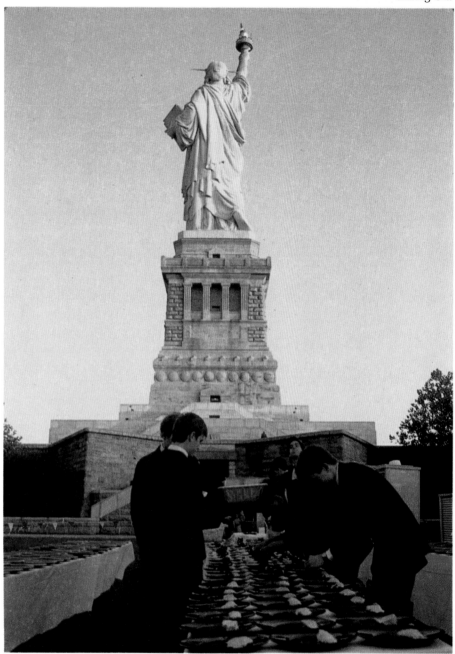

A small social affair catered by Mister Sean Driscoll.

college graduate. We have artists, actors, writers, stock brokers, and they use this work to support their day life. They're all very intelligent. It's not necessary for them to have experience when they come to us. I'm after the mind first."

Driscoll has a staff of three people running the booking department at Glorious Food. For butlers and waitpersons, they maintain a color-coded file to indicate the exact experience of each, and exactly where each one has worked with Glorious Food before. "We do a lot of repeat business," Driscoll says. "Clients appreciate it when the same crew comes back every time."

"Anything in food now attracts young people. The average age of our staff is 27. And our kind of work calls for youth—on an average night we have five different jobs which

can vary, as tonight for example, from a small dinner for 120 at the Met, to a cocktail party at Saks, to a couple of private dinners in homes. We must *never* show the strain of the work. But effortlessness takes a lot of effort."

Driscoll feels that off-premises catering (which is what Glorious Food does) "is only going to get larger and larger, because household staffs and corporate dining staffs have become less and less. And over time, people have realized that the job can be done, very successfully, this way.

"We do," he says, "deal with a lot of detail. In truth, we treat it like a show, an opening night on Broadway. Like a show, our business is a three-hour commodity, and there's nothing to take home afterward but a memory. We want to be sure that it's a very *beautiful* memory." ●

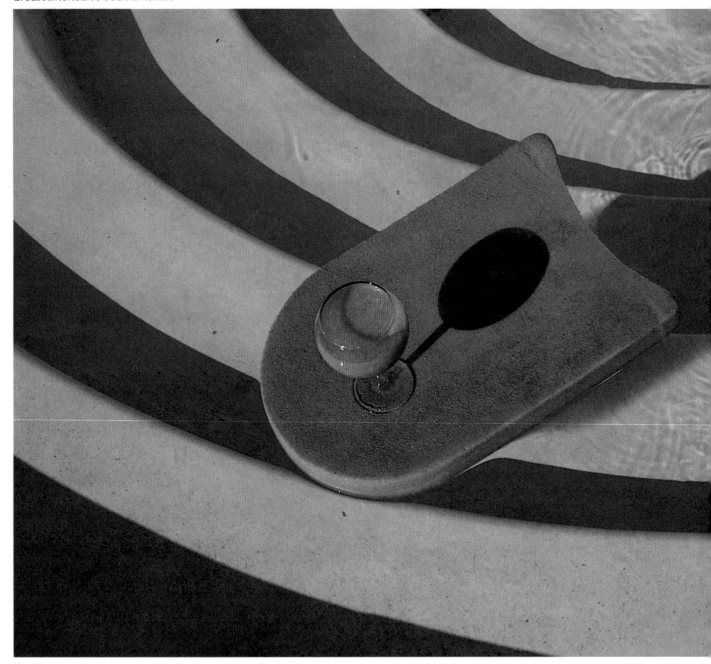

The Spa pool at the Sonoma Mission Inn in sparkling sunlight, and a glass of something juicy, all courtesy of California.

SPA FOOD

In the 50s there were "fat farms"—luxurious places in sunny climes like Florida or California, where, for a very high price, overweight matrons would go to shed pounds put on during the busy social season. There they would eat minimally, go to a few exercise classes (huffing, puffing and groaning all the while), and be pampered with facials, steambaths and vigorous poundings by formidable, stern-faced Northern European masseuses. A stay at a fat farm was usually something to be grudgingly endured for the rewards it brought at the end: a good complexion and a slimmer, firmer body that

would hopefully not look too bad on the beach at Nice or Majorca. And, more likely than not, any lessons learned about nutrition at the fat farm would be quickly and happily forgotten as soon as the stay was over.

Today, 30 years later, we have "fitness resorts"—places like the Sonoma Mission Inn, La Costa and The Golden Door in California, Gurney's Inn in Montauk, New York and Canyon Ranch in Tucson—which are as emblematic of the 80s as fat farms were of the 50s. Trends that began in the 70s— Cuisine Minceur, stress management seminars, concerns about the effects of choles-

terol, sodium, fiber, sugar, caffeine and additives in the diet, the zealous pursuit of physical exercise, high-tech fitness equipment, the popularity of unusual ethnic cuisines (such as Japanese, Indian, Mexican and Thai) and a burgeoning market for exotic fruits and vegetables, as well as our never-ending quest for slimness—have combined to make the regime of today's fitness spas an inevitability.

The best of the current spas offer classes in nutrition and stress management, a low-fat, low-cholesterol, sugar-free, low-calorie diet (for women, usually 800 calories a day

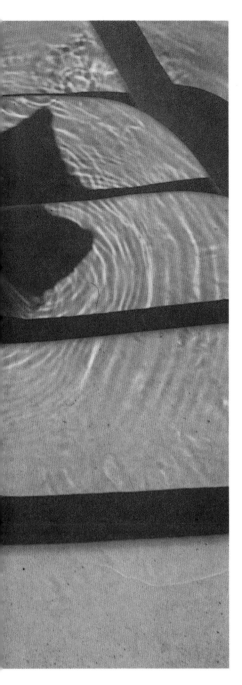

edible flowers, dressed with a walnut oil vinaigrette, all artfully arranged on a black lacquer plate. Spa food is based on the freshest raw ingredients, cooked and seasoned to bring out their natural goodness, and exquisitely presented. Frying and sautéeing are taboo; instead, foods are steamed, grilled, roasted or poached. Reduced stocks, arrowroot, vegetable purees and essences of lemon or lime are used to thicken sauces. Flavor comes from fresh herbs and spices, chopped garlic and assorted capsicum peppers, not salt. The coffee served is decaffeinated, but freshly ground and properly brewed. The influence of ethnic cuisines is apparent in the Japanese minimalist approach to presentation and in the ingredients—fresh coriander, enoki mushrooms, papayas and mangoes, curry power, cumin. Red meat is used in moderation, if at all; the emphasis is on whole grains, fish and plenty of fresh fruits and vegetables. Mineral water is downed in great quantities—at least six glasses per day at most spas. In fact, many spas recommend that the first day be devoted to cleansing the body of toxins by consuming only fresh fruit, nuts and seeds. But after that guests rarely feel a sense of deprivation. A typical day's menu at the Sonoma Mission Inn, for example, might consist of the following: Breakfast—assorted fresh fruits, cinnamon-orange poppyseed bread with honeyed apple butter and herbal tea or decaffeinated coffee; Lunch—chicken coriander tostada with refried beans and tomato salsa, and pineapple-lime sorbet; Dinner—asparagus spears with lemon dressing, grilled shrimp and vegetables with dilled yogurt sauce, and blueberry mousse topped with whipped "cream" made from nonfat skim milk.

Those who can't afford the $3,000 or so for a week at a spa can now enjoy spa cuisine at many restaurants, including The Four Seasons in New York City, where chef Seppi Renggli consults with nutritionists from Columbia University for advice on creating healthful meals. Renggli's innovative dishes have proven enormously popular—even with what used to be called the three-martini lunch crowd. For the same amount of calories in three martinis (about 450), a diner can feast on Renggli's chicken gumbo and a timbale of bay scallops in spinach—and still have 7 calories to spare. ●

for the first five days and 1,200 thereafter). Jacuzzis, saunas, herbal body wraps, outdoor activities like tennis and hiking, workout rooms with state-of-the-art equipment—all in exquisite settings. Small wonder that visits to spas are no longer dreaded but, rather, eagerly anticipated. And the food served is a major reason for spas' appeal.

If the term "spa food" calls to mind a few sad lettuce leaves on a plate, seasoned, perhaps, with a squirt of lemon juice, think again. At a typical spa of the 80s, that same salad is likely to be endive, arugula, watercress and radicchio with fresh herbs and tiny

THE FOUR SEASONS' MARINATED BAY SCALLOPS

Diets of denial have become the ultimate of esthetic indulgence .

Serves 4 as a first course
Calories: 81
Cholesterol: 13.4 g.
Fat: 2.24 g.
Fiber: 1.2 g.
Sodium: 79.7 mg.

Ingredients:
Yellow pepper puree:
2 medium-size yellow bell peppers, seeded and coarsely chopped
1/2 small onion, coarsely chopped
1 small clove garlic, crushed
A 1/2-inch piece fresh or dried hot pepper
1 1/2 teaspoons walnut oil
1 1/2 teaspoons red wine vinegar
1 1/2 teaspoons fresh lemon juice
Scallops:
6 ounces bay scallops
1/2 cup fresh lemon juice
2 fresh jalapeño or serrano peppers, halved and seeded
3 tablespoons fresh lime juice
Freshly ground black pepper
1/4 cup chopped fresh cilantro

Method:
1. Put all the ingredients for the yellow pepper puree in a small heavy saucepan and bring to a boil over moderate heat. Cover and cook over low heat for 30 minutes, stirring several times, until the vegetables are very soft. Uncover and cool slightly.

2. Puree the pepper mixture in a blender or food processor. Press with a wooden spoon through a fine sieve. Cover and refrigerate until ready to use.

3. Combine the scallops, lemon juice and jalapeños in a small, non-corrodible bowl. Refrigerate overnight, stirring several times. The acid in the lemon juice will "cook" the scallops.

4. Drain the scallops. Divide them among four coquille shells or small dishes.

5. Add the lime juice to the yellow pepper puree and spoon it over the scallops. Season with freshly ground pepper to taste and sprinkle with the cilantro.

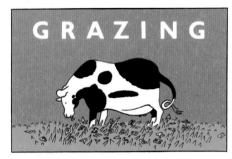

GRAZING

A Footnote To Strawberry History

In 1712 a French naval captain named André Frezier was sent to South America to report on Chilean coastal defenses and when he came home, he bore armloads of the big-berried, pineapple-flavored Chilean strawberry plants. In his enthusiasm, he had selected only the most beautiful, the most vigorous, the most flower-filled plants to transport back to France. He had unwittingly selected only females. The plants transplanted happily enough—they bloomed profusely—but for 30 years they bore no fruit. And then, by chance and by mistake, some foundlings of the Virginia variety were set in amongst them. The South American spinsters mixed and mingled with Virginia's dandies and a union was consummated in the beds of France.

Ruth Epstein, editor, *The American Festival*

Good Enough To Eat To sell, a product must look good, but it better not look phony. However, photographic food stylists need some tricks to keep food looking delectable under hot lights.

Not allowed: whipped, dyed mashed potatoes masquerading as ice cream; marbles in a soup bowl to buoy up the vegetables. What is allowed are non-melting acrylic ice cubes, at $60 and up, in beverage ads (photographers often use vodka for water, too—no little bubbles form); drops of glycerine, applied with a hypodermic, as beads of "water" on a luscious pear. What's a la mode? Rich, Rembrandt colors, reds and blacks, for backgrounds; foods that don't touch each other on a plate. Oriental foods, especially, require this breathing space on the platter, while Latin foods often tend to mingle.

Philosophy Of The 80s
"My mother was a good recreational cook, but what she basically believed about cooking was that if you worked hard and prospered, someone else would do it for you."

Nora Ephron, author, in *Heartburn*

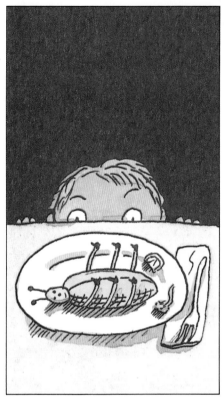

In Which Case Look In The Door But Turn Your Steps Elsewhere Before jettisoning the word "gourmet" as an adjective entirely from our vocabulary, we culled the following from a book called *The Official Gourmet Handbook* (Contemporary Books, 1984). "It is *not* a real gourmet restaurant," the book says, if:
- wine bottles are hanging overhead
- there's a game or quiz on the placemat
- there's a placemat
- you're asked if you want coffee with the entree
- the lighting is bright enough to read the menu
- you are offered a choice of salad dressings, one of which is creamy French
- posted on the wall near your table is a picture with instructions on how to perform the Heimlich Maneuver to help someone choking to death.

Food Of Love We spend over $4.5 billion on [chocolate] annually. If chocolate be the food of love, munch on. As ever-young Claudette Colbert said when confessing her lifelong habit, "I'd give my soul for a Tootsie Roll."

Mira Stout, writer, *Vanity Fair*

A Tiny Fork, A Wedge Of Lemon And Thou Consider the oyster and you may find it the prototypical food for today. Oysters have a benign flavor. They can be eaten without a knife. There is not very much of them. They do not need to be cleaned, or cooked, and in a pinch can serve as their own plates, to save on dishwashing.

Insect Digest

Although entomophagy—insect-eating—is a common practice in many parts of the world, it is anathema to most Americans, who tend to think of insects as filthy, vicious, disease-carrying monsters. But try for a moment to put aside your prejudices and take a look at insect-eating rationally and in a new light.

As arthropods, or organisms with jointed legs, insects are actually first cousins to lobsters, crabs and other eminently edible creatures of the sea. Grasshoppers have the same shell-like exoskeleton, the same jointed legs, and the same frightening antennae as lobsters do, and what's more, grasshoppers eat nice, clean grass, instead of garbage and dead fish from the muddy ocean floor. Furthermore—and I hate to bring this up—most of us eat insects all the time without realizing it. The lettuce we nonchalantly throw into our salads is prime grazing ground for aphids, and flour and rice make cozy homes for all sorts of weevils and beetles. Even the Food and Drug Administration considers a few bugs in our food OK.

Now, consider the advantages of eating insects. Most important of all, they're nutritious. Ounce for ounce, the average termite contains twice as much protein as sirloin steak, and has fewer calories and less fat, besides. In fact, studies show that termite protein has more of the amino acids essential to our diet than protein from any animal. In addition, insects are readily available in almost any part of the world. And if the species you like doesn't happen to be around, there's no reason you can't import a couple and breed them like cattle. Finally, insects could be the most abundant source of food on earth, a simple solution to the world's hunger problems, if only we would learn to be a little less finicky. With as many as five million species scurrying about, there's no reason to ever worry about making the same dish twice.

Instead of complaining so much about insects destroying crops and infesting our houses, and insecticides making food unfit to eat, we might do well to heed the advice of an anonymous entomophagous sage: "If you can't beat 'em, eat 'em!" And if you find yourself saying "Okay, okay, I'll eat insects, but how do I cook them?", peruse *Entertaining With Insects*, a cookbook recently published in—where else—California.

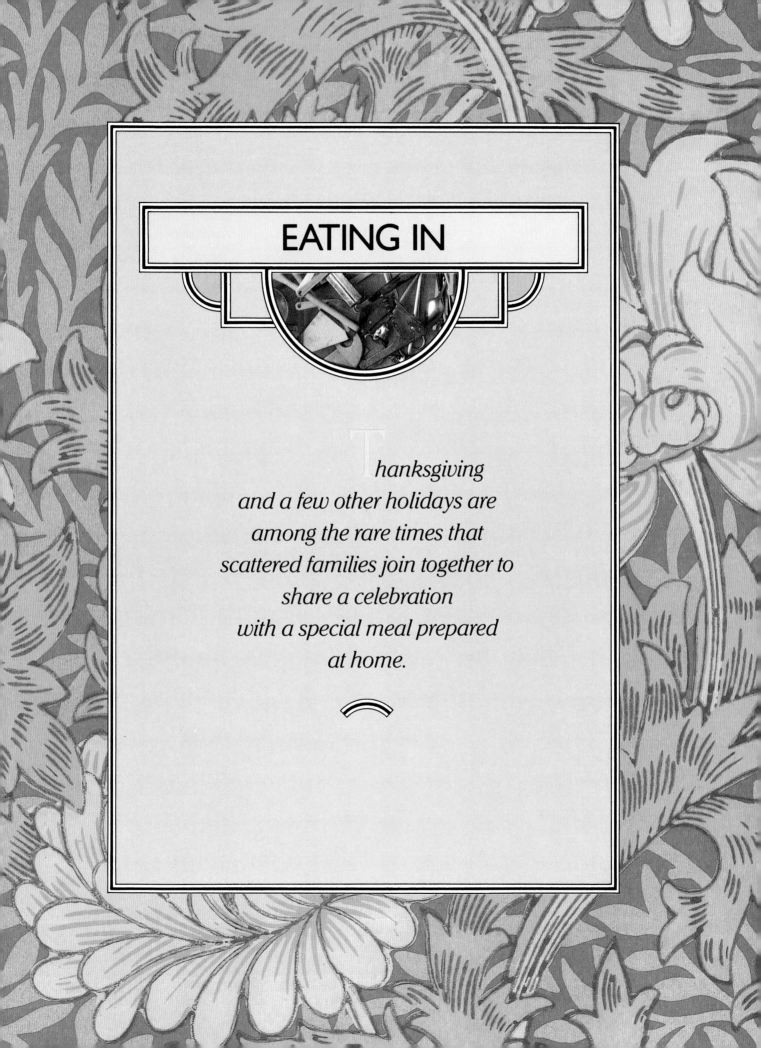

EATING IN

Thanksgiving
and a few other holidays are
among the rare times that
scattered families join together to
share a celebration
with a special meal prepared
at home.

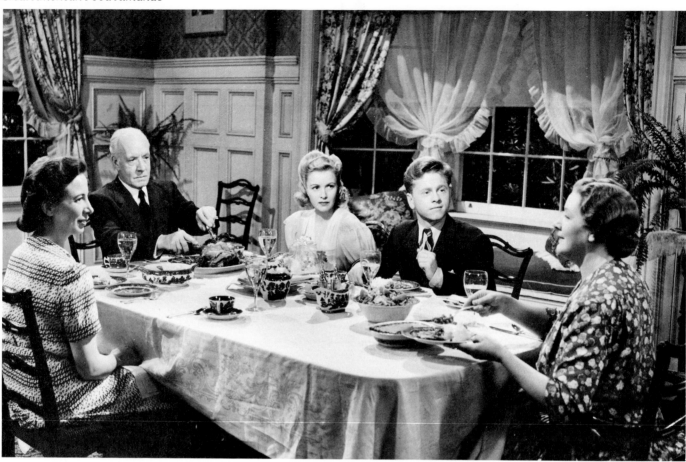

Famous film families feeding: above, Andy Hardy (Mickey Rooney) and his strict but doting parents set a model for the 30s.

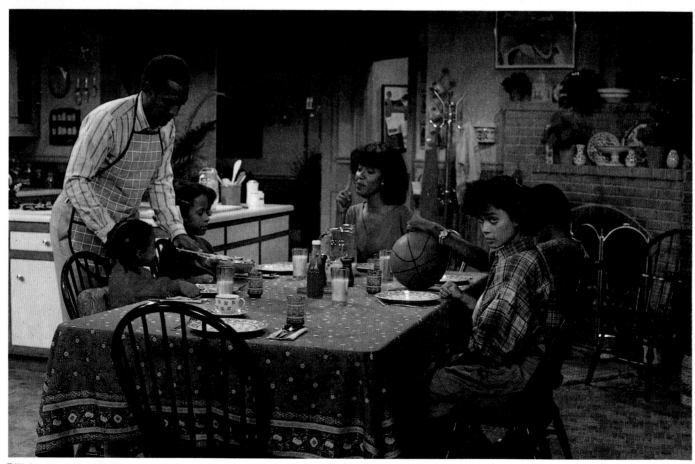

Bill Cosby and his TV clan stand for unity and caring in the busy two-career family of the 80s.

FOOD AND THE FAMILY

One of the best loved, most visible families in America has dinner together almost every night. Three girls, ages 6, 12 and 17 (and a fourth, when she's home from Princeton) join their mother, father and 15-year-old brother at a nicely-set table in their spacious, gracious, Brooklyn brownstone kitchen. Cliff and Clair Huxtable run a tight ship, and family meals—most especially dinner—are a cornerstone of their lives.

The close-knit, ordered family existence on The Cosby Show may not be the national norm, but the #1 rating of this television mega-success indicates that it certainly is the American ideal.

Millions of real family members may grab a burger on the way to the Planning Board meeting, or take a solitary turn at the microwave to zap a slab of something into edibility, but nobody claims that it's fun. Some sociologists sense a yearning for traditional family values: Wesley Burr, professor of family sciences at Brigham Young University, posits that "the 'me' generation of . . . the 1960s and 70s is moving back to family orientation."

Just what is a family?
The Census Bureau states that "a family requires the presence of two or more persons related by birth, marriage or adoption," and according to their latest figures, the United States has 62.7 million family households, including single-parent ones.

The average family size (who says statistics paint any picture of reality?) is 3.23. How often does the family (including little .23, who presumably has a small appetite) eat together?

According to the Better Homes and Gardens Consumer Panel Inquiry into Food, dinner, by far the most popular family meal, is shared by 80.3 percent of families five to seven times a week. One quarter of the panelists are cooking *more* than they were several years ago. The BH&G panel represents 7,450,000 subscribers in all parts of the country, and as such is a good indication of the eating patterns of the great American middle class: those who are modestly to very well off.

What is the family eating?
While certain statistics are readily available—Americans ate 209.2 pounds of vegetables per person in 1984—that doesn't really break down into what Mom, Dad and the kids (remember little .23?) each ate. It's just a mean—and meaningless—average. Fifty-nine of those pounds were canned or frozen vegetables, and the rest were fresh, including home-grown produce. Don't forget that waste—peels, spoilage—is counted too. Also a great deal of the 142.9 pounds per person of fruit (bananas led, followed by oranges and apples) was peeled, or discarded altogether as over the hill. And despite a lot of self-congratulation about new nutritonal awareness, Americans in the mid-80s actually eat fewer fresh vegetables and approximately seven less pounds each of fresh fruit than in the 1950s.

Keeping the family trim is a weighty concern. The BH&G survey found that over 80 percent of their panelists were very concerned about calories, and 65 percent had changed their cooking and serving methods to lower the intake. More fish and seafood, less beef and pork, are appearing on the table. But the latest update for *Trends*, published by the Food Marketing Institute, reports that beef is still a main course favorite, a good bit more popular with men than with women. Taste is the main reason cited for choosing a favorite main-dish food (41 percent), followed by ease of preparation (27 percent). Nutrition was important to 23 percent, and economy to only 20 percent. *Trends* reports that 9 percent say their households are reducing meat intake, and 9 percent are upping vegetables. It's not clear if these households are the same.

P at and Ken O'Malley of Duxbury, Massachusetts, have seven children. The youngest three—Brian, 16, Don, 18, and Patsy, 20—all live at home. Family members get their own breakfasts (cold cereal, juice, raisin toast or rolls) and eat lunch out. The kids eat in the school or college cafeterias. Ken eats on the job; he is a carpenter, and Pat packs his lunch (thermos of soup, two sandwiches, fruit and cookies) most days. Pat works from 9:00 A.M. until 2:00 P.M. as a part-time bookkeeper. Lunch for weight-conscious Pat is fruit brought from home.

Pat does all the shopping. She doesn't have a microwave, but relies on her freezer a good deal. Often she won't decide the dinner menu until around 4:00 P.M. "I arrange things to thaw easily," she says. "I buy hamburger and make and freeze the patties myself—I hate that boxed stuff. Pork chops and other meat I'll trim off all fat. My husband is an ice cream freak and we have it almost every day, but that's okay because I think it's good for the kids." Tonight's dinner? "Baked chicken breast with rice pilaf and broccoli, and butterscotch brownies."

This family eats dinner together around 6:30, for about 45 minutes, six nights a week. "We need to be together one time a day," says Pat. "We say grace, catch up on what we're all doing, and we miss the kids who are away terribly."

On the other hand, some families don't factor in the shared meal at all. Upsetting as that may be to those of us who see lunch or dinner as the high point of the day, other things are more important. Food is only fuel to stoke the jogger or tennis player, and a necessity for growing kids, but no big deal. What sociologists call "food events" are supremely unimportant to these people.

" I baby-sat for a family in Florida for almost three months," reports 16-year-old Alison, "and they never once sat down at the table together. The mother kept fruit, milk, cold cuts and cheese for sandwiches, and I fed the 8- and 11-year-olds." Alison adds they were all lean and athletic, and pleasant enough to one another, even though they didn't seem to know each other very well.

All this was very different from the way Alison was brought up. The second of four children of a psychiatrist father and journalist mother, Alison is used to family meals as structured affairs: nutritious and delicious, noisy and cosy. All of the children, two boys and two girls, have been able to cook from an early age. These teenagers make teen-age food—brownies and pizza—but the brownies are made from scratch, not a package, and the pizza dough is made in a food processor. The kids'll cook when an enthusiasm *strikes, but not on a general basis. Occasionally, when the parents leave them to their own devices, they do, as brother Ben puts it, "live out of a potato chip bag."*

The trend toward ethnic
Ethnic and regional food appeals to 85 percent of families. The leader? As you'd expect, Italian is the winner—after all, spaghetti and meatballs is as American as apple pie. More than half in the BH&G poll like Mexican and Chinese food; German and Tex-Mex are popular too. The approval of 12.9 percent of respondents goes to French cooking, in a photo finish with the cuisine of—Poland.

Naomi Wong is a divorced mother in San Francisco with two girls: Sophie, 10, and Betsy, 7. That makes her one of the 5.9 million single mothers (out of 6.7 million men and women) who is head of household. She estimates that she and the girls eat together five nights a week. On weekends they usually go to Dan, their father, either in the city or with him to his mother's suburban house.

"With no other adult around," she says, "I cater to their narrow tastes. When my former husband lived here, I'd do curries and elaborate Chinese food. But I don't really cook interestingly for children—there's just no response."

Naomi also felt that Dan set the tone at their dinner table and was much stricter than she is without him. "I don't insist on formal manners, but they know that at other people's houses there is no commenting on food, no saying 'yuk' and no food throwing! But the wrong fork or a dropped chopstick is okay."

"Family life can get dreadfully routine," says Naomi. "I make an effort to have guests, use the best china, make something special like chicken and broccoli with more seasoning than usual. That renews our appetites."

Are husbands manning the stove?
Indeed they are. In the BH&G survey, nearly 50 percent had cooked in the last four weeks, on an average of five times. Cooking meat and barbecuing are preferred, but the main reason given for cooking at all is, "My wife is working." Most stressed that "quick and easy" recipes are the ones they would try.

Jim Kraemer of Madison, Wisconsin, cooks four nights a week for his 16-year-old son, Ethan. Jim and his wife Carolyn always cooked together for the family or took turns, but now Carolyn, who has a full-time job, goes to law school four nights a week. Perhaps because his parents are quite skillful in the kitchen, Ethan doesn't cook, but this only child has a sophisticated palate: Swordfish with lime butter is his favorite dish. Fridays and Saturdays Ethan is with his friends, and the parents go out or entertain. Sunday dinner is the most important meal of the week for the Kraemers, and it's usually an elaborate one. "This family occasion is precious to us," says Carolyn. During the week, says Ethan, his father prepares "easy stuff—roast chicken, broiled fish and couscous."

Who is feeding the little ones?
The New York Times recently reported that nearly *half* of American women with children under a year old worked outside the home last year. Nearly two-thirds of all mothers with children under three now work, and the number of mothers returning to work within a year of childbirth has nearly doubled since 1970. Most of these parents need to work, and few can afford the luxury of a nanny or sitter. Someone has to care for—and give lunch and snacks to—the 7.8 million children. Corporations such as Campbell Soup, Hoffman-Laroche and Wang Laboratories offer good day care from enlightened self-interest—to attract and keep the best workers—but quality care, including nourishing food in pleasant surroundings, remains a worry for most of the nation's young parents.

Help from the deli
We carry home a lot of convenience food, especially from the delicatessen. Over half the supermarket shoppers queried buy deli and other take-out items. Packaged foods designed for microwaving are bought by 28 percent of shoppers; these shoppers tend to be young and affluent, including both the Baby Boomers and their elite subspecies, the yuppies. Southerners buy the most salad bar offerings, and Easterners the most delicatessen.

Broadening the base
Dr. Wesley Burr of Brigham Young University feels that though trends show a definite drift toward conservatism and a lessening of the divorce rate, "We Americans are nevertheless becoming an ever more varied and pluralistic society." Our religious diversity certainly affects family eating styles. Buddhists, Amish, Orthodox Jews and Sikhs sit down to different food from most of us, but they still live in families.

Betty Cooney, a Seventh Day Adventist, is delighted that the natural food, largely vegetarian diet followed for years by her 600,000 American co-religionists is right on target for certain of the newly health-minded. A typical meal for Betty is wheat pilaf with spinach salad and spaghetti squash, and that is the way she has fed her daughter and son.

"That doesn't mean," she says, "that we won't grab the occasional hamburger." ●

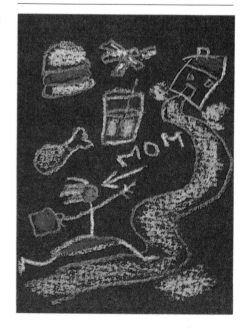

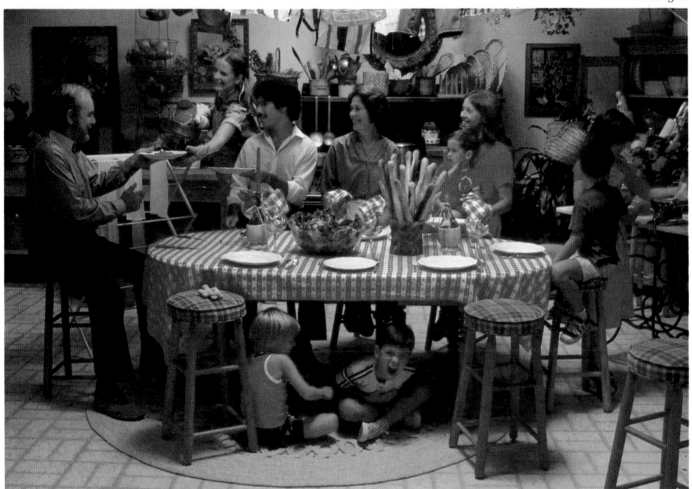

Simple is best when communal sharing has priority, and no one protests if the children ingest fun rather than food.

On The Ritual Meal

Judith Olney

f, when grown, a child is to remember the nurturing parent/mother cum food kindly, then it is necessary to establish a repetitive pattern in the course of the child's culinary development, a timed sequence of meals appearing in regular, dependable order that settle a ritual aspect in his mind.

When life used to turn on seasons and revolve around the getting and growing of food (and in some few places it still does) ritual meals and feasts paced regularly through the socioeconomic year. But in these days of plenty, we have lost that interdependent feel of feast-or-famine-together brotherhood. There is no particular need to rejoice and celebrate the fertility of land when spring brings an end to winter's want of food. There is no communal sharing in autumnal harvest or little imperative for the cooperative putting up of nature's plenty to see us through the dark season. And so those times and places of communal need and necessity, those occasions so often resulting in rit-

ual feast and celebration, are largely lost to us.

If one has not had the good fortune to be born privy to an ethnic or cultural heritage rich in Hanukkahs or saints' days, then the most successful and memorable drilling of food, scene, circumstance into the childish mind probably occurs in our main food-allied holiday, Thanksgiving. Awakening in a small bed, the outer world still gray, the child snug in the warmth of his covers first realizes the penetrating odors of the turkey, and perhaps the most important sensory impact here is the olfactory, for he is deluged with the aroma for hours on end before he eats. The smell perfumes the time, the day, over a period of protracted waiting until the actual eating of the bird itself is almost anticlimactic. Then, too, he sometimes remembers other aspects of the occasion—the overeating, overextending restless surfeit of the day.

For a ritual to be set, however, the established holiday or the full feast proper is

hardly necessary. One dish can do it—the pot-au-feu, the whole meal stew, the Lancashire hot pot, the New England boiled dinner, red beans and rice—any one dish where elements stew and intermingle into a powerful, cohesive whole suffices. Or a simpler soup that demands and provides the full, dominating focus of a meal and against which the accompanying food is mere ornament—a crouton or cracker, a light salad, a piece of cheese or small dessert. But it must be a soup or stew that appears and reappears with regularity, once a week in certain season and most often winter. And it will not be contrived cooking, but rather some old favorite or known, familiar dish, perfected through centuries and eaten by generations that pleases most and that, in turn, will speak to us most clearly down through the haze of time and culinary dross. It is, in the main, not our hit-or-miss attempts at culinary grandiosity or the dishes tried for effect, impressing one time but soon out of mind, that are remembered. And it is to such simple feasts that we should invite relatives and close or longed-for friends over and over again, not necessarily pushing on to greater gastronomic heights but inviting them to share in what is most comfortable, for comfortable foods, like comfortable old clothes and houses, are most contenting . . . fit best . . . become most.

This repetition is a small thing, a small even easy matter, a simple choosing of some dish (after children come to the maturity needed to accept such things) that all enjoy. A simple bean soup, a thick minestrone, a potato noodle soup, a boiled dinner with dumplings—anything that tastes pure, cleanly pure and of itself, so that the very purity of the bean, the onion, the potato, the plump dumpling fixes in the mind and remains there embedded. From such meals are familial archetypes made.

People say, speaking back the generations, "I remember how my grandmother used to fix spetzli. No one could make spetzli like my grandmother."

I ask, "Have you tried?"

And the answer is "No," or "Yes, but it was not the same . . ." and there a budding tradition/ritual falters, stops.

But we must gird up, allow for our own diminishing senses, allow for ever-changing time and space and place, and attempt the re-creation for our children's sake. And it matters even more if there are cherished roots and origins. This, you say, was the dish your Irish grandfather liked best; this came from great-grandmother's Bavaria; that is what they ate in our African homeland; or even, this came with us from the North or South. And if there is no established tradition, no ritual to support and maintain, here and now start one. And if there can be some simple task involved, making noodles, cutting sippets of bread, setting table in some "special" way for this meal and this meal alone in which a child can involve himself, so much the better.

Again, there must be repetition. Memorable meals or dishes always involve repetitive ritual.

"When I was sick, Mother always fed me ____."

"For Sunday dinner we always had ____."

"Every Friday night Mother fixed ____."

And even in the simplest ritual meal there should be a moment of drama,

planned for and acted upon . . . a transcendent moment.

Stop time and the day. Shorten the dining table, compacting and enfolding the participants together. Carry on the soup tureen, place it at the table's center, whisper something, and when people are hushed and bent to hear, with all eyes fixed, slowly remove the cover. Let the steam rise, the savory odors flood the room and drown those who await in heady delight. Flourish on the croutons. Make Chinese rice cakes and drop them into the soup at the last moment so they hiss and sizzle. If the dish has a crusted surface, break it with dramatic gusto. Carry on the roasted joint to sputter and rest at table, rather than in the kitchen, before carving. Make everyone wait.

Use the best silver. Tuck snowy napkins under chins; tie on bibs. Let the family eat in bathrobes for this our family treat. Chant a special prayer. Listen to the same classic music. Allow the children a wine goblet filled with cold water and a spoon of wine "just this meal," then toast each other. Sing, joke, dance about the table—whatever it takes to shake the normal dinner time from its settled course of daily complacency.

Foster contentment and well-being. Use the time to heal and mend and nurture. Charm the eaters, willing the occasion well and fiercely into their very minds and being, and then repeat the glad ritual again and then again, for if one would establish confluence with the past, there is no better way to do it than to say, tonight we eat what I ate as a child, what my father's father ate, and his father before him, for in such a way are ancient bonds maintained and new links forged for future. ●

Judith Olney is a cookbook author.

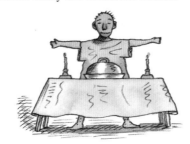

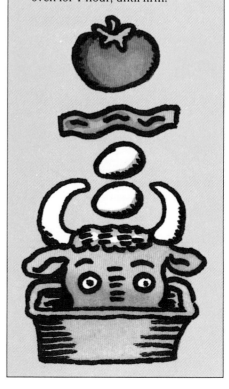

ANN LANDERS' MEAT LOAF

Reputedly this is the most frequently requested recipe in the English language. While the finest restaurants labor to create fantasy, the world yearns mostly for meatloaf!

Serves 6

Ingredients:
2 pounds ground round
2 eggs, beaten
1½ cups breadcrumbs
¾ cup ketchup
1 teaspoon Accent
½ cup warm water
1 package Lipton onion soup mix
Salt and freshly ground pepper, to taste
2 strips bacon
1 can (8 ounces) Hunt's tomato sauce

Method:
1. Preheat the oven to 350 degrees.
2. Mix together all the ingredients except the bacon and tomato sauce. Blend thoroughly.
3. Put the mixture in an even layer in an oiled loaf pan. Smooth out the top with a spatula.
4. Lay the bacon down the length of the meat loaf and pour the tomato sauce over.
5. Bake in the middle level of the oven for 1 hour, until firm.

Who's Coming To Dinner?

Barbara Kafka

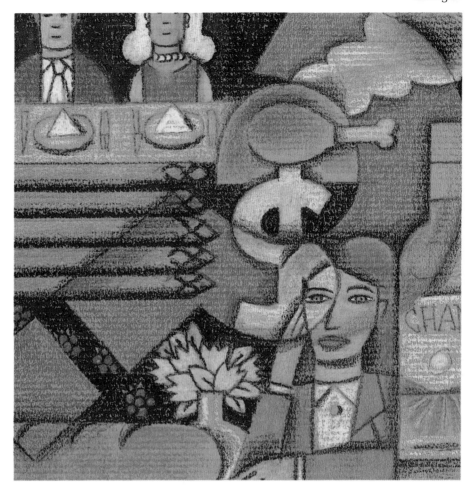

Most of the time I don't consciously plan a meal. It just happens. Particularly when I am in my habitual hurry, a series of automatic questions seems to pop into my head followed by answers and summed up with the beginnings of work to get dinner on the table. Correction occurs only when I am set back by a sudden sense of distaste: "that's really awful" or "creamed chicken after crème Germiny, yuck." However, the internal computer was not always so efficient and, for those of you for whom it is not automatic as yet, here goes the basic list:

Was it really tonight I invited the X's?

What's the date anyhow?

Did I invite anybody else?

That makes ten, right?

Did I include us when I counted?

Now I only get eight. Whom did I leave out?

It is eight. Eight's a terrible number; that man/woman thing never works.

Should I invite another couple? Remember: six or ten. Never mind, Anne will just have to sit next to me and the other end of the table will work out somehow.

When can I get home to cook?

Is there anything in the house?

Who is allergic to what? Didn't he say his wife couldn't even eat mussels she was so allergic? I wonder if that means lobster too? Better play safe.

Do I have any money with me? Anyhow, I have a supermarket checkcashing card.

Maybe there's some bread in the freezer.

Is it hot because I've been running around like a nut, or is it just hot? Hot! Well, then, who wants a great hot soup? Who said I was making a soup? Well, it is always easy. Just think of something else. Cold soup's nice. If I don't get home until six it won't be cold.

What else can we start with? Have I seen anything recently that was nice? Asparagus. Everybody likes asparagus. If I just get a few sea scallops and sauté them with the asparagus, some butter, lemon, and some parsley, that should be light, not too hot, and even slimming.

What will we drink? A gewürztraminer should hold up to the scallops.

Booze first? I hate it when they get to the table drunk. Does that mean another wine first? After all, unless you're German, gewürztraminer is a little weird all by itself. I don't have enough wine glasses for a wine before dinner, a wine with scallops, and something with the main course. I won't wash glasses in the middle of dinner.

Well, if I start with the Chandon—I think there are three bottles left—that can go with the scallops as well. If there's any left, it can go with dessert.

Are there eight unbroken champagne glasses left? How Herman managed to break three the last time he was over I will never know. If there aren't, it will just have to go in goodness knows what glasses.

I guess that takes care of the first course. It should be fancy enough—so that I don't have to have a fancy main course, just a roast. It can be cooking while we're eating; nice and easy; my favorite kind of meal.

Can I get away with a chicken? I love a good roast chicken, lemon and garlic inside. The Thatchers have never been to the house before. Maybe they will think I'm being cheap. I'd better stick with a leg of lamb. Then I can do some of my potatoes in olive oil and garlic that everybody loves. They go in the oven at the same time as the lamb. That will be perfect. Salad and cheese plus a simple dessert and I'm home free.

Now let's see. What do I have to get: red wine for the meat and cheese, asparagus, lettuce for salad, the meat, bread, new potatoes, lemon and scallops. Oh, good heavens, do you think mussels means scallops? Too bad, I can't go through it again. If she can't eat it, she can't eat it.

Now, what about dessert? I'm so tired. I'll buy some cookies and hope they have some good fresh raspberries. Nobody can be insulted by raspberries and cream.

Do I have coffee? I must. If not we'll do without.

All I have to do is run into the house, turn on the oven to 450°, set the table, put the wine in the fridge and start to cook. It will be quick and easy, about a half hour's time before the guests arrive. If I remember to pick up flowers on the way and I want to change, I'll need another half hour. ●

Barbara Kafka is a restaurant consultant, author and contributing editor of *Vogue*.

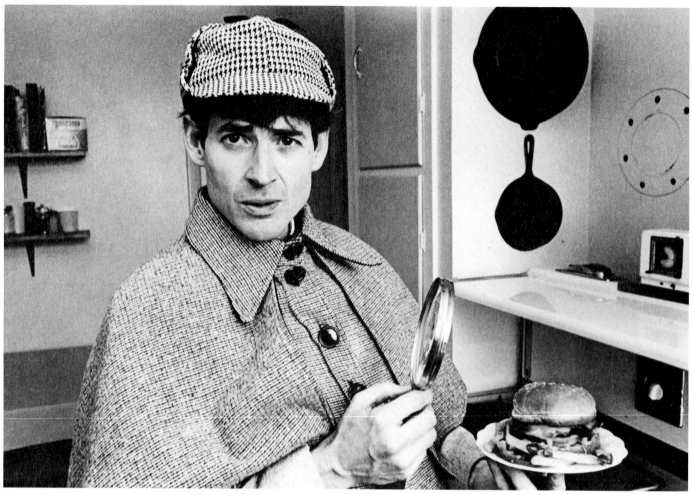

Master food detective, Ian Dengler, in his sleuthing outfit. Your choice of food, from hamburger to cranberry mold, tells him who you are.

Clues In The Cranberries

Ruth Reichl

Most of us subconsciously realize that the foods we choose say something about us; some people even speak of "ordering well," which implies that the whole process is a kind of test. But few people think about food choice once the menu has been removed, and very few even consider the question outside the restaurants. Very few, that is, except for Ian Dengler, who thinks about little else.

"Food choices," he once told me, "are like handwriting. You have to collect at least five or ten items in any given meal before you can make sense of it, but if you've got enough items, collected in order, no one can hide his social background from you."

When he says "you," he actually means "me." There is probably no one else in the country who has done such specialized research on who eats what, and why. Academics don't agree—they think Dengler's research doesn't fit into any classifiable pigeonhole. What I say is

that you can't argue with results, and Dengler can tell more about people from the food they eat than they are happy to have him know.

Actually, Dengler didn't set out to study food; he started with a simpler subject. Sex. "I wanted to study cultural and popular traditions as a scientist. But I found that I couldn't interview anyone about sex; there was nothing that I could believe. You see, I am primarily interested in understanding the problems of social change, but I wanted to study outside of literate society, and outside of the great. Some people call this folklore or ethnology, but those are not precise fields, and I wanted to do it scientifically."

Dengler was still studying sex when he was asked to teach a course in food history. ("No one else in the UC history department wanted to do it," he admits.) He suddenly realized that it was the perfect field of research for him. "And when I looked around for a standard meal model, Thanksgiving was obvious."

Aunt Birdie's Thanksgiving dinner

My grandmother, who is known to all as Aunt Birdie, was 100 in March. Ian Dengler asked that I interview her for him. "I'm particularly interested in the Thanksgiving meal she remembers from her childhood," he said, "because although Thanksgiving came into being during the 1850s, the foods were not standardized until about 1890. I don't have any other informants old enough to have been around in that formative period."

The Dinner

(Ian Dengler's analysis in parentheses.)
Oysters on the Half Shell, Served on Ice with Lemon. *(Oysters were very popular at the turn of the century. Ice was expensive before refrigeration, so the family was clearly well-to-do and lived in an East Coast city.)*
Chicken Broth with Noodles. *(The soup is German; the kind of soup is Jewish. And you see that at this point the meal was*

still being served in the nineteenth-century system called "service à la russe.")

Celery, Olives and Nuts Served in Glass Dishes. *(This was typical at the turn of the century; in those days nuts had to be shelled and roasted at home.)*

Cranberry Mold with Small Pieces of Orange. *(Cranberry sauce only became common after the advent of canning, in the thirties. The idea of a mold, once again, implies wealth and elegance.)*

Roast Turkey with Chestnut Stuffing and Gravy. *(The stuffing once again denotes the family's German background.)*

Fresh Asparagus with Hollandaise Sauce. *(Before the advent of frozen foods, the wealthy were offered a lot more hothouse vegetables in the market, year-round, than are commonly available now.)*

Candied Sweet Potatoes. *("No mashed potatoes?" he asked. I called and asked, and Aunt Birdie said that they did not have them when she was a child. "Good," said Dengler. "There was a point when Americans decided that mashed potatoes were an important festive food, but I rather suspected that it was later.")*

Pumpkin Pie and Apple Pie. *(Jews never ate mincemeat. The fact that there is no mincemeat pie, and the chicken-noodle soup, are the only clues that this is probably a Jewish family.)*

Café Noir. *(Her family clearly belonged to the epicurean tradition.)*

Rhine Wine. *(Before 1935, wines were simpler in their presentation. Most people tended to think of wine as either red or white. The Rhine wine shows both sophistication and, once again, the German background.)*

Ian Dengler summed up the background of this family as follows: "A well-to-do family from New York, and probably German-Jewish. But this is a family that is very well assimilated into American culture; your grandmother was at least third-generation American, with sophisticated tastes."

Aunt Birdie concurred: "My father was a traveling man and he liked a good table, so my mother always lived up to a holiday. Whatever anybody was supposed to have, she had. Both of my parents were born in this country, but their families came from Germany. Thanksgiv-

ing seems about the same to me today, but it is less friendly. In those days, everybody was invited to somebody's house. The parade used to come right by our house, and everybody would come to watch it. Of course, they always stayed for dinner."

William Farley's Thanksgiving Dinner

The following Thanksgiving dinner is that of a friend whom I interviewed and whom Dengler placed—without ever meeting or talking with him—within 100 miles of his home town.

The Dinner

Turkey—*"It was cooked properly."*

Whipped Potatoes—*"Made with real potatoes, real milk and real butter."*

Mashed Turnips and Squash—*"These were both plain. Everybody helped himself, and then added as much butter as he wanted. There was always plenty of butter on the table."*

Boiled Onions—*"No sauce."*

Bread Stuffing.

Gravy—*"Of course."*

Squash Pie—*"The crust was always a little undercooked."*

Pineapple Pie—*"My aunt always brought that."*

Milk, Coffee and Tonic to Drink—*"Tonic?"* I asked. *"You mean like Schweppes?" "No," said Bill, "you know—tonic—like Pepsi and ginger ale."*

Sweet Potatoes—*Bill forgot to mention*

these, but when I asked if they had them, he said, "Oh yes, of course."

Ian Dengler commented as follows on the menu: "This is a typical New England dinner. Plain mashed vegetables are typically served and spices are scarcely used. And look at the lack of green vegetables!

"This is not at all an orgasmic food experience—all he's told you is what's wrong with the food, or what's not wrong with it. But not once has he said that anything was wonderful. Nobody there gives you the quality of personal taste.

"From the nomenclature I'd say that this was rural, not urban New England, because that is the one area of the country where there is no standard nomenclature. In that part of the country they are often petty to the point of naming dishes after members of the family. The point is not that the terms 'tonic' or 'squash pie' or 'whipped potatoes' are standard—they're not—but neither is anything else.

"There's nothing elegant about the meal, but it's a standard, lower-middle-class dinner. I'd say your friend is from somewhere around the northern border of Massachusetts, and I'd say that his family has enough of a tradition to be fairly well established in this country.

"And why didn't you ask him about those pineapple pies?" ●

Ruth Reichl is the restaurant editor of the *Los Angeles Times Magazine.*

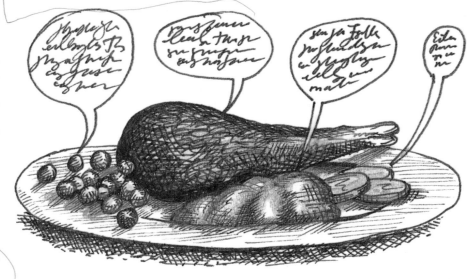

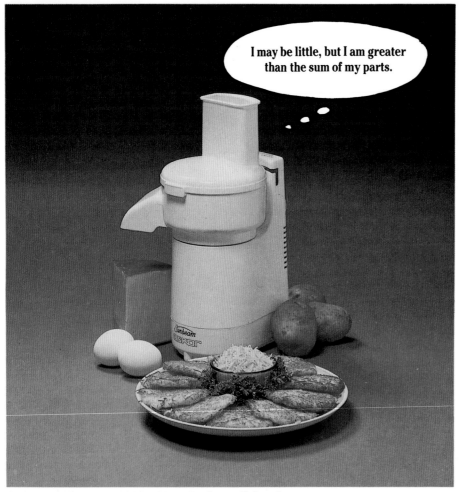

Oskar the food processor: leading edge in small electrics

What's New In The Kitchen

According to a report in the April 1986 issue of *entrée*, the gourmet housewares industry trade magazine published by Fairchild, the small appliance industry had some ups and downs in 1985. Up were food processors (by 53 percent over 1984), hand mixers (27 percent), electric knives (16 percent), microwave ovens (12 percent), can openers (7 percent) and toasters (2.1 percent). Down were toaster ovens and stand mixers (both by 6 percent), fry pans (12 percent) and coffeemakers (23 percent). Blender sales remained the same.

Manufacturers of these items, in an effort to lure buyers, have come up with ever more attractive features for their products. To wit:

Microwave ovens

Three years ago, only 28 percent of American households owned microwaves. Today, microwaves are in 44 percent of all American households, and in 60 percent of all two-career households. Three segments of our populace account for a 91 percent increase in sales during the last two years: young singles households, grandma-and-grandpa households and low-income families. Re-searchers are predicting that by 1990, microwaves will be in 80 to 90 percent of all American homes. As of 1985, microwaves were the largest selling major appliance in any given year to date.

Today's models are smaller and less expensive, averaging $175 to $250, down from about $600 only a few years ago. Some can now brown food, and one company, Vivalp, has come out with a compact "Micro-Toaster Oven" which bakes, broils, toasts, microwaves and defrosts.

Food processors

Less than ten years ago, the food processor was the newest must-have kitchen appliance and the Cuisinart was the sine qua non of the business. Dozens of companies tried to beat Cuisinarts at its own game and get hold of its juicy market share, but none—not even the Robot Coupe—succeeded.

Then in 1984, Sunbeam introduced Oskar, an acronym for Outstanding Sunbeam Kitchen All-Rounder. Over a million Oskars have been sold to date, accounting for one third of all the food processors sold in the U.S. and making Sunbeam the new market leader. This pint-sized food processor, suitable for a small family, sells for a small price (generally from $50 to $80) and takes up less counter space than a toaster. Retailers have found—happily—that even customers who already own a standard-sized food processor are buying Oskar as well, to do smaller jobs.

Oskar has become the hottest kitchen appliance of the 80s—in the words of Tim Davis, former editor of *entrée*, Oskar "has been to small electrics what the Cabbage Patch Kid was to toys and Diet Coke to soft drinks."

Yet Cuisinart still holds title to the concept and the name of that company remains a part of our language.

Coffeemakers

"Eurostyling" is in. This translates into sleeker, slicker designs of the type pioneered by Braun and Krups. And compact space-saving models abound.

Many manufacturers are making thermal carafes for their coffeemakers as an alternative to the usual glass carafe sitting on an electric warming plate. Thermal carafes are easily portable and maintain the heat of the brewed coffee, obviating any need for re-heating which tends to make coffee bitter.

Stop-brew mechanisms—allowing you to stop the machine during the brewing process, pour yourself a cup and restart the machine—are another innovation.

Toasters

High styling, as exemplified by companies like Vivalp, Maxim and Rowenta, is very much in evidence. Microchip controls now make the perfectly browned piece of toast a happy reality, and bigger slots mean that we can toast a bagel, muffin or croissant as easily as a slice of bread.

Ice cream makers

Gone are the days when making ice cream meant buying rock salt and cranking furiously (for hours, it seemed). Now, with the Donvier or Simac's Il Gelataio, we can throw the ingredients into the machine, turn it on, walk away—and have freshly made ice cream or sorbet in 20 to 40 minutes. Total Donvier sales, nation-wide, were 500,000 units in 1985, making it a phenomenal success in the small-appliance business. ●

Conversation With A Cookware Merchant

Alan Shefter, co-owner of Kitchen Bazaar, one of the nation's leading cookware retailers in Washington, D.C., has seen enormous changes in the business during the past 15 or so years. For one, people have become better educated and increasingly sophisticated about cooking.

He remembers an amusing incident of way back, when he noticed a customer inspecting a soufflé dish with apparent perplexity. "What's this for?" she demanded peremptorily.

"Why, that's a soufflé dish," Shefter said, and proceeded to explain about the egg whites and the copper bowl and the cheese and all.

"Oh," said the customer, "I don't need one of those. I am not a gourmet like Julia Beard."

"Something like that would probably never happen today," Shetfer says. "Everyone knows James Beard and Julia Child. People love to browse in cookware shops and dream of all the great food they are going to cook."

Alan, I have heard that a lot of the small cookware shops are falling on their swords by the hundreds and going out of business at a horrendous rate. Is this true?
Well, yes and no. Some of those who opened up in the big 60s boom have fallen by the wayside—that's true enough. But these were the people who started a little store more as a hobby than as a way to earn serious money. There is a lot more to retailing than meets the eye.

The American palate has been whetted for fine food and is no longer satisfied with hot dogs and hamburgers. . . . People will continue to cook and go to cooking schools. Though the smaller ones have fallen away, the more efficient ones have adapted to the times by offering evening classes and the kinds of foods people want to cook.

Are you worried about the increasing sales of cookware through mail-order catalogues?
No, not really. They have their market and we have ours. We have a mail-order catalogue, too. The catalogues serve a specific segment of society which doesn't want the hassle of going to a shopping mall. Others love to go shopping, and think of it as entertainment. They like to feel and touch before they decide to buy. Then they like to carry their purchases home with them and use them immediately.

Is it mostly women who come into your store?
No. More men are cooking for relaxation than ever before. They are good customers for gadgets and more expensive equipment. Both men and women are looking for true labor-saving appliances.

I think there's an increased interest in time-saving equipment. This began with the advent of the food processor, which was originally used only by very serious cooks. Today people want to cook elegant, great food, but they have time limitations.

What is the average age of your customers?
You would think it would be those between the ages of 20 and 50, but for us [it's] all ages. Young people come in to get something for their parents, and older people buy for their children and grandchildren.

As far as we're concerned, it's a grand business to be in. But you have to know customers, and what they want.

Once, I saw a woman looking at one of our latest gadgets, a bagel cutter. I could see right away that she didn't know what it was. I made a guess and told her it was for cutting muffins. "Oh," she said. "And will it cut bagels, too?"

What are your hottest sellers?
Well, the Donvier Ice Cream Maker has been a terrific hit all over the country.

The Mouli mincer is hot now. It has a four- or five-ounce capacity and will chop a clove of garlic, a small amount of parsley or a sliver of gingerroot, as well as grating cheese and grinding coffee. It works well, serves a definite purpose and doesn't take up a lot of room.

We are also doing well with a new knife-sharpening machine with diamond wheels.

The gift/cookware industry seems always ready to rip off any idea that looks like a winner. Do you think this is so?
It is probably true, but no more so than other industries.

I've read that Sunbeam has had to go to court to protect its Oskar food processor against copyright infringement. What do you think about this?
If a manufacturer takes an existing idea and improves it, it will ultimately help the customer. The Oskar was successful because it didn't look complicated and people thought it would be good to have an appliance that they could use often. If another company makes it into a better product, that's good for everyone. If it is changed only to steal, that's bad; but you can mostly trust the customer to buy intelligently. ●

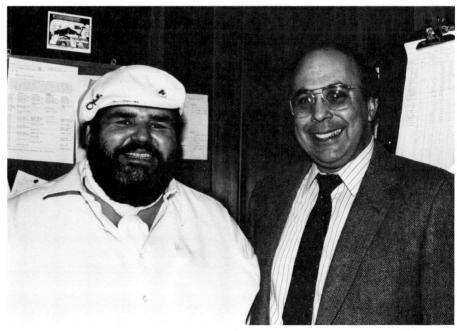

Alan Shefter, cookware merchant (right), with his famous friend, Chef Paul Prudhomme

Decisions, Decisions

Hilary Philips

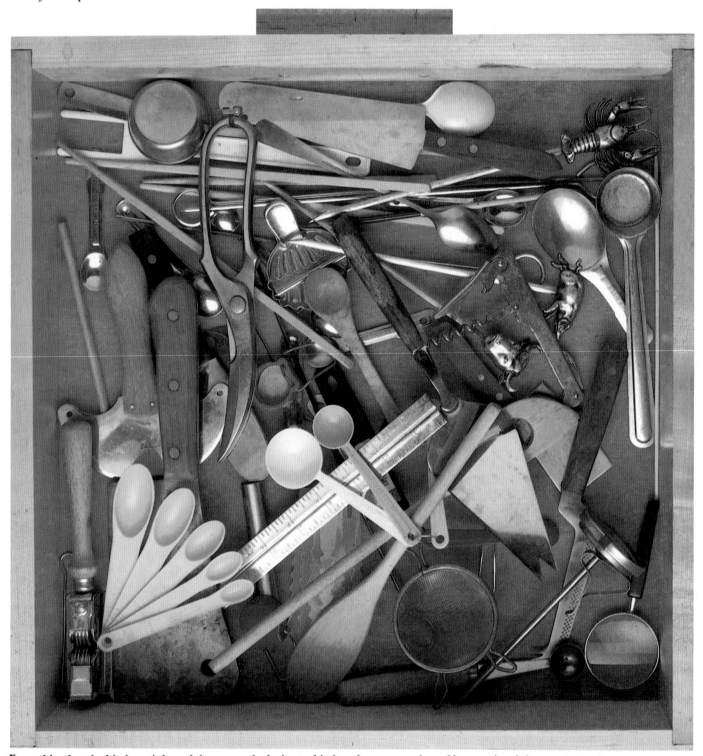

Everything but the kitchen sink, and then some, lurks in our kitchen drawers, orphaned by ennui and the new technology.

A few days ago the kitchen was painted. This meant that everything *had* to be taken out of the cupboards. It was a nuisance but not too much of a problem. The problem was in putting it all back. Wrestling with a four-foot-long fish poacher, it dawned on me that not once in lo these many years have

I ever had the opportunity to cook a four-foot-long fish. Once someone brought me a fish that was four-feet-two-inches-long and not knowing whether to lop off the poor dead creature's head or tail, I cut it in half. This spoiled the effect completely. I decided, quite impulsively, to pitch the fish poacher. When I buy fish these days, I

reasoned, I buy enough for two people. It still doesn't seem quite proper to serve fish for ten, and besides, only rarely do I invite ten for dinner. What then should be done with the fish-filleting knife, the oyster knife and the clam-opening knife too? I have gotten the clam knife stuck under the top of the kitchen drawer a thousand times.

Sometimes I have used it for stabbing the frozen pastry of Stouffer's chicken pot pies. The clam knife has never made the acquaintance of a clam. It probably never will. The ten clay pots haven't been used for years either. Nor has the Crock-Pot, the fondue pot, the waffle-maker or the crepe pan. Sometimes the kids use the precious omelette pan for frying bacon. Its once sacred, slick surface has long since disappeared.

I am looking at the toaster and the convection oven and realize that I don't need them, now that I have a compact microwave oven. Come to think of it, I don't need the stove either. The mixer, the juice extractor, the minipimer and two dozen knives have also obsolesced and been replaced with the food processor. The $450 pasta machine and the $350 ice cream machine seem to sneer at me as I cook pasta only in the form of under-300-calorie frozen fettuccine to go with chicken in red wine. Homemade ice cream is made in the Donvier, but everyone is on a diet, so no one actually eats it. Still it is comforting to know that there is some homemade ice cream in the freezer. It makes me feel motherly.

I don't know what to do about the tart tins and rolling pins and cake pans and cheesecake pans and pâté molds and angel food cake molds and ring molds and bread pans and ravioli tins and six different sizes of soufflé dishes, ramekins and cookie presses not to mention pastry bags with all those fancy tips for making birthday cakes. Now all the stuff we used to cook at home is cheaper to buy from the local take-out store—and faster, too—and we don't have to eat up all the leftovers.

I am puzzling over the preserving kettle and all those canning jars that get washed from time to time and put back—always empty. If I actually counted, I think there are ten different sizes of casseroles and no end of saucepans, frying pans and all the copper pans that are faithfully polished every three weeks. To ponder how many man-(woman) hours have been spent polishing the copper is to boggle the mind and dazzle the imagination. And always, when the copper is cleaned, it rains, so it instantly becomes tarnished again. There are two sizes of apple-corers and one gadget for disemboweling a pineapple. There are measuring cups and spoons, stirrers and whisks, spatulas of wood, metal and plastic, bowls and strainers, sieves and salad spinners. I think I'll keep the salad spinner—perhaps one of the strainers too.

It dawns on me that all I really need these days could fit into a space that is very small indeed. In fact, come to think of it—do I need a kitchen at all? Eureka. All I need is a telephone for ordering from the local Chinese takeout. I could use the kitchen as an office or a consulting room, a home entertainment center or a gymnasium, a library or a workshop. I was thinking about all these possibilities as I washed every blessed thing and put each one neatly back in its appointed place until the next time the kitchen is painted. ●

Hilary Philips is a freelance writer.

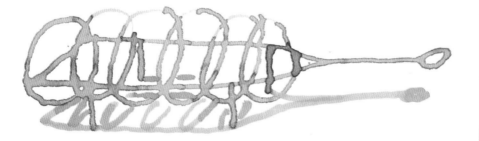

EDNA LEWIS' HAM BISCUITS
Biscuits are hot today.

Makes about 18

Ingredients:
3 cups sifted flour
1 scant teaspoon salt
2 2/3 teaspoons cream of tartar
2 teaspoons baking soda
2/3 cup lard
1 cup plus 2 tablespoons buttermilk
1 cup finely chopped country ham

Method:

1. Preheat the oven to 450 degrees.

2. Sift the flour, salt, cream of tartar and baking soda into a large bowl. Work the lard into it with your fingertips or a pastry blender until the mixture has the consistency of coarse cornmeal.

3. Add the buttermilk all at once, scattering it all over the dough. Fold in the ham. Stir vigorously with a wooden spoon for 2 to 3 minutes until the dough stiffens slightly.

4. Transfer the dough to a lightly floured surface. Sprinkle about 1 tablespoon of flour over the dough and gently flatten it out with your hands into a thick, round cake.

5. Knead the dough for a minute by folding the outer edge into the center, giving a light knead as you fold the sides in to overlap each other. Turn the folded side face-down and dust lightly with flour if needed. Use flour sparingly; too much will make the dough stiff and the biscuits tough.

6. Using a floured rolling pin, roll out the dough to a thickness of 1/2 inch or a little less. Prick the top of the dough all over with a fork.

7. Dust a biscuit cutter or the rim of a small glass with flour. Press the cutter into the dough and lift it up quickly, without wiggling. Cut the biscuits close together to avoid having big pieces left over to be rerolled.

8. Place the biscuits 1/2 inch apart on a buttered, thick-bottomed cookie sheet. Bake for about 13 minutes, until golden. Let the biscuits rest for 3 to 4 minutes before serving.

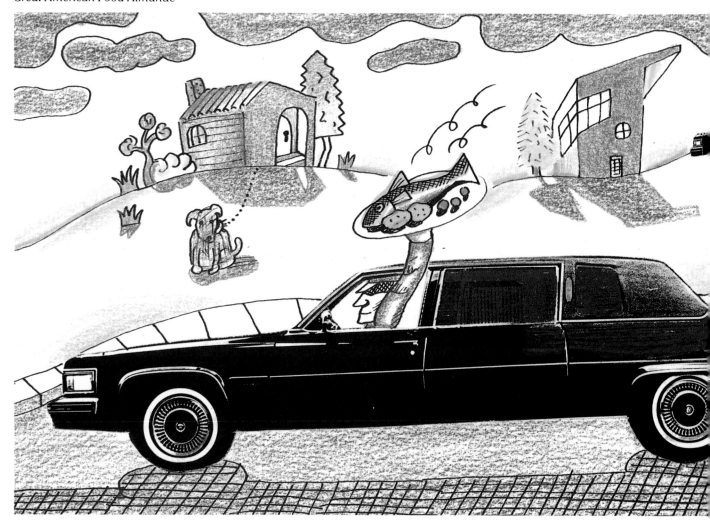

Eating Out While Eating In

Until recently, if you'd ordered 'dinner to go' at Michael Foley's posh Printer's Row restaurant in Chicago, you'd have been told "We're not in the take-out business." But before the year is much older, Foley's Printer's Row will be doing take-out, joining some of the nation's most expensive restaurants, the Quilted Giraffe in New York, The London Chop House in Detroit, L'Espalier in Boston, in what may be the most rapidly expanding area of the restaurant business.

Take out is nothing new. Messengers carrying bags of lunches to offices are part of the everyday scene in the nation's major cities. Fast food, with its pizza trucks and fried chicken wagons, is now a part of any urban and suburban scene.

What is new is that upscale restaurants are beginning to cater to clientele who can't or don't want to leave busy offices along with people who want to take home a little something for dinner. It is, of course, part of the lifestyle revolution brought about by two-career families whose members often may have more disposable income than time or ambition for cooking.

Ralph Brennan of the Brennan family of restaurants in New Orleans, has been testing a take-out menu for his Mr. B's restaurant, and hopes to put the concept into practice before the fall season. In Boston, Steve Elmont of Creative Gourmets has been experimenting with takeaway products to meet the needs of what he sees as "a market niche made up of people who want to trade up from deli sandwiches, but down from regular restaurant meals."

But while the pizza and fried chicken arrive in their sometimes limp cardboard or polystyrene containers, the posh new venturers in the prepared meal business are taking the high road with expensive packaging and custom delivery service.

The London Chop House, for instance, will dispatch its gourmet fare via stretch limousine. Take-out dinners arrive in foil-lined, insulated zippered boxes protected by colorful insulated shopping bags wearing the restaurant's logo.

New York trend

New York's Woods, famed for its new American cuisine, has two take-out units called Out of the Woods, adjoining its restaurants. Restaurant and takeaway stores share a kitchen. Owner Zeus Goldberg calls the added outlet "a way of maximizing operations without building more space."

Vienna Park, another of New York's poshest white tablecloth restaurants, has opened three shops under the Fledermaus marquee. The units feature many of the Vienna Park specialties and include tables along with machines to sell wines by the glass. Average checks at the Fledermaus run $5.50 to $7.50 against $40 and upward at Vienna Park.

Buffalo to go

Take out at The London Chop House in Detroit is an integral corner of the restaurant, offering every item on the menu, whether it be northern Michigan buffalo with morel mushrooms, frozen hazelnut soufflé, lobster bisque, tartar sauce or the chef's special salad dressing by the quart.

Lanie Pincus, who runs the restaurant with her husband Max, says they put in take

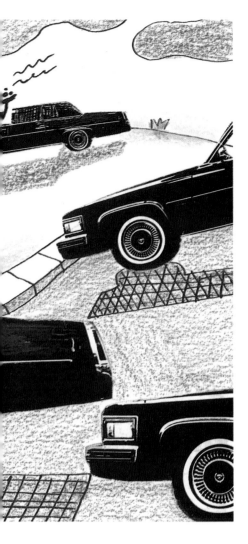

out for several reasons. "There were a lot of people who couldn't afford to eat at the restaurant. Now they can enjoy our food in their homes."

For Michael Foley in Chicago, his new retail shop "will allow us, as a small, fine dining restaurant, to get our product out there, and to make certain things we don't do any more, such as country pâtés. We're very well equipped, so that we want to create an apprenticeship program and build a good cooking base here at Printer's Row. Having a little shop next door will allow us to produce and sell dishes we wouldn't normally serve at the restaurant because they're not our style.

"The shop will have a more casual specialty menu, pasta, pâté and pastry and we'll also be able to sell our base work stocks, sauces and dressings that we can put up in packages. It's another way to add cash flow.

"But this type of shop must be set up for take out. You produce a higher volume off your walk-in take out that from your walk-in sitdown business. We will have 12 stools set up so that people will be able to come in for

espresso, cappuccino, a light simple meal, breakfast, lunch or early dinner, but we wouldn't be able to pay for the space with just sitdown customers."

Easy pickup

"Working couples want it quick and easy, something that they can have delivered or pick up on their way home at night." Ilene Sobel, proprietor of The Market of the Commissary in Philadelphia, says she's working on a major delivery program to service those needs. The Market is the newest link in the five restaurants founded by entrepreneur Steve Poses. It offers even more choice than its supply source, Poses' upscale cafeteria, The Commissary. The Market is located around a corner from The Commissary kitchens, but their back doors adjoin to facilitate delivery. Customers, as many as 1,000 a day, can choose from 12 salads and 10 entrees at The Market.

Take out is hardly limited to the big cities. La Camembert in Mill Valley, California, is a suburban restaurant whose traveling list covers the full gamut of the restaurant's specialized charcuterie menu. Chef-owner Steve Wilkinson of the Fine Bouche in Centerbrook, Connecticut, opened his combination patisserie and charcuterie shop several months before his restaurant was ready. "We took the idea from places we'd enjoyed in Europe after we saw a need for a small, quality-oriented food shop in this area. We felt we could attract customers to come in and browse, those who preferred to entertain at home and those whose budgets excluded dining in the restaurant.

"When we had tournedoes on the restaurant menu, we'd use their tips for Stroganoff or Beef Niçoise for the carryout. Duck breasts at dinner gave us duck legs for cassoulet or an oriental duck salad and the ham that we sell in the shop gave us bones for a rich split pea soup, a staple take-out item.

"Many of our customers are retirees or working people who enjoy good food but don't have the time or skill to make it themselves. We don't advertise, except for Christmas or Easter specials, and we do very well by word of mouth. We've also been helped by TV ads for convenience foods such as Lean Cuisine which has helped people to think beyond the TV dinner and pizza as their options for dining at home." ●

Mort Hochstein, food reporter, Market Watch

Hunger In America

On Memorial Day weekend of 1986, U.S.A. for Africa, which was so successful in raising funds for starving people in Africa, joined hands with Coca-Cola to organize Hands Across America in an effort to help hungry and homeless Americans. At 3 P.M. EST, 5½ to 6 million people joined hands for 15 minutes to bring the plight of the needy to the public's consciousness. The event, which began in New York City and ended in Long Beach, California, covered a distance of 4,000 miles, and raised about $35 million, with California leading in donations. The existence of hunger in one of the richest nations in the world shocked and shamed many people who had been unaware of the enormity of the problem until groups like Hands Across America brought it to light. Some hard facts:

- The poverty line for a family of four is $11,000 a year, which leaves about $2.50 a day with which to feed each family member.
- The number of Americans living in poverty jumped from 24.5 million in 1978 to 35.3 million in 1983. Almost 13 million of those have incomes of less than $5,500 a year.
- The poverty rate for children under six is 25 percent—far higher for black and Hispanic children, 51 percent of whom the government considers at "high risk" for poverty and hunger.
- According to the Department of Agriculture, in 1980, 21.1 million people received food stamps; for 1985, that figure was 19.9 million. Food stamp benefits have decreased from a maximum of about $63 per person per month in 1984 to $45.61 in 1986.
- According to a statement by the Physicians' Task Force on Hunger in America in April, 1986 "The problem of hunger in the U.S. is now more widespread and serious than at any time in the last 10 to 15 years. . . . Hunger in America is a national epidemic." ●

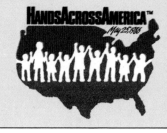

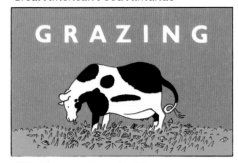

What's My Line? Egg Peeler

Barbara Dale-Avant, who works for Atlantic Food Inc.'s cooked-egg division, in Hemingway, South Carolina, holds the record for number of hard-boiled eggs peeled per minute, according to *The Wall Street Journal*. Her best total was 48, which means that she dawdled away exactly 1¼ seconds on each egg. And her boss, Wilbur Ivey, is not a man to tolerate bits of shell among the eggs, which are shipped to East Coast restaurants. To get these perfect results, he is willing to allow 3 seconds per egg, but that's only when peelers are first starting on the job.

"A real clumsy person couldn't do this," remarked one of Avant's fellow peelers, somewhat unnecessarily. Another confided that the members of the six-woman team (who together once peeled 10,000 eggs in an eight-hour shift) sometimes throw eggs at each other, recreationally, although Mr. Ivey does not entirely approve. On the other hand, he is clearly no spoilsport, as he is credited with devising the initiation rite for new egg-peelers: He slips a raw egg into a recruit's first batch.

A Smaller Bite In America currently, food eats up an average of 17 percent of total income, down from 19 percent in 1970.

Remember Fuzzy Peach Skins? Where Did They Go? To some extent the fuzz has been bred out of peaches by their growers, and additionally a de-fuzzing process is included in most fresh-peach packing operations these days.

They Probably Think The Moon Is Made Of Bleu Scientists at the Lawrence Livermore Laboratory named three of their recent nuclear-explosion tests after cheeses: "Cottage," "Camembert" and "Roquefort."

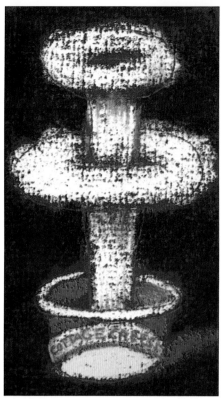

Another Man's Poi·son? Poi, a kind of puree made of fermented taro root, is a traditional Hawaiian delicacy whose popularity among natives often mystifies visiting mainlanders.

But Hawaiians are as particular about their poi as Bostonians are about their baked beans. Different types of taro are grown on each island, and the poi made from each differs in color and character. Molokaians, for example, favor poi made from reddish lehua taro, while Honolulu natives prefer poi from their own island.

Future Schlock Here are some new food products we can all look forward to: a taco shell filled with ice cream and topped with chocolate and peanuts, a butter substitute made from polyester, noodles shaped like the state of Texas, tofu baby food, tofu hot dogs, mesquite-flavored hot dogs, pizza-flavored hot dogs filled with cheese.

Just A Sliver For Me, Thanks, I'm Dieting As part of Texas's sesquicentennial celebration in 1986, Duncan Hines commissioned a cake, Texas-style—that is, very, very big. The cake contained 93,108 eggs, 2,425 gallons of water, 647 gallons of oil, and 31,026 boxes of (naturally) Duncan Hines yellow cake mix. It had three layers made up of 20,000 three-pound cakes, served 300,000, measured 80 by 110 feet, and weighed 90,000 pounds, including the icing. "This is one monster cake," declared Franz Eichenauer, cakemaster of the ceremony.

Moon Pies?

In the Northeast, where clams are abundant, one of the most popular (and toothsome) ways of preparing the tasty mollusks is in a clam pie.

It seems that every region from Maine to Long Island has its own variation, and the people of Chatham, on Cape Cod, are no exception. They feel that the key to making a truly great clam pie is to do it the night after a full moon. When the moon is full, residents head for the beach, where they dig up bushels of giant sea clams, which are about four times as big as the quahogs favored by most New Englanders.

To make the pie, minced fresh clam meat is first combined with milk, flour, seasonings and onions that have been sautéed with salt pork. The filling is then baked in a double-crust pie. Sometimes, vegetables or potatoes are added.

Hold The Escargots

When 502 teenagers were asked to describe their "fantasy meal" in a 1985 Gallup poll, the results were as follows:

The overwhelming favorite first course was salad (44 percent), with shrimp cocktail a distant second (15 percent). Caviar and escargots interested only two percent and one percent.

For a main course, it seems that red-blooded American teenagers like red meat. Forty-four percent named steak as their favorite entrée, with lobster coming in second (20 percent). Although we tend to think of teenagers as burger and pizza junkies, only two percent and one percent would choose those as their fantasy entrée.

Potatoes, baked or otherwise, were the number one choices for a side dish—with 25 percent choosing baked and 19 percent others.

Pie and cake tied for first place as the dessert of choice, but the big surprise was that chocolate mousse, the second choice, edged out ice cream by two percent.

As might be expected, carbonated soda was the favored beverage.

COOKING SCHOOLS

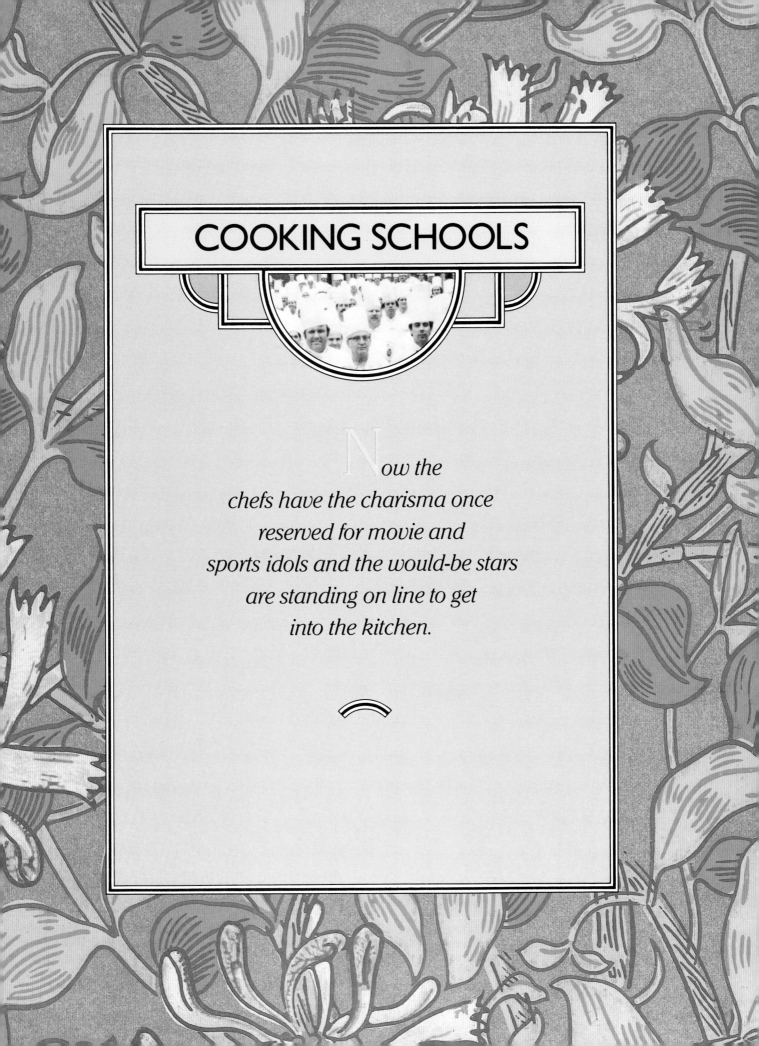

*N̲ow the
chefs have the charisma once
reserved for movie and
sports idols and the would-be stars
are standing on line to get
into the kitchen.*

THE OTHER CIA

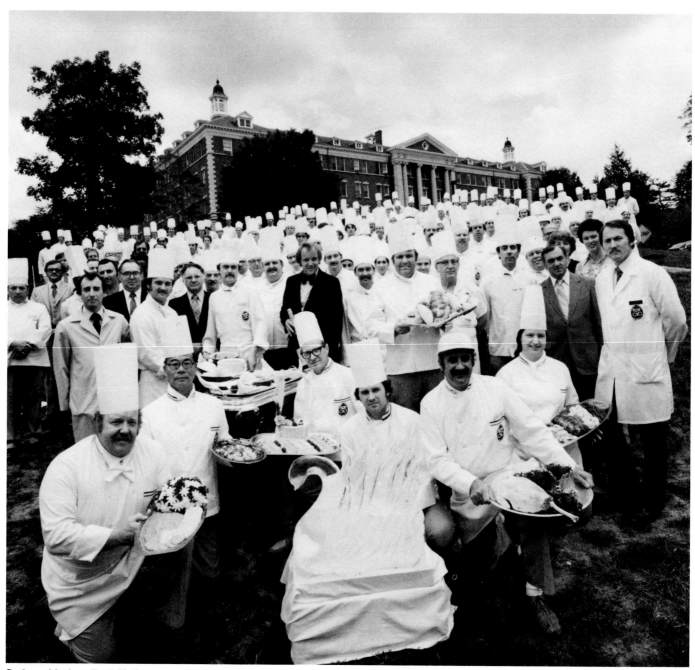

Gathered before Roth Hall, once a Jesuit seminary, faculty and staff of the Culinary Institute of America display their art

Is there a sight more truly splendid and up-lifting than that of a couple of hundred healthy, smiling American professionals, all decked out in dress uniform, in serried ranks assembled for their group picture on the steps of a venerable academic building? There they stand—bright, keenly alert, eager to serve their country, their white aprons as stiffly starched as nuns' wimples, their white toques worn at jaunty angles above bright eyes and gleaming teeth.

Aprons? Toques? Well, yes, chefs' toques, for this is the family of the Culinary Institute of

America, set upon the banks of the Hudson River at Hyde Park, New York, and 40 years old in 1986. This CIA, operating in the Victo-rian Gothic halls of what was once a Jesuit seminary, boasts 17,000 graduates dis-persed to fine restaurants, hotels, clubs and the like internationally. The current crop of 1,850 full-time students takes a two-year course in the fundamentals of cooking and baking, instructed by a faculty of some 90 chefs and other professionals in the food ser-vice industry. Graduates of the CIA do not smile *only* because they've had a happy time

on a pretty campus. They smile because they know that each of them has an average of five jobs to choose from, at home and abroad, upon graduation.

Their prospects today are a measure of the enormous growth in their field since the school's founding in 1946 as the New Haven Restaurant Institute, at New Haven, Con-necticut, "to raise the standards of food preparation and serving and to train veterans for vital roles in the restaurant industry." The school today is operationally self-supporting, with an annual budget of about $21 million.

More than 80 percent of the students receive some form of financial aid, and can be reasonably confident of being able to pay it back. Starting salaries are in the $20,000–$30,000 range, out there in the world of well-trained sous chefs. Nobody, not even possibly the *other* CIA, knows what master chefs can bring down annually, but the best-informed guesses come at $60,000–$75,000 annually, and then some. And as America eats out more and more, and demands more and more in terms of quality, bright neophytes—whether from the elite Culinary Institute or from the many other professional training schools around the country—can expect to find well-paid work and splendid prospects for advancement. Confirmation comes from the Bureau of Labor Statistics, which forecasts two million new jobs in the industry by 1995, an increase of 38 percent since 1982.

What must the student ante up to get in on this bonanza? The CIA offers a 21-month program for an Associate's degree at $12,198. Admissions office: (914) 452-9600. The Cornell University School of Hotel Administration, one of the grandfathers in its field, grants a BS degree upon completing four years of study in hotel and restaurant management for an annual tuition cost of $10,500. Call (607) 257-6376. Briefer programs are offered by many schools. The New York Restaurant School, for example, offers a 20-week course in cooking and management for $5,500. Call (212) 947-7097. And the California Culinary Academy has a 16-month program in cooking skills for $11,000. Call (415) 771-3536.

Food service is a hands-on industry, and a great many aspirants prefer to grow in the business by starting at the bottom and working up. This is what most current successful restaurateurs did in creating their careers, and nobody in the field will discourage young people from that old and rocky road. It is one of the last apprenticeships left in our society, and it works. But neither will anyone discourage professional education as it flowers now in a time of demand which, by all estimates, has not yet begun to peak.

Meanwhile, the people of America who eat say to the eager young people in their toques and aprons: Serve your country now, and please hurry up about it. We're hungry! ●

MARTIN JOHNER AND GARY GOLDBERG'S CHOCOLATE "FETTUCCINE" ALLA PANNA

The New York Culinary Center invents a new taste treat.

Serves 12

Ingredients:
Chocolate "fettuccine" (crepes):
6 eggs
1¹/₃ cups half-and-half or light cream
1¹/₃ cups water
¹/₄ cup sugar
¹/₄ teaspoon salt
6 tablespoons clarified butter, melted and cooled, plus additional for greasing the crepe pan
1³/₄ cups presifted flour
¹/₄ cup unsweetened Dutch-process cocoa

Chantilly cream:
2 cups heavy cream, well chilled
2 tablespoons confectioners' sugar
2 teaspoons vanilla extract

Dark chocolate sauce:
5 ounces semisweet chocolate, coarsely chopped
1 ounce unsweetened baking chocolate, coarsely chopped
¹/₄ cup sugar
¹/₂ cup brewed espresso coffee, hot
2 tablespoons almond-flavored liqueur
2 tablespoons unsalted butter

Method:
1. To make the crepes, put all the crepe ingredients in the container of a blender or food processor and process until smooth. Let the batter rest for at least 20 minutes, covered.
2. Brush a 6-inch crepe pan with a small amount of clarified butter. Heat the pan over moderately high heat until a drop of water sizzles on contact.
3. Pour ¹/₄ cup of the batter into the pan, swirl quickly to cover the pan bottom and return the excess to the bowl.
4. Cook on one side until the edges brown lightly. Flip and cook for 15 to 20 seconds. Turn out onto a plate. Repeat until all the batter has been used.
5. Let the crepes cool. Cover, if holding for later use, but do not refrigerate.
6. To make the chantilly cream, combine the ingredients in a chilled bowl and whip until soft peaks form. Cover and refrigerate.
7. To make the chocolate sauce, melt all the chocolate in the top section of a double boiler set over hot (but not boiling) water. Dissolve the sugar in the hot espresso, add to the melted chocolate and stir to blend. Add the liqueur and butter and blend well. Remove the sauce from the heat to stop further cooking. Warm the sauce in the double boiler just before serving.
8. To assemble: Cut each crepe into thin strands about ³/₈-inch wide with a very sharp knife. Separate the strands carefully, toss them gently with your fingers so that they resemble fettuccine noodles, and place them in a large, shallow serving bowl. Carefully form a well in the center of the "fettuccine" and spoon the chantilly cream into it. Using two wooden spoons, toss the "fettuccine" until it is coated with the cream.
9. Serve in individual bowls, ladling the warm chocolate sauce over each portion.

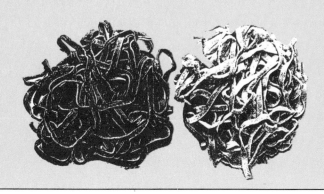

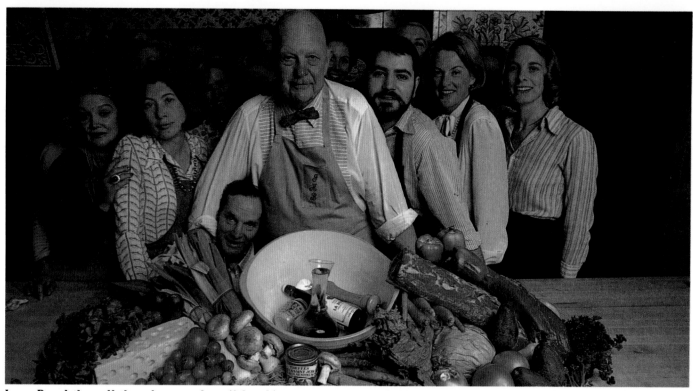

James Beard, the godfather of so many beautiful cooking events, led the field in training you and me in the culinary arts.

SEPARATE FIVE EGGS

About cooking schools, there's the story about a student embarked on learning the mysteries of the soufflé. "First, separate five eggs," the instructions begin. Obligingly, the student picks up two eggs and puts them at the far left of the counter, then picks up three more and puts them at the far right.

That is, at least, a start, but it calls urgently for instruction in basic fundamentals and certainly that is the place to begin with serious amateurs. But how this is done varies enormously: Cooking schools come in many forms, ranging from those that never suffer the student to touch the ingredients, to those that require the students to do all the separating, chopping and stirring. The reward, whichever the type of instruction, is the tasting of the food at the end of the class.

James Beard held what were purportedly among the very first modern cooking classes for the layperson, above Manhattan's famed Lutèce restaurant almost 30 years ago. When he first started teaching, there were only a handful of cooking schools in the country. Today there are some 800 of them registered with the International Association of Cooking Professionals, a society which Julia Child, appropriately enough, helped organize ten years ago. It was Julia Child's television cooking "classes" that taught two generations of Americans not only how to cook but how to have fun at it too.

The nature of cooking schools has changed. In the early days, most classes were held in the mornings and the majority of the students were housewives. Now even the *word* "housewife" seems quaintly old-fashioned. These days, many women are working and those who choose to stay at home are, for the most part, much too busy to be attending cooking school. Therefore, it is the evening classes that are drawing the crowds and these also include many more men who are taking up cooking as a hobby.

In general, the tone and style of the teaching is serious and emphatically practical. The courses are less focused on whole meals and menus than on how to prepare fresh ingredients quickly. It is a direct reflection, of course, of the changes in society which find very few people able to afford the leisure time to accomplish and present elaborate meals with multiple courses.

Today's schools range as hugely in quality as they do in type—from the one-woman-one-skillet sort of operation, (which is not, per se, wanting in quality, though fewer and fewer of these small schools survive every year), to the kind of outfit that has several classes going on simultaneously. Among the best of these large schools are L'Academie de Cuisine in Washington, Peter Kump's New York Cooking School and Tante Marie's, Mary Risley's school in San Francisco.

The touring stars of the schools circuit work very hard in making their rounds—Jacques Pepin for example is on the road for as much as 32 weeks of the year; Marcella Hazan and Giuliano Bugialli teach both here and in Italy. Others also attract students who like to see their favorite food in its natural setting: Diana Kennedy teaches at her permanent home in Mexico, Jane Butel holds week-long classes in the cooking of the Southwest in Santa Fe and also at a new kitchen in Woodstock, New York. Yet others follow their leaders across the globe.

Lydie Marshall, whose specialty is French cooking, and Elizabeth Andoh, the authority on Japanese cooking, both teach close to home in New York. Joanne Pruess does something no one else is doing—she holds classes in a grand kitchen at Kings supermarket in Short Hills, New Jersey. Arlene Feltman organizes cooking demonstrations by visiting celebrities at Macy's in New York and these have proven so popular that she is now taking the show on the road. The most magnificent setting for a cooking school, however, is the Mondavi Winery where the Great Chefs' series of classes is held.

While it seems that we are increasingly eating away from home or buying prepared meals to eat at home, it is, nevertheless, clear that the pleasure of cooking and entertaining at home is still an important part of many of our lives. As long as the interest is there the cooking schools will be there too, to teach the skills and techniques necessary to prepare fine food. ●

Domestic Cooking Schools

Alaska
A Moveable Feast
(907) 479-4375

Alabama
Bonnie Bailey Cooking School
(205) 967-7002

Creative Ideas For Living
(205) 877-6000

Market Place
(205) 534-1116

Southern Living Cooking School
(205) 877-6576

Arizona
Look Whose Cookin'
(602) 835-4676

California
Badia a Coltibuono
(415) 346-0890

California Culinary Academy
(415) 771-3536

Cantonese Gourmet Cooking School
(415) 221-5804

Chateau de Saussignac
(415) 939-5974

Cooking with Susan Rhoades
(415) 283-1207

Epicurean
(213) 855-7000

Great Chefs—Robert Mondavi Winery
(707) 963-9611

Inner Gourmet Cooking School
(818) 441-2075

Judith Ets-Hokin Culinary Company
(415) 668-3191

Kanora Kitchen Crete
(415) 928-8786

Le Cordon Rouge
(415) 331-3663

Le Kookery Cooking School
(818) 995-0568

Let's Get Cookin'
(818) 991-3940

Ma Cuisine
(213) 655-3880

Menus Cooking School
(415) 574-7788

Microwave Cooking Center
(818) 987-1701

Mission Gourmet Cooking School
(415) 657-8062

Mon Cheri Cooking School and Caterers
(408) 736-0892

Montana Mercantile
(213) 451-1418

Phyllis Ann Marshall Cooking School
(714) 646-3206

Piret's Perfect Pan School of Cooking
(619) 576-3805

Specialty Cuisine Workshops
(916) 587-2048

Tante Marie's Cooking School
(415) 788-6699

The Tasting Spoon
(213) 250-3919

Unique French Cuisine
(619) 438-7777

Colorado
Broadmoor Cooking School
(803) 632-6810

Les Chefs D'Aspen
(303) 925-6217

Connecticut
The Ann Howard Cookery
(203) 678-9486

The Complete Kitchen
(203) 655-4055

The Happy Cookers
(203) 242-9322

Hay Day's Cooking School
(203) 227-4258

The Silo Cooking School
(203) 355-0300

District of Columbia
Kitchen Bazaar
(202) 355-0300

Delaware
Creative Cooking—The Cooking School
(302) 475-0390

Florida
Bobbi & Carole's Cooking School
(305) 667-5957

Cuisine Classics Cooking School
(813) 349-7626

Lively Kitchen Inc.
(813) 792-0487

Mary Starnes' Cooking School
(904) 837-2832

Pot N' Pan Tree Cooking School
(305) 586-4410

Someone's in the Kitchen with Mimi
(904) 733-3024

Sue Sutker's Creative Cookery
(813) 877-8625

Georgia
Chef!
(409) 956-9368

The Cloister Wine and Cooking School
(800) 732-4752

Cook's Corner, Inc.
(404) 231-1872

Peggy Foreman's Cooking School
(404) 876-7845

Ursula's Cooking School
(404) 876-7463

Illinois
Charie's Kitchen
(312) 446-4066

Chez Madelaine
(312) 325-4177

The Cooking and Hospitality Institute of Chicago
(312) 944-0882

Cooking in France
(312) 246-5845

Gourmet's Oxford
(312) 246-5845

La Cucina Italiana
(312) 328-4443

La Venture
(312) 679-8845

Oriental Food Market and Cooking School
(312) 274-2826

Proper Pan
(309) 692-6382

Quincy Steamboat Company
(217) 222-2351

What's Cooking
(312) 986-1595

Indiana
Country Kitchen School
(219) 484-1893

The Eight Mice Cooking School
(317) 447-5255

Louisiana
Betty Lyons—Food and Table Consultant
(504) 486-2658

Cooking Inc.
(504) 626-1824

Lee Barnes Cooking School and Gourmet Shop
(504) 866-0246

Tout de Suite a la Microwave Inc.
(318) 984-2903

Wok & Whisk Inc.
(504) 769-5122

Massachusetts
Creative Cuisine—Cambridge School of Culinary Arts
(617) 354-3836/354-3888

Peggy Glass
(617) 964-8171

Maryland
L'Academie de Cuisine
(301) 986-9490

L'Ecole/Baltimore International Culinary Arts Institute
(301) 752-4710

Maine
Creative Cooking
(207) 772-6606

Michigan
Mid-West Cooking School
(313) 585-9550

Minnesota
Byerly's School of Culinary Arts
(612) 929-2492

Thrice
(612) 228-1333

Missouri
Dierbergs School of Cooking
(314) 532-8884

Halls Plaza Cooking School
(816) 274-8200

The Pampered Pantry
(314) 727-5088

Mississippi
The Everyday Gourmet Inc.
(601) 362-0723

Nebraska
Lincoln Cooking Company
(402) 488-6514/483-6106

Nevada
Truffles
(702) 329-6995

New Jersey
Annie's Kitchen
(201) 756-9328

Cooking at the Kitchen Shop
(201) 836-0833

Cooktique
(201) 568-7990

Carole Walter/Food and Baking Professional
(201) 325-0119

The Cooking Studio
(201) 575-3320

The Uncomplicated Gourmet Inc.
(201) 666-8070

New York
A La Bonne Cocotte
(212) 675-7736

Carol's Cuisine, Inc.
(718) 979-5600

The Chocolate Gallery
(212) 582-3510

Cordon Rose
(212) 475-8856

Culinary Center of New York
(212) 255-4141

De Gustibus at Macy's
(212) 534-2178

The French Culinary Institute
(212) 807-0936

International Pastry Arts Center
(914) 666-2325

Karen Lee's Chinese Cooking Classes and Catering
(212) 787-2227

The Kings Chocolate House
(718) 848-8564

Kitchen Privileges Culinary Center
(516) 466-4884

New York Cooking Center
(212) 947-7097

Peter Kump's New York Cooking School
(212) 410-4601

Sunrise Cuisine
(718) 273-3187

The Wire Whisk Cooking Center
(516) 757-5050

North Carolina
Cooks Corner Ltd.
(919) 272-2665

The Kitchen Cupboard
(919) 756-1310

The Saucepan
(919) 763-6430

The Stocked Pot & Company
(919) 722-3663

Ohio
American Chef Institute
(614) 224-9503

La Belle Pomme
(614) 463-2665

Lazarus Creative Kitchen
(513) 369-7556

Zona Spray Cooking School
(216) 650-1665/656-2665

Oklahoma
Creative Cookery
(405) 840-1716

Gourmet Gadgetre Ltd.
(405) 248-1837

The McCartneys Kitchen
(405) 722-7770

Oregon
Cloudtree & Sun
(503) 666-8495

Cook's Nook
(503) 484-5725

Hot Pots Cooking School
(503) 764-2000

Pennsylvania
Charlotte Ann Albertson Cooking School
(215) 649-9290

Cook's Nook Cooking School
(412) 946-3120

The Garden
(215) 546-4455

Jacqualin Et Cie
(215) 794-7316

Kay's School Of Cookery
(412) 683-2500

Kitchen Kreations
(717) 697-0501

The Kitchen Shoppe Cooking School
(717) 243-0906

continued on page 232

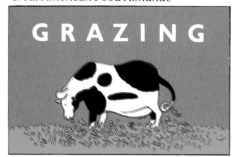

GRAZING

Non-Poetic License

Last year, the state of Wisconsin decided to redesign its license plates. Reflecting the state's primacy in dairy farming, many of the more than 46,000 entries proposed continuing the slogan, "America's Dairyland," which has identified the state's plates since 1979.

Others carried the theme a bit further, suggesting tags shaped like cows or milk cans, and there was even one—which didn't make it into the final rounds of judging—for a tag shaped like a slice of Swiss cheese with the slogan, "State of Udder Beauty." But the snappiest entry of all was submitted by none other than Governor Anthony S. Earl. The governor was inspired, no doubt, by New Hampshire's inspirationally patriotic slogan ("Live Free or Die"), and concerned, perhaps, by falling consumption of dairy products. His slogan? "Eat Cheese or Die."

Please Chew Your Food Carefully Santa Monica restaurateur Michael McCarty notes that the cost of restaurant insurance has risen 300 percent in the last year. No wonder the check has increased too.

It Came From The Sea On the third Thursday in August, the town of Beaufort, North Carolina holds its annual Strange Seafood Exhibition.

The start of the two-hour long event is heralded by the sound of a whelk shell, blown by no less than the director of the North Carolina Maritime Museum.

The strange seafood includes periwinkles, mullet roe, dog clams, triggerfish, stingrays, pinfish, coquina clams, eel, sea urchin roe, and other even more odd denizens of the deep. They are prepared by local volunteer cooks in over 40 ways.

Getting Our Priorities In Order
"Who would have thought that anybody would ask $25 for a pint of sorbet? They never would have done that with plain old sherbet."

Maggie Waldron, public relations executive. *Food Watch*

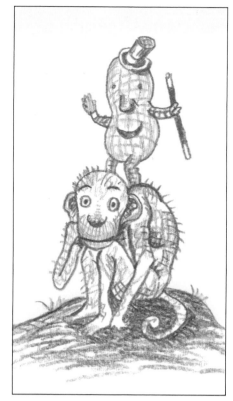

I Could Really Go For A Nice Dried Beef And Cream Cheese Pinwheel Right About Now When Gallup polled 1,509 Americans about which finger foods they would be interested in eating (and, we hasten to add, gave the respondents a list of nine from which to choose), baked potato skins with sour cream and scallions generated the best response (39 percent). Raw vegetables with blue cheese dip (30 percent) was closely followed by (who dreams up these dishes, anyway?) dried beef and cream cheese pinwheels (29 percent). At the bottom of the list were deep-fried zucchini and cauliflower with tarragon sauce and deep-fried chicken wings with barbecue sauce.

Finding The Best Deal For an extra $85 a day, Cedars Sinai Hospital in Los Angeles will not only serve you a luxury menu; it will also call your favorite restaurant to duplicate the chef's recipes and send its cooks to your home to instruct *your* cooks. "We have the best patient occupancy rate of any nonpublic hospital," says Ron Weiss, Director of Food Services.

Midwest prices are more reasonable. A seven-course gourmet dinner is $20 at St. Joseph's in Fort Wayne, Indiana. "We like to believe some people come here because of the food," says Paul Marki, food service director.

And at Mount Sinai Hospital in Minneapolis, a mere $4 extra will get you wild-rice soup, skewered marinated vegetables, Chateaubriand and a glass of wine. Guests can join for $12.

Peanutrivia

Quiz: If four monkeys eat four sacks of peanuts in three minutes, how many monkeys will eat 100 sacks in one hour? (Answer below.)

• The inventor of peanut butter was a St. Louis physician who ground up peanuts in 1890 to serve as a nutritious and easily digested food for his elderly patients. Sadly, this hero's name has been lost in the mists of time despite efforts by peanut researchers to unearth it and honor him by name.

• Over two *billion* pounds of peanuts are produced—and consumed—by Americans annually, half of which becomes peanut butter while the other half gets divided almost evenly between the salted kind and that which goes into candy.

• Enough peanut butter to cover the entire floor of the Grand Canyon is consumed annually by Americans.

• It takes 540 peanuts to make a jar of peanut butter.

• By the time he or she finishes high school, the average American schoolchild will have eaten 1,500 peanut-butter-and-jelly sandwiches.

• Adult consumption of peanut butter is mainly at breakfast, on either toast or an English muffin.

• Nearly half of all confectionary products sold in the U.S. contain peanuts.

• Botanist George Washington Carver discovered more than 300 uses for peanuts, including shampoo and shoe polish.

Joke: Why did the elephant quit the circus? Because he didn't want to work for peanuts.

Answer to quiz question: Five.

Another Great Leap Forward Milk can now be purchased in a pouch, which if dropped on the floor will—bounce.

Not To Be Sneezed At One single ounce of black pepper is enough to season 1,440 fried eggs—but that doesn't stop us from consuming 75.9 *million pounds* of the stuff annually in this country. Sales of hot spices in general are exploding, with red pepper spices up 61 percent over a decade ago, black and white pepper both up 34 percent and dried ginger up 39 percent.

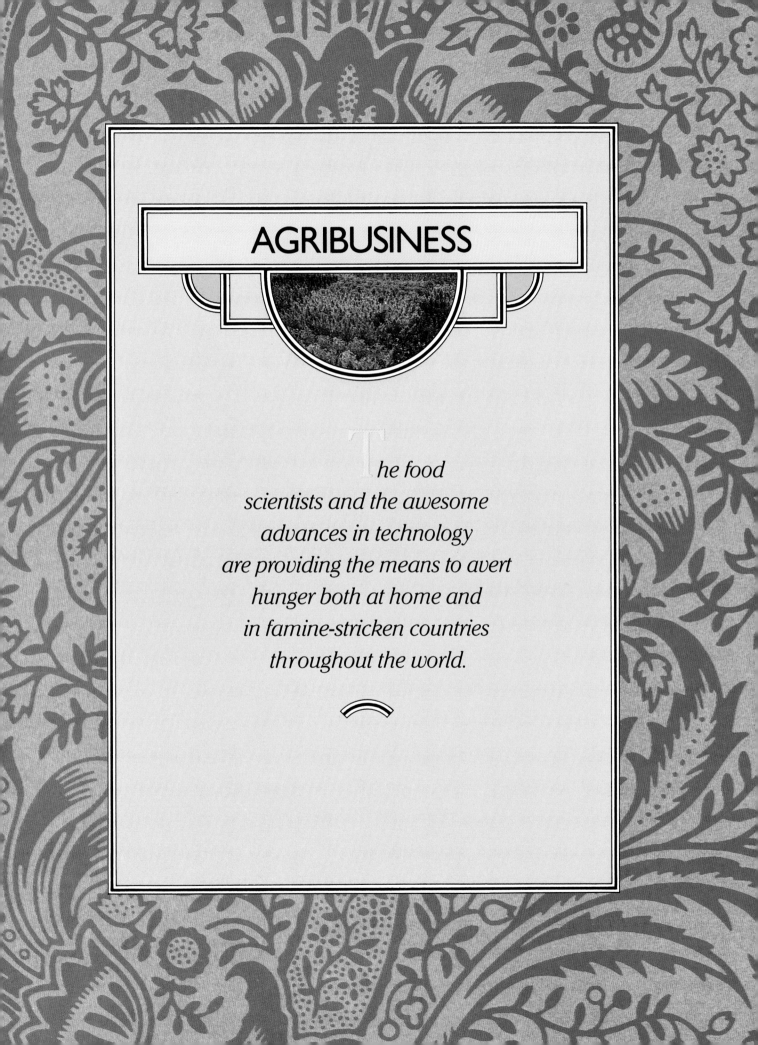

AGRIBUSINESS

The food
scientists and the awesome
advances in technology
are providing the means to avert
hunger both at home and
in famine-stricken countries
throughout the world.

AGRIBUSINESS

Oh, to live on a farm, where the work is honest, the land is good and life is simple and rewarding. We like to imagine ourselves as men and women of the soil, but this vision lies far from the truth. Only 2.5 percent of the population lives on farms, and a small minority of those farms are family-run. The twentieth century has spawned a remarkable change in the way food is grown, a second agricultural revolution of sorts. Today, food production is agribusiness, not agriculture, and it's high-tech business at that.

Witness some of the changes that have come to the process of growing food just in the last two decades: New methods of irrigation have turned marginal land, even deserts, into flourishing oases. Intensive breeding has produced such wonders as the square tomato that can be picked mechanically without bruising and other breeds that can ripen even in the chilly autumn of northern states. "Supercows" have been bred to churn out as much as 30,000 pounds of milk a year, compared to an average of 13,000 pounds for a normal cow. The ova, or eggs from just one of these milk machines can be extracted from the ovaries, fertilized *in vitro* (in a test tube or dish), and implanted into a dozen other heifers, each of whom will give birth to one more supercalf. There's

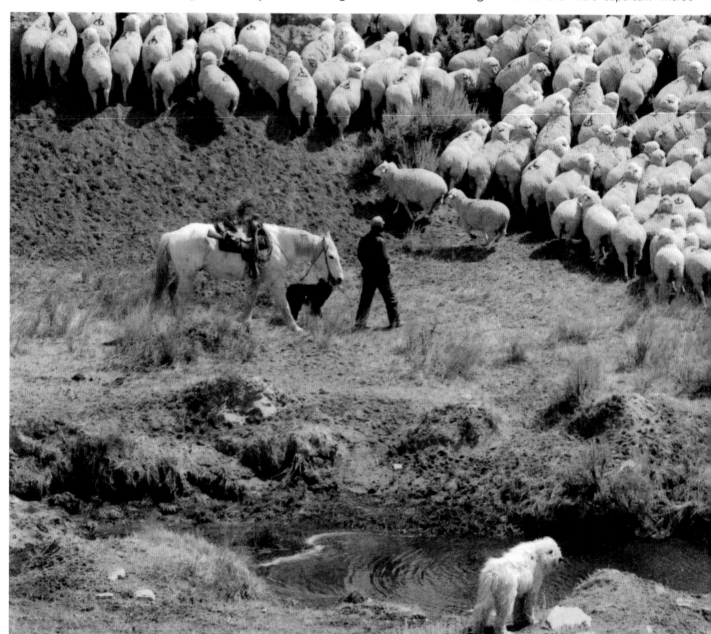

It may be "agribusiness" these days, but many basics endure: the watchful sheep dog, the herdsman riding, not a Ford, but a faithful Scout.

even a low-fat breed of cow, now, in Texas.

Genetic engineers have become so adept at manipulating bits of DNA in crops that they can introduce the genes that code for resistance to some diseases into the seeds of highly productive, but unresistant strains. Farmers are experimenting with crops that are new to us, like quinoa, a delicious grain high in protein that has been grown by Indians of the Andes for centuries. We can even

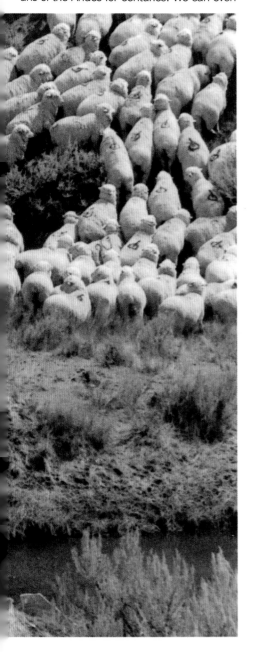

grow plants in water.

The aim of such agronomic marvels was to bring prosperity to farmers, and to satisfy the American dream that our fruited plains could feed the hungry people of the world. And so they have, but with a terrible vengeance. American farmers are now drowning in the wealth of their own productivity.

A combination of a worldwide glut of farm commodities, a strong U.S. dollar, and the collapse of the federal government's byzantine farm subsidy program threatens the well-being of more farms than did the Great Depression. Huge quantities—some 10.4 billion pounds—of milk products bought by the federal government from dairy farmers sit unused in vast underground caverns in Minnesota in cold storage, while 4 to 6 billion bushels of wheat, corn, barley, oats and soybeans lie unsalable in silos around the nation. Retail food prices are rising at the slowest rate in nearly two decades, and far below the general inflation rate, while agricultural commodity prices fell 20 percent in 1985.

Good news or bad news?
That may sound like good news to the consumer, but it means finding a new job to hundreds of farmers. Banks are likely to foreclose on seven percent of U.S. farms in 1986, most of them with annual incomes of $40,000 to $500,000. Even California, which offers up $14 billion annually for some 250 crops, is feeling the squeeze. The wide diversity of specialty crops, such as avocados, almonds and grapes, which long protected the state from slumps when one or two commodities were hit, are now contributing to the problem. Such specialty crops are subject to wide price fluctuations, and, as one California economist remarked, the world doesn't exactly need almonds to survive.

But according to some experts, a far worse crisis than economic woe looms. Farming, as most farmers now practice it, they say, threatens both the farmers' livelihood and the nation because it is ethically, environmentally and ecologically destructive. "Conventional agriculture wastes land and it wastes people," says author Wendell Berry.

Strong words, but a look around the countryside confirms that agriculture is no longer the pure, wholesome practice it once was. Farming's deep dependence on chemical

fertilizers and pesticides is bankrupting farmers while poisoning groundwater and affecting the health of farm workers. For example, in California's San Joaquin Valley, one of the most bountiful cornucopias in the nation, polluted agricultural runoff has caused gross and twisted mutations in birds living in Kesterson Wildlife Refuge. Plowing and irrigation practices send 6 billion tons of irreplaceable topsoil washing into the oceans every year. Feeding livestock low doses of antibiotics, a technique that farmers, and particularly the drug companies, tout widely as a means of increasing production, is creating strains of "super bacteria" that are beginning to infect people.

Once more, to the barricades!
To some experts, like plant geneticist Wes Jackson and horticulturist Booker T. Whatley, it's high time for the third agricultural revolution. Jackson heads the Land Institute, a privately funded research farm along the Smoky Hill River near Salina, Kansas, while Whatley teaches at the Tuskegee Institute, in Montgomery, Alabama. In their minds, the farm of the future will work with nature instead of battling it.

Farmers will practice polyculture; they'll grow a strange, variegated mixture of crops, combining fruits and vegetables and honey on a Whatley farm. Or, at the Land Institute, the Maximilian sunflower, whose roots make a natural herbicide, will grow with giant wild rye, a Siberian perennial. Gone will be the heavy dustings of pesticides and fertilizers. According to the Rodale Research Center, another private institution, farmers could already start switching to "regenerative" (what most of us would call organic) farming methods, using no herbicides and manure instead of inorganic fertilizers, and enjoy net returns 10 to 25 percent higher than with conventional techniques within three years.

One result of this third agricultural revolution will be a completely new array of foods offered up on market shelves. Already, Americans are regularly eating such homegrown exotica as kiwi, lychees, carambolas, wing-beans and soybeans. But even more important than providing a tempting new variety of foods, agriculture of the future will assure that our richly fruited plains and amber waves of grain will continue to feed this nation, and maybe even the world. ●

HIGH TECH IN THE BARNYARD

"Hello, Ethiopia—you say you need more milk for your hungry children. Tell you what we're going to do. We're going to send you a Holstein-Friesian cow, a daughter of Fernhame Ned Oceana of Hadley, Mass. 'Ned' produces 23,000 pounds of milk a year—rich in butter fat. Give this daughter a shot of ovulating hormone—she'll produce a lot of ova. Then give her a dose of prize bull semen—that could cost $250—flush out the fertilized eggs and transplant them into 15 or so of your ordinary cows. In nine months you will have a dozen or so calves that will become supercows. And soon you will have more milk than vats to hold it—as we do."

The message to Ethiopia may be invented, but Fernhame Ned Oceana is for real. So is the embryo transplant technique used on her. Ned's owner has turned down offers of more than $100,000 from breeders anxious to get her awesome milk-producing reproductive apparatus.

We take you now to Manitowoc, Wisconsin, where dairyman Jon Matthias has 42 Ned-type supercows in the 23,000-pound-a-year class. He picked 28 of them and flushed them for fertile embryos; 226 of these were top-grade and, when transplanted into mongrel cows, resulted in 207 pregnancies. Matthias expects 250 calves from his 42 cows in just one year. He sells some of his pregnant cows here and abroad for handsome prices—and to keep his barn walls from bulging.

Recently, veterinarians found that they could freeze embryos in nitrogen and ship them anywhere in the world—ready to thaw and implant into native cows. This method is both better and cheaper than shipping pregnant cows, because the native mother and her implanted calf will be immune to native diseases which might fell a Wisconsin cow.

Now—are you ready for this? Timothy Williams, a scientist in cowboy garb at Colorado State University takes a fertile cow embryo and slices it in half with a micro-manipulator, so that the recipient mother will deliver twins—two supercalves for the price of one. Some bold experimenters abroad have even sliced embryos into four parts, and had successful implants in three out of four of the foster mothers.

The technique of embryo transplants also holds great promise elsewhere in the barnyard—as against the old-fashioned one-on-one "natural" method. Already the embryo transplant business in the U.S. grosses $25 million a year, and as it expands from cattle to include goats, sheep and swine, forecasts are that it will become a billion-dollar-a-year business by 1993. Inducing twinning in ewes, using the same embryo-slicing technique used on cows, could well be, for example, the salvation of shepherds of the U.S. Our per capita consumption of lamb chops and mutton is remarkably low, attributable, we can assume, to the high cost of rearing the woolly flocks. If the productivity of ewes can be doubled, we're told, costs would drop and consumption would soar.

Recent work with a bovine-growth hormone, another highly effective form of genetic engineering, is promising. This hormone, derived from the pituitary glands of cows and then cloned, can boost milk production by as much as 40 percent. One day a medium-sized dairy farm may consist of only a dozen super-supercows.

Not content to tinker only with animal hormones, researchers are now experimenting with a combination of animal and human hormones. In a laboratory at the University of Pennsylvania, microbiologist Myrna Trumbauer, working with a projection microscope, manipulates a hollow needle to pierce a mouse ovum and inject human growth hormone. The ovum came from an ordinary mouse, fertilized by an ordinary male mouse, but a certain percentage of the litter will grow to be supermice—twice the size of their litter-mates. Mice are preferred in the laboratory because of their fast gestation and maturation, but the next step is obviously the barnyard. The process is one form of gene-splicing and supersheep, supercattle, perhaps superchickens all loom on the horizon. One species that may be the last to be tinkered with, however, is the pig: over the centuries, pig farmers have bred the largest strains of pigs by selective breeding—mating the largest porkers with the largest sows until today's pigs are possibly the maximum obtainable size—but don't bet on it.

Recently, breeders have learned how to examine fertilized ova to determine what sex they will become. This is important to dairymen: A bull on a dairy farm is a third leg—just another mouth to feed—while beef ranchers prefer males. Male ova can be sorted out by the dairy breeders and female ova can be discarded by the ranchers.

It all sounds a bit like playing God, but so far there have been no reprisals from On High. ●

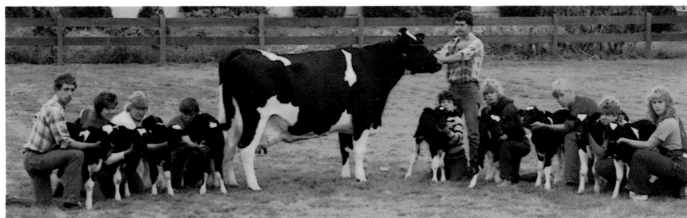

Thanks to recent advances in bovine genetic engineering, these cute little calves will—in only a few months' time—become supercows.

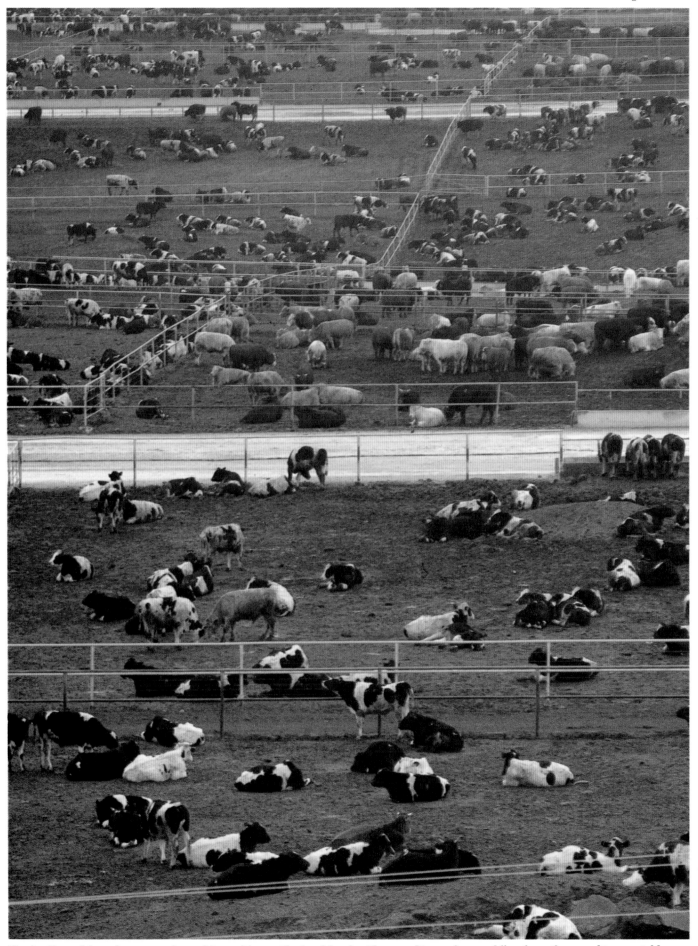

The feedlots of America are restless with nutrition on the hoof, beef cattle reared to run lean and firm from the corral to your table.

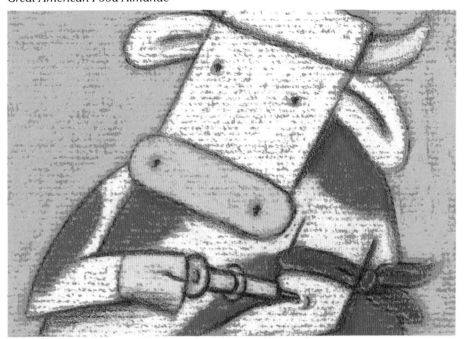

Wonder Drugs And Meat

In 1949, Dr. Thomas Jukes, then head of nutrition and physiology at a division of American Cyanamid Corporation, made a discovery that changed dramatically the process of raising meat. Jukes and his colleagues fed young chickens feed that happened to contain low levels of the then newly discovered antibiotic tetracycline. To their astonishment, the chicks began gaining weight at rates 10 to 20 percent above normal.

Everybody's doing it

Since then, feeding animals antibiotics has become common. Drug industry and agricultural spokesmen claim the drugs not only speed weight gain, but also allow more animals to be cultivated in less space. Growers routinely feed their animals levels too small to do much more than provide a few ounces of prevention. But all those little doses add up to a lot of medicine: Livestock consume 40 percent of the antibiotic production, an estimated $250 million worth a year.

The effects are not all beneficial. Increasing numbers of scientists have been charging that doctoring animal feed is creating strains of drug-resistant bacteria, "super-bugs" that can infect people, and make attempts to cure them with standard antibiotics much more difficult.

Naturally, the drug industry is lobbying hard against any efforts to curb the dosing of animals. In 1974, the European Common Market banned tetracycline in animal feed; but when the U.S. Food and Drug Administration tried to follow suit, the agency was blocked by congress. The FDA's failure was due, in part, to intense lobbying, and also to

a lack of direct evidence that drug-laced feed can be blamed for drug-resistant bacteria. The drug industry's major claim is that superbugs are cultivated more by physicians being too free with prescriptions for antibiotics than by the puny doses given to animals.

That particular line of defense has recently broken down. Health officials from the Center for Disease Control in Atlanta tracked down what they believe is an indisputable link between more than a dozen cases of food poisoning and drug-resistant salmonella bacteria in meat. In 1983, 18 people in four midwestern states came down with acute food poisoning. All of them required hospitalization, and one died. Every one of them got the bacteria from meat.

Sifting the evidence

The CDC's medical sleuths concluded, ironically, that 12 of the 18 people became ill when they began taking antibiotics for other illnesses. Drug-resistant salmonella in the meat didn't make them sick immediately. Instead, the bacteria remained, undetected, in their intestines. Other species of bacteria, which normally inhabit the human gut without ill effects, competed with the salmonella for nutrients and kept the virulent bugs in check—until victims began taking antibiotics. The drugs killed the beneficial bacteria, leaving the salmonella to flourish.

The clincher for the case came when the CDC discovered that ten of the victims had eaten hamburger meat bought at eight different grocery stores, but which originated in a single feedlot. That feedlot routinely dosed its cattle with antibiotics. ●

FRANK PERDUE'S TWENTY-FOUR CARAT GOLD-PLATED CHICKEN

We all secretly knew that the tough man dined at home like an emperor—no plastic forks for him either.

Serves 4

Ingredients:
3–3 1/2 pounds Perdue lower-fat chicken
1/3 cup finely chopped shallots
1/2 cup finely chopped fresh parsley
2 tablespoons olive oil
2 teaspoons fresh lemon juice
1/4 teaspoon dried thyme
Salt and freshly ground pepper
1 book gold leaf (twenty-five 3 1/2-inch sheets, see note)

Method:
1. Preheat the oven to 350 degrees.
2. Rinse the chicken and dry well with paper towels.
3. Combine the shallots, parsley, oil, lemon juice and thyme in a small bowl. Season to taste with salt and pepper.
4. Loosen the chicken's breast and leg skin by gently inserting your finger through the thin membrane between the skin and the flesh.
5. Stuff 1/2 cup of the herb mixture in an even layer under the loosened skin. Brush the remainder inside the body cavity and spread a thin layer over the wings and back.
6. Truss the chicken and place it on a rack in a roasting pan. Open the book of gold leaf and press one page at a time onto the skin, overlapping the sheets, until the entire bird is covered.
7. Roast the chicken for 20 minutes per pound, turning to brown it evenly, and basting every 15-20 minutes with the pan juices. The chicken is done when the juices run clear yellow when the thigh is pierced with a fork.

Note: Gold leaf is completely edible, and may be purchased at bookbinders' supply houses. (If finances are tight, this chicken is very good without the gold leaf.)

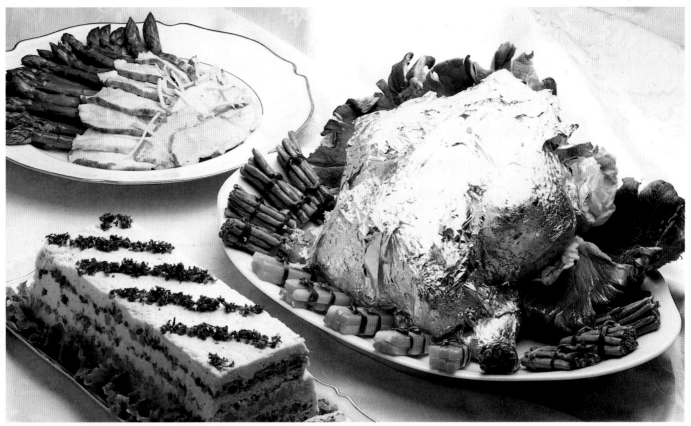

Like chicken *and* gold? Baste your bird in 25 sheets of edible good leaf.

Fat City: Or How To Convince The Public To Pay More For Less

For the past 50 years, farmers and ranchers have been doing their best to fill our demand for tender, juicy beef, plump, rich chicken and succulent pork. Breeders culled their herds and flocks with care to select only their prime animals, the ones that put on the pounds, and marbled all that nice flavorful fat into the meat.

Now, suddenly, we want to be healthy. No more greasily delicious barbecued ribs; so much for bacon every morning. Per capita meat consumption has plummeted and meat growers are hurting. What are all those ranchers to do?

Talk a thin line, for one thing. In January 1986, Holly Farms and Perdue Farms, the leading chicken marketers in the U.S., introduced "low-fat" chicken. Gone are the days when they boast their fowl are the plumpest and juiciest. Now we have Frank Perdue himself, that scion of the chicken ranchers, appearing on television to state that he hates pudgy poultry. "Fat legs and chubby thighs," says he, "really turn me off."

Just how svelte and low-fat are these fryers, anyway? They're actually the same old chickens you've always bought, but with the "leaf" or abdominal fat removed for you. "It's more a matter of convenience," says a spokesman for Holly Farms. "We're just getting rid of the fat. People don't like to pull it out." It would seem that Holly and Perdue, who between them represent one quarter of the $4.4 billion fresh chicken industry, are waging their marketing wars on the newest battleground of fat. And for this, you get to pay an additional 10 to 15 cents a pound.

Beef growers can't be far behind in the wooing of the newly health-conscious public. The National Cattlemen's Association has begun an ad campaign to convince consumers that beef and pork really aren't all that high in fat—honest. But in reality there are only two ways to reduce the fat in meat: change feeding practices, or change breeds. In cattle production, for example, the industry standard is a cross between the glossy black, cantankerous Angus and the more tractable brown and white Hereford. The resultant piebald hybrids are grazed on the open range, anywhere from six months to a year and then shipped off to feedlots for fattening. There, they are fed a rich diet of grain before slaughtering and some feedlots increase weight-gain even more by injecting the cattle with hormones.

Now, an obvious means of cutting down on fat content is to quit feeding cattle grain, a method that feedlot operators are reluctant to employ, since it would cut sharply into their profits. The other way to reduce calories is to develop new breeds of cattle that, pound for pound, put on proportionally more muscle than fat.

That's exactly the kind of steer a group of Texas ranchers is starting to breed. Called a Braler, it's a cross between the Saler, a breed originally imported from France, and the feisty Texas Brahman. The meat of the Braler has been declared by the USDA to be 58 percent lower in fat than that of an Angus-Hereford.

Although you probably won't see Braler steaks on meat counters for a couple of years, leaner beef is already out there, usually bearing the label "lite," "leaner" or "lower fat," which means it's 25 percent less fatty than other products in the same category. Lean beef enthusiasts say it's actually more flavorful, if somewhat tougher, than the fatty stuff. Not convinced, one health-conscious, beef-loving New Yorker tried a taste test between identical cuts of USDA Choice and "leaner" beef. To her disappointment, the healthy stuff was "bohhring," and twice the price, besides. Once again, the American consumer gets to pay more for less. ●

YESTERDAY'S SEEDS FOR TOMORROW

One of the many complaints the Third World has against the U.S. is our refusal to sign an international concordat to form a central bank for the sharing of seeds, rootstocks and genetic plant tissue—an agreement already signed by 140 nations. Our refusal is a complex issue involving both the right of U.S. companies to protect their breeds under patent laws, and concern that politics, in the future, might control scientists' access to the new international seed bank (in contrast to an existing, much smaller storage system, largely backed by the U.S., open to all).

Regardless of what the resolution of this issue should be, the key words today are Hybridization, Genetic Engineering and Agribusiness. When the Pilgrims arrived here there were no indigenous crops to speak of; the Indians' maize and beans had been traded up from Central and South America. All other crop seeds and roots since then came from Third World regions of Africa, Asia and South America. In this century, we began to develop hybrid seeds from the straight strains, achieving high-yield crops that made us the world's breadbasket. The main hitch is that hybrid seeds—unlike the straight strains—can't reproduce themselves, and must be bought every year from Uncle Sam's seedmen—at their price.

Illusion in Our World

Along with the development of hybrid seeds came a shrinkage in the variety of the crops we grow. Out of 20,000 edible plants, most of the food we grow comes from only 20 species: wheat, rice, corn and potatoes alone provide the bulk of the world's food intake.

Isn't that risky? The entire U.S. corn crop is based on only four strains: Each ear of corn is a brother or cousin of the ear next door. A blight could wipe out a quarter to a half of our total crop. Many of us would call that living dangerously.

The citrus canker bacteria plague of 1984–85, during which Florida growers had to burn millions of trees, is another example: Modern varieties of orange and grapefruit have no resistance to the infection, nor can the bacteria be controlled by any known pesticide. Food scientists must look to China and South America for the immune ancestral varieties—if they can still find them.

Enter the new buzz-words of the 1980s: Genetic Engineering and Gene-splicing.

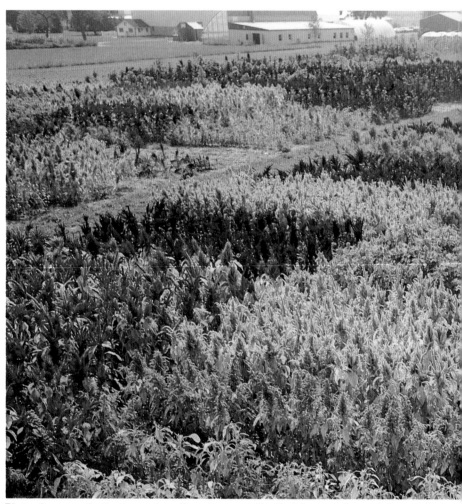

Plots of amaranth plants create agile patterns at the Rodale experimental farm, where

Multi-national giants—Shell, Arco, Monsanto, Ciba-Geigy, Pfizer—are now deeply committed to the $7 billion seed business, and their vast research facilities dote on the gene-splicing challenge. Aside from the scent of big profits, some of their work may well turn out to be *pro bono publico*. For example, if you can splice in resistance to pests, fungi or blights, you may eliminate some toxic chemicals from our farms and save some lives among farm-workers. But unlike the medical profession, which rushes to print with every tad of its research findings, agribusiness research and the fruits thereof are strictly proprietary—and profitable.

Nutrition from the Third World

Another, still largely untapped route toward maximizing food volume, lies in greater use of some Third World foodstuffs that have the potential for better nutrition. Yes, we glommed onto the soybean—unknown to us a generation and a half ago—and now it is our third largest crop. But what about the many other underutilized species that once fed millions? Many have higher protein and amino acid content than our prized wheat, corn and rice, but were ignored in our drive for machine-cultivation—not that they couldn't be re-engineered for a tractor-oriented economy. Several species spring to mind: bambera ground-nut, marama bean, winged bean, tepary bean, moth bean, quinoa and amaranth.

The latter two are worth a fresh look. Quinoa (pronounced keen-wa) is a grain grown by the Indians of the Andes and it contains up to 20 percent protein—about

Listening To Plants Grow

For a while, rumor has been abroad in the land that plants thrive when we talk to them. Recently, the tables have been turned and now the plants are talking to us. Scientists are employing magnetic resonance scanners similar to those used for diagnosing disease in people, to pick up faint radio signals emitted by plant atoms when they are in an intense magnetic field. The signals are translated into computer images enabling researchers to watch roots carrying water and to see seeds germinating. Their knowledge will give genetic engineers an inside view of how plants grow and provide an early warning system to detect potential trouble as disease processes appear in the root system before showing up in the leaves of the plant.

All this high-tech plant research is not as far out as it may first appear. The more knowledge there is, the more the seed technology can advance. Seeds can be engineered with built-in fertilizers and insecticides that will be appropriate to many different growing conditions.

There will be 12 billion new mouths to feed in the next decade so the greater the yield from each plant, the less danger there will be of catastrophic famines. Already the genetic engineers are developing seeds that will grow in sandy, arid soil and can survive when irrigated with salt water. ●

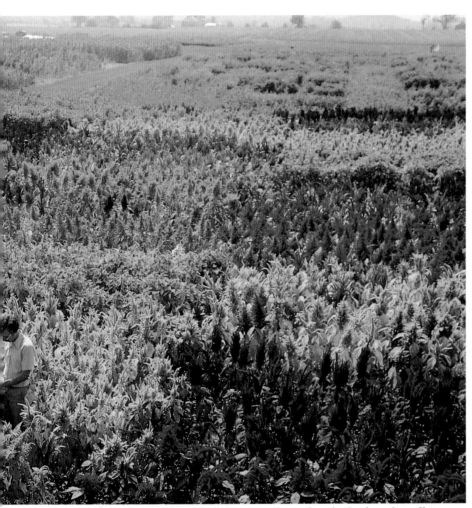

researchers work to give this Latin American wonder a place in the American diet.

twice that of most grains—and the essential amino acids lacking in our major cereal crops. It is said to "look like canary feed, is cooked like rice and has a squash-like taste with nutty overtones." It's a high-fiber food with no cholesterol and can be used as a meat substitute.

The New World had it first

Then there is amaranth, also from south of the border. Before Christopher C. arrived, it was a basic food in the New World. Thousands of acres of Aztec and Inca farmland grew this grain and 20,000 tons of it were sent annually as tribute to Montezuma's palace in what is now Mexico City. Aztec women ground the seed, mixed it with honey or (horrors!) human blood and patted it into the shapes of snakes, birds, deer and gods to be eaten during ceremonies at the Aztec temples. This so unnerved the Spanish Conquistadors that they banned the rituals—and amaranth—so this valuable grain faded into obscurity. Some is still grown, however, in Mexico, Guatemala, Peru and Bolivia.

Enter Rodale, the food and environmental wizards of Emmaus, Pennsylvania. They knew that amaranth had a protein content far higher than wheat, corn and rice and of a higher quality, with twice the lysine of wheat. It can be used as a breakfast cereal, or cooked or milled into flour. It lacks gluten and thus must be blended with wheat flour to make baked goods "rise." When heated, the grains pop and taste like nutty-flavored popcorn. Rodale has re-engineered it for machine cultivation, and is growing fields of it in Emmaus. ●

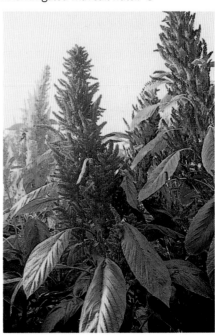

Amaranth: more than a pretty face

WATER BABIES

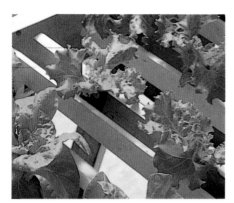

Every cook's dream: grit-free lettuce

Hydroponics—a very new and formidable word in the English language—does not refer to the nine-headed monster slain by Hercules. Neither is it a disease or a means of lifting sea planes into the air. Rather, it is an ingenious method for raising crops in flowing water, without a speck of dirt or soil anywhere and at many times the rate of productivity currently possible in conventional farming.

The new word, a marriage of the Greek "hydor" (water) and the Latin "pons" (bridge) means what it says. The farmer secures his baby plants in long metal troughs and sends a steady stream of nutrient-enriched water flowing around the tiny roots. Plants are so pleased with this nursery care that they grow, in their literal water-bridges, at an astonishing rate. One farmer in Salisbury, Connecticut is now producing 20,000 heads of lettuce by this method every week, all 12 months of the year.

The Salisbury hydroponics enterprise, aptly named AgrowNautics, Inc., was started in the late 70s by a refugee from Wall Street, G. Graham Davidson, Jr., who had a vacation home in Lakeville, Connecticut. He became disturbed by the fact that most of the produce available in New England came from far-off states and arrived wilted and not very nutritious. Puttering around in a rented greenhouse, he found that with plastic troughs, water, chemical nutrients and fluorescent lamps he could grow lettuce, spinach, tomatoes and cucumbers—without getting dirt under his fingernails and without bending over. His findings lured in some venture capital and today his crops, in clear see-through bags labeled Lakeville Lettuce, can be found in supermarkets and restaurant kitchens within a 50-mile radius of Salisbury.

More or less simultaneously, big food companies were studying dirtless farming, which by now was being called "controlled environment agriculture." The ideal environment, after all, does consist of light, temperature, humidity, carbon dioxide, growing media, water, nutrients and space. The ideal one-square-inch space required for a seedling must be expanded, automatically if possible, to 20 square inches at the end of its 22-day maturity cycle.

Such challenges would of course intrigue food scientists. Sure enough, after two years of study, General Mills leaped into the nutrient-laced waters of hydroponics. In De Kalb, Illinois, near the Chicago and Milwaukee markets, the food giant equipped a two-story 200-by-250-foot building with all the controlled environment gear needed to grow spinach, bibb, Boston and leaf lettuce year-round. They calculate that the output of that building equals the yield of 100 acres of land in the West or Midwest—independent of such factors as rain or shine, heat-wave or blizzard. And with no dirt, no bugs, no fungi, no chemicals.

Growing leaf vegetables is one thing; getting them to market looking freshly picked and with all nutrients intact is another. So General Mills devised a packaging technique using polyethylene bags into which the lettuce is dropped with its roots intact, inflated and heat-sealed so that the humidity inside the bag remains constant for three to six weeks in the supermarket—regardless of how the produce manager handles or mishandles it.

Such creativity in the corporate world did not go unnoticed: The General Mills package—patented under the name "Pillow Puff"—won the Institute of Food Technologists Award "in recognition of an outstanding food process . . . a significant advance in the application of food technology to food production."

As one might expect, other big corporations sniffed the air and grabbed for a piece of the $650 million-a-year salad greens market and other hydroponic profit centers. One hears names like Whittaker Corporation, Control Data, Pepperidge Farms and General Electric, wheeling and dealing for slices of the hydroponic pie—some successfully and some not. Weyerhaeuser, the West Coast lumber baron, entered the hydroponic produce field in Rapidan, Virginia with a seven-acre plant, complete with computerized technology, to grow lettuce for the Washington, Baltimore and Richmond markets, and, the company says, tomatoes, cucumbers and other specialty vegetables are soon to come on line.

Descending from such corporate heights to cottage-industry levels, we hear some heartening stories:

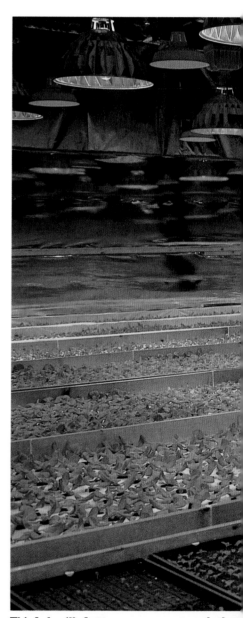

This Lakeville Lettuce panorama upends the

¶ Amid the burned-out buildings and rubble-strewn lots of the South Bronx, Gary Waldron, a former controller at IBM, grows herbs hydroponically and sells them to the top restaurants in the New York area, and, via air express, to restaurants across the country, who claim that nowhere else can they get such variety and freshness. (See overleaf)

¶ In Bridgeport, Connecticut, immigrants from Afghanistan, Laos and Cambodia are being trained to run solar-heated hydroponic greenhouses, built by the city on land donated by General Electric to grow strawberries, tomatoes, cucumbers and basil year-round, for the area's restaurants and supermarkets. One foodstore chain has agreed to take their entire tomato output.

¶ Across the East River from Manhattan, in Queens, a one-acre project called Aqua Farms uses waste heat from a power plant, plus hydroponic greenhouses, to grow tomatoes, lettuce and cucumbers that can be in the stores as fast as the traffic lights on Second Avenue will allow. The half-acre lettuce patch can produce a million heads a year; the tomato plants form a huge waist-level field; cucumber vines reach ten feet to the roof.

Where is this liquefication of the vegetable kingdom likely to take us? Will Frank Perdue develop a ducken? Will cattle be fattened in cornmeal-laced swamps? Will soggy cereals become the rage? Stay tuned . . . ●

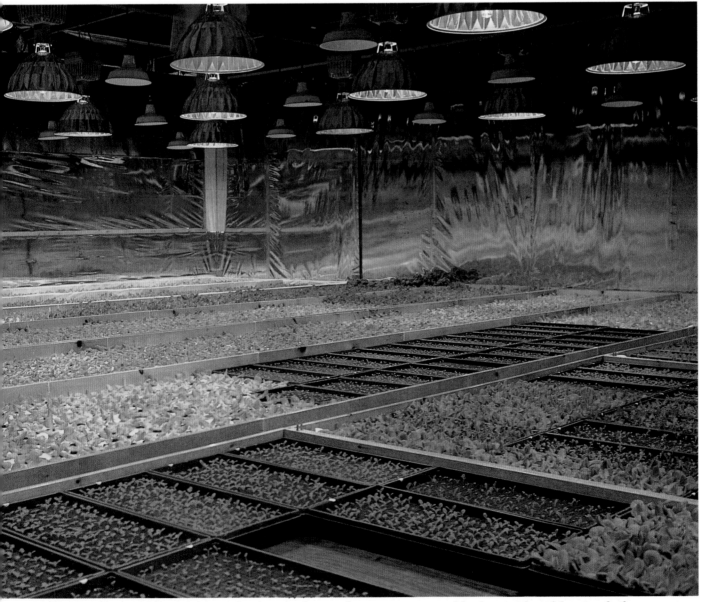

conventional garden: wall-to-wall lettuce, spinach, cucumbers and tomatoes, roots soaking in a nutrient-rich watery bath.

Who Is The Most Successful Farmer In The South Bronx?

Gary Waldron, a 43-year-old former IBM executive, built a glass house that became a $1.5 million business in the most unlikely spot in the world—the South Bronx, a neighborhood that you know well from pictures of the ruins of London after the war.

One day in 1980 he stood in a devastated empty rubbish heap between two crumbling, abandoned, derelict buildings and viewed what was to become his pasture: an empty concrete lot filled with bulging garbage bags and strewn with slashed tires and empty-mouthed, crushed washing machines mourning on one side.

He put two thoughts together. Here is a location 15 minutes away from the heart of one of the world's greatest cities, New York, and here too is a towering problem: an army of unemployed and unemployable, uneducated youth that loiters idly with nothing to do and few hopes for the future.

High inspiration

The solution was obvious from the start. He would grow mushrooms to supply the huge potential market and to do this he would turn the idle youths into horticulturists. What's more, he'd make them stockholders in his company.

How could such a dream turn into reality for a young man who had, himself, grown up in the South Bronx?

The son of a steelworker, Gary Waldron managed to escape the squalor of the area. Trained as an accountant, he made the leap into the buttoned-down business world. He became a controller at IBM, a company that has been derisively described by some as the world's largest Boy Scout troop. But it is this quality that is in some ways also its greatest strength. IBM, like many large conglomerates, has developed a social conscience, taking up where the old robber barons and railroad royalty left off. IBM encourages its executives to take a year's leave of absence, on full pay, to nurture noble causes. Gary's cause was passed upon as being noble.

And so his vision blossomed. Finding staff was no problem. In addition to the unemployed youths, their aunts and uncles were looking for work too, and they found it with Gary Waldron.

They cleared the lot and built a greenhouse—a craziness that can only make you gasp at the audacity and the folly. Gary and his helpers built the glass house and took turns guarding it when they were not being paid to work. On Sundays they brought the whole family to see what they were up to. The babies came in strollers. The little kids came and so did the big ones. The grandparents beamed. The turnover of staff and the absentee rate was phenomenally low—much lower than in the corporate world across the river.

After a year Waldron returned to IBM, but only for six days. He quit, because, as he later explained, "At IBM I was an invisible man in a big company. Security wasn't as important to me as a challenge."

A dive to the bottom

He took a $40,000 drop in salary, threw off his three-piece suit, rolled up his sleeves and went back to work in the Bronx. His superiors at IBM may have viewed his decision as a leap into lunacy, but his wife supported him—a bit grudgingly at first but eventually enthusiastically. She got herself a job and his three kids cut out all the luxuries and didn't complain—at least not too loudly.

The first corporate office of Gary Waldron's Glie Farms was a "bombed-out" building. He suggested to the absentee landlord the means of getting his hands on a sizable tax break if the building was turned over to the city. The landlord leapt at the chance. Gary quickly got some small grants and loans to fix up the building—enough to keep the rain off the papers and the telephone.

But by 1982, after only two years, he was close to being finished—washed up on the rocks that had inspired him.

No one said it would be easy.

It wasn't.

At that time a new possibility occurred to him: In addition to selling mushrooms, he began to sell herbs in small pots to garden centers. It was cheaper to grow fresh herbs than mushrooms—but there wasn't enough money in it. Not enough to survive. "I had 20 employees," he recalls and, "I had to lay off all but three." The telling of those hard times, familiar to all who have ever tried to start a small business, still causes pain. He fiddles with his cuff. Looks away.

It was then that he hit on the idea of going to the restaurants with the herbs. There are plenty of fresh mushrooms around, but he was the only one with fresh herbs.

He began knocking on the delivery doors of a few restaurants in Greenwich Village. Astonished, he discovered that he and his tiny staff could sell every leaf of fresh basil, thyme, rosemary and oregano that he could supply. The laid-off staff returned.

Green grows the Bronx

Today, Glie Farms has 70 full-time employees. The original greenhouse has grown into 14,000 square feet of lush cultivation—and a center of technological innovation. The "farm" has attracted new businesses to the Bronx and now thrives in a newly erected industrial park financed by the Port Authority of New York. It doesn't look like a farm. From the outside there is nothing to see but a vast, windowless building surrounded by slate-gray, packed-down earth and a chain-link fence, surmounted by multiple strands of barbed wire. At a glance, it could be a power station or perhaps a small prison. It isn't in an area where you would even think of taking a leisurely stroll.

But it is thriving.

Many, though not all of the 28 varieties of Glie Farms herbs are grown hydroponically. This is a process in which the plants are installed in long metal gutters and fed by a constant computer-controlled flow of nutrient-enriched water.

And Gary is now experimenting with new seed varieties in plants around the world. In the Puerto Rican plant, he employs a Mennonite farmer from Pennsylvania, a childhood friend from the days when the Fresh Air Fund made it possible for him to escape, in the summertime, from the very place to which he has returned.

Gary Waldron's son Mike has pinned a sign that he made himself inside his father's office door. "My dad's #1," it reads in a broad hand, "From his #1 son, Mike."

Gary Waldron is a nice man, a funny, quiet, honest, gentle man. He is something of a genius too. ●

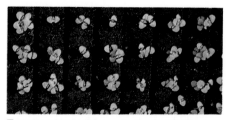

Fragrant herbs bloom in the South Bronx.

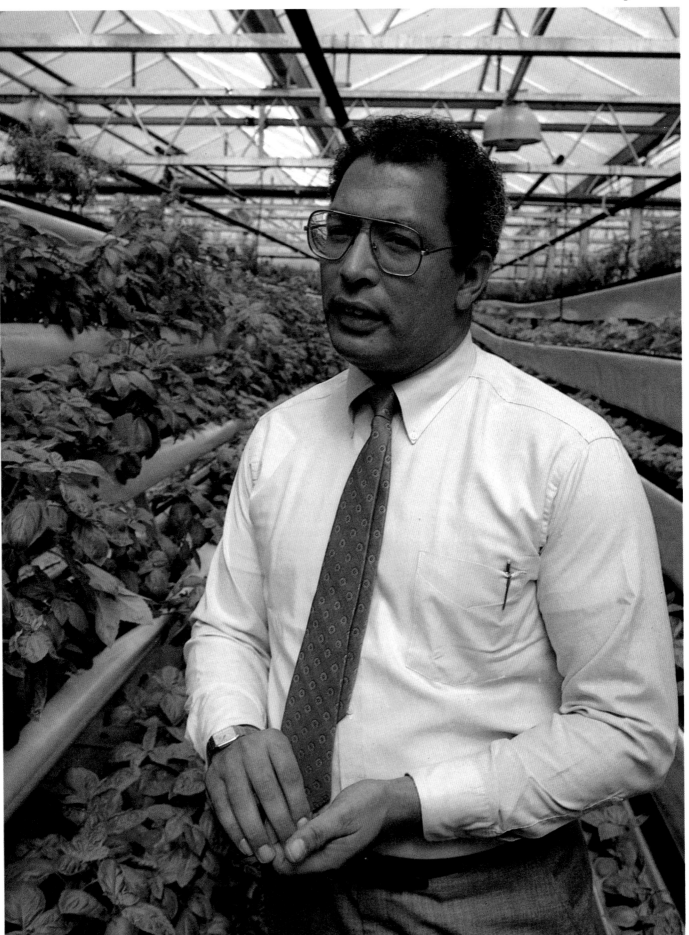

Gary Waldron, voluntary IBM exile, sniffs the sweet smell of success in the 14,000 square feet of Glie Farms herbs.

EXOTIC FRUITS AND VEGETABLES

If You'll Eat It, We'll Grow It

The English, who enjoy a joke on themselves, quip about their culinary arts: "England has three vegetables, two of which are Brussels sprouts"—and as Calvin Trillin says "cooked as long as Parliament remains in session."

We Americans, in the past, have had similar restraints on our choice of fresh fruits and vegetables at the supermarket: peas, beans, broccoli, carrots, cucumbers, potatoes, cabbage, peppers, spinach, turnips, citrus, bananas and some seasonal fruits. But now, especially if we live in southern Florida or California, the picture is changing: Scores of fruits and vegetables with strange names and shapes and delicious flavors are being spread out before us. What's happening?

Credit the kids

Immigrants are happening. Waves of them continue to arrive, from Southeast Asia, from Africa and India, from Cuba, the Caribbean and Central America. We can almost hear the children of the earlier arrivals saying: "Mamma, how come you cooked so well back home and here your cooking is so blah?" So Papa sent home for seeds and soon Mamma was cooking good food again.

Air freight is playing a part too. Importing perishables from Chile, New Zealand, Central America and other far-off places no longer presents problems, although in some cases there are U.S. Department of Agriculture and Environmental Protection Agency problems about their importation—bugs, fungi, pesticides and that sort of grief. However, the main explosion in exotic fruits and vegetables here is due to the skilled farmers among the hundreds of thousands of immigrants who have come to our shores. They, and some native Floridian and Californian agronomists are determined to get many of the 3,000 tropical fruits and vegetables into commercial production here.

In southern Florida, growers are actually tearing out citrus groves and putting in jakfruit, longan, carambola, lychee, atemoya and mamey. One part-time farmer has a single mamey tree (mamey is the Cuban national fruit) that yields a thousand dollars per harvest; high fences and fierce attack dogs are factored into the selling price of the yield.

Dr. Noel Vietmeyer, an eminent food scientist, was recently taken to a South Miami market: Xtra Super Food Center. His eyes and mind boggled. "Here," he said, "is the produce of the world"—red, yellow, white, green and speckled, long, thin, round, flat, bumpy, smooth, rough and fuzzy—piled high on counter after counter. This one market sells more than 400 different kinds of fresh fruits and vegetables a year.

One of the reasons for this explosion is demographics: While the U.S. population has grown 17 percent since 1970, the Hispanic population increased 87 percent and the Asian 127 percent. U.S. growers read such statistics and moved quickly.

By any other name

This boom is not, however, entirely without precedent. Back in the 30s, some growers speculated that the alligator pear might have a future. An ugly duckling, tough-skinned and unlike any pear we'd ever seen, it wasn't easy to sell at first. But when people got inside it and tasted it, its popularity grew. Changing its name to avocado didn't hurt either. A generation or so ago bananas and pineapples were considered exotic specialty items.

Or, take kiwi. This brown, fuzzy fruit was first successfully bred in New Zealand in the 60s after a difficult gestation. It's loaded with vitamin C and ships easily, so it began to trickle into the health-conscious U.S. Earlier it was called Ichang gooseberry or Yangtze berry, reflecting its Asian origin, until an American importer suggested a name-change. A New Zealand farmer came up with "kiwi," after the island's famed flightless bird. This kiwi took off: The island exported 50,000 tons in the last recorded year. California growers are rapidly taking over kiwi production, now that we realize it is not just a small suede potato.

As with the Yangtze-Ichang gooseberry metamorphosed into "kiwi," we can expect some nomenclature revisions when our Florida and California grower-magicians get together with Madison Avenue marketing magicians. Middle America is not notably Latino-oriented, or even Orient-oriented, and the fact that many of these exotic goodies are often ugly roots or strange-looking doesn't help. But there are exceptions: Snow peas sound comfortable to and on the Amer-

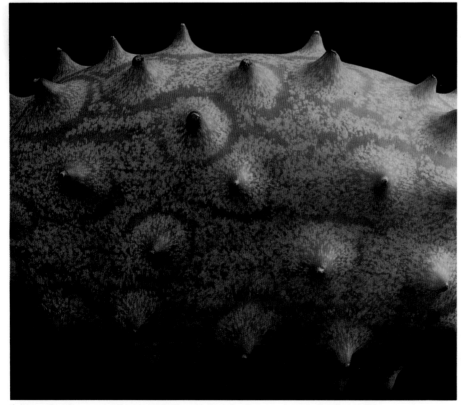

A lunar landscape to the eye, the horned melon's taste is out of this world.

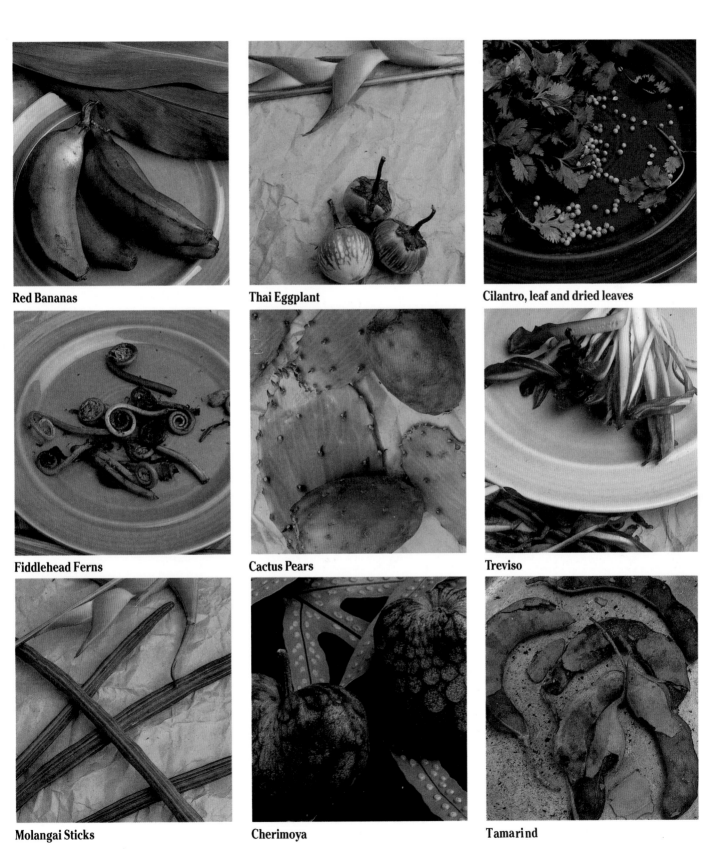

Red Bananas

Thai Eggplant

Cilantro, leaf and dried leaves

Fiddlehead Ferns

Cactus Pears

Treviso

Molangai Sticks

Cherimoya

Tamarind

ican tongue, so they come in from Guatemala and Honduras in plane loads of 50,000–60,000 pounds a week. And winged beans, those nine-inch protein-rich pods originally from the Philippines and now a big crop in Florida, that can be steamed, stir-fried or eaten raw with a dip, have no language barrier either.

By whatever name, some great taste sensations are moving into your supermarkets.

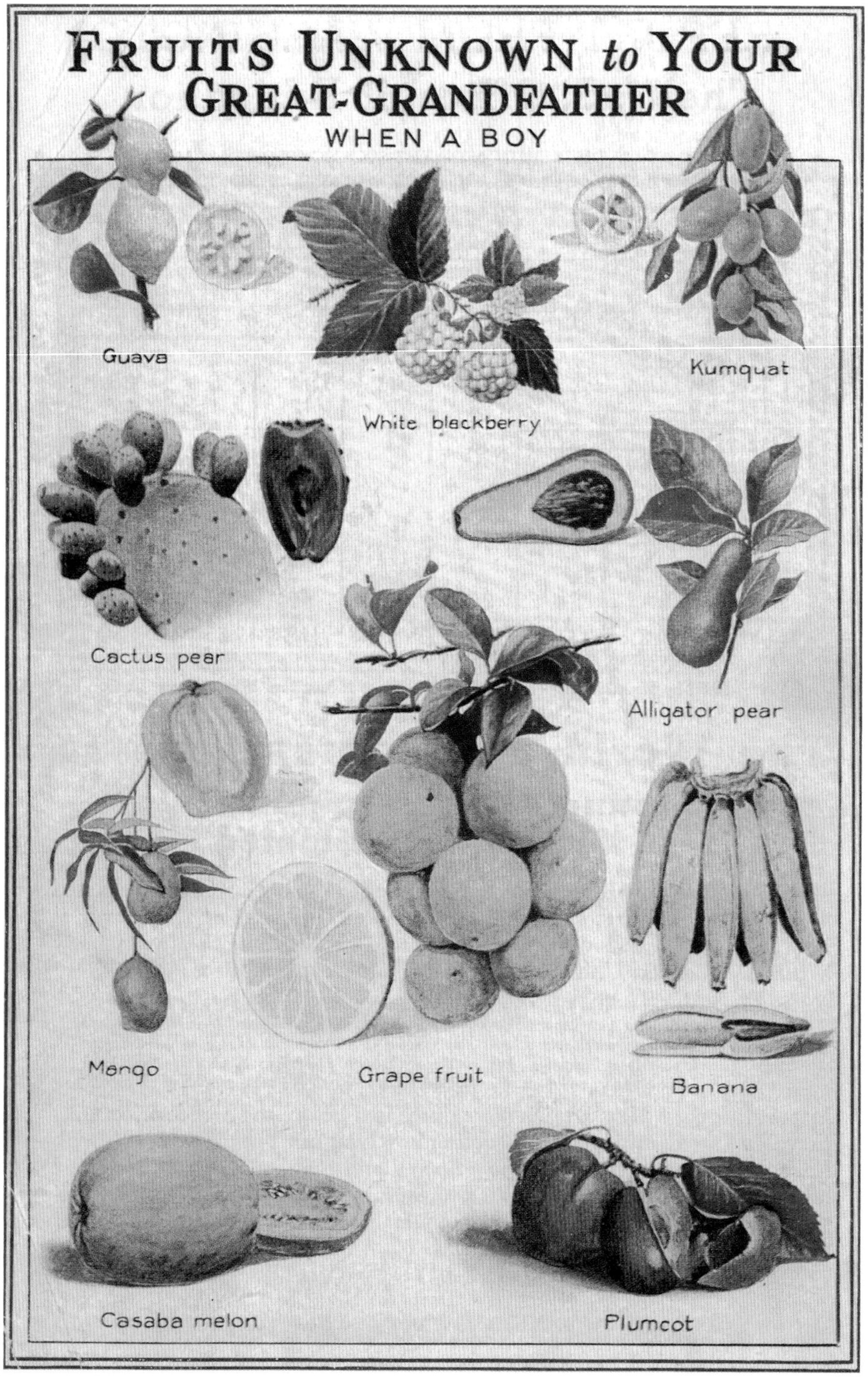

FRUITS UNKNOWN *to* YOUR GREAT-GRANDFATHER
WHEN A BOY

Guava
White blackberry
Kumquat
Cactus pear
Alligator pear
Mango
Grape fruit
Banana
Casaba melon
Plumcot

A Mini-Sampling Of Exotic Foods

Atemoya/Sugar Apple
From South America, now Florida. Banana-pineapple custard-flavored dessert fruit.

Carambola/Star Fruit
From Malaysia, now Florida. Used in salads, jellies, desserts.

Ceriman
From tropical America. Eaten raw or in ice-cream, milkshakes.

Cherimoya/Custard Apple
From Peru, now Southern California. Flavor of pineapple, banana, strawberry, papaya.

Jakfruit
From Southeast Asia. A huge tree-fruit (up to 60 pounds) with a unique musky flavor. Eaten cooked or raw; seeds are boiled like chestnuts.

Jicama
From Mexico. An ugly root, but sweet and crunchy as an apple.

Kiwi
From New Zealand, now California. Exotic in the 60s, now a staple; brown, fuzzy-skinned, bright green inside; high in vitamin C content.

Longan and Lychee
From China. Tasty either dried or fresh.

Mamey
From Cuba. Eaten fresh or in shakes.

Pummelo
From the Malaysia–Indochina region, now big in Florida. Headed for stardom.

If you'd like to know more about such exotica as calabaza, mamey, feijoa, pepino, guanabana, or malanga, you might enroll in some evening Spanish courses and get friendly with your neighborhood bodega proprietress. Or read *Uncommon Fruits & Vegetables: A Commonsense Guide* (Harper & Row) by Elizabeth Schneider. Meanwhile, *bon appétit!* ●

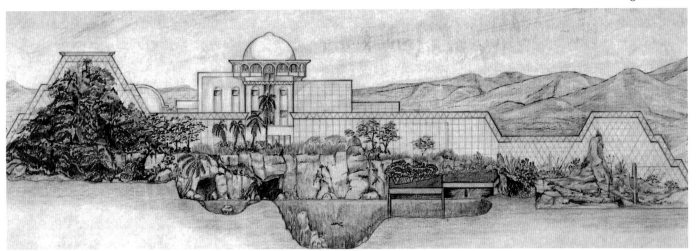

Duplicating earth's own ecosystem in miniature, Biosphere II will be home to eight pioneers near Tucson, Arizona.

Biosphere

It is, on the face of it, a fantastic concept. Imagine a vastly glorified greenhouse, covering an area of land the size of a football field, and filled with a wonderland of trees and crops and animals. The life within is completely closed off from the outside world by panes of plastic and glass, yet butterflies flit among cabbage flowers inside as a breeze bends laden heads of wheat, and a gentle rain falls from a glass-enclosed sky. In 1989, four men and four women—Biospherians, as they're called—will enter just such an enormous steel, glass and plastic structure, known as Biosphere II, situated in the Arizona desert near Tucson. They will seal themselves inside for two years without receiving or removing materials. They will live self-sufficiently, communicating by various means of information exchange.

Sound like an episode of Buck Rogers? Not so: Biosphere II is quite real. It began as the brainchild of the Institute of Ecotechnics, a London-based international ecological development firm, and is now in the final planning stages at the Environmental Research Laboratory (ERL) of the University of Arizona, whose scientists specialize in developing controlled environment agriculture—self-sufficient farming complexes that allow food to be grown on marginal land. The ERL has constructed such complexes all over the world, growing shrimp on Mexico's arid western coast at Puerto Peñasco and cultivating cucumbers in a greenhouse in the sands of the Arab sheikdom of Abu Dhabi.

But Biosphere II is not just an agricultural project; it is an attempt to model, on a small scale, the complex and interacting parts of the ecosystem of our own planet. More than half of the structure's interior will be occupied by five major scaled-down mimics of biomes, the ecologically discrete regions that cover what the ERL's director, Carl Hodges, likes to call Biosphere I—the earth. A rain forest biome, complete with dangling lianas, birds, insects and even a small stream, will spring from the desert environment to brush the very top of Biosphere II's 80-foot ceiling. Fish and plankton will swim in a 35-foot-deep ocean with wind-driven waves lapping a sandy shore, while lizards will scurry between cacti in a biome that replicates the Arizona desert. "There won't be any jaguars or elephants, of course," says Hodges. "And I'd just as soon leave out the snakes."

These different environments are possible in such a small area, he says, because the sunlight and humidity in different regions of Biosphere II can be regulated. Like a real rain forest, the miniature biome will be kept warm and humid, while the desert will be hot during the day and cool at night. With the help of a computer, the Biospherians will be able to monitor the environmental conditions inside, and they will adjust a complex array of shutters built into the Biosphere's dome to control the amount of sunlight striking each biome.

The remaining one-half to three-quarters of an acre not covered by a biome will, by necessity, be devoted to raising food for the Biospherians. Scientists at the ERL, as well as the Biospherians who have already been chosen, are planning precisely what will be grown, and how to do it. Using techniques and knowledge developed over the past two decades in part at the ERL, the small plot of cropland inside Biosphere II will be 20-60 times more productive than most land in the U.S. today. Every need conceivable must be considered before complete closure in 1989, from how many plants are necessary to produce sufficient oxygen, to what kind of food and how many calories the inhabitants will eat. Thus far, chicken, rabbit, fish, goat's milk and many cereal grains have made it onto the menu, as well as a tremendous variety of beans.

If Biosphere II succeeds—if the Biospherians can indeed maintain themselves inside their miniature world—Hodges sees a galaxy of possible uses for more Biospheres. He would like high schools to have them, for example, so that students can learn firsthand about the delicate interplay of ecological systems. Already NASA has expressed an interest in the project as a possible prototype for space stations. Some people even see Biospheres as a way to colonize inhospitable planets to escape the ills of over population and habitat destruction on earth. But Hodges disagrees with that vision. "I don't see it as an escape vehicle," he says. "The mental image of it being a way to get away from problems at home doesn't appeal to me."

Because Biosphere II is so small, any perturbation of its ecological balance will show up far more quickly than a comparable upset in the ecosystems on earth. The ERL planners are considering, for example, raising the level of carbon dioxide ever so slightly—not enough to adversely affect the Biospherians, but enough to mimic the changes in our own atmosphere that have been brought about by burning of fossil fuels and destruction of rain forests. Such global parameters, as scientists call them—things that affect the working of the entire planet—can, for the first time, be tested in Biosphere II. For Hodges, this grand and beautiful structure will represent "another biosphere to talk to, to understand our own."

But perhaps the people with the most to gain, at least in the short term, will be the Biospherians themselves. They are embarking upon a strange and marvelous adventure, where the human and non-human biological worlds are utterly dependent upon each other. Imagine having your own private forests and savannah and desert to wander through. It is indeed a fantastic concept. ●

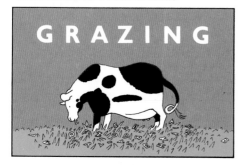

GRAZING

The Platters Will Do It Everytime

As anyone who has recently eaten in a noisy, trendy—and usually yuppie—restaurant can tell you, background music is out and foreground music is in. One company, AEI, which claims to be the leader in the foreground music field, has 23,000 customers (primarily restaurants and clothing stores). For a monthly fee, they are supplied with a special tape deck with a motor powerful enough to withstand 10,000 hours of running time, and a library of six tapes. AEI categorizes its tapes as "hot," "medium," "mild" and "mixed tempo" and reports that the most popular tape is one called "Timeless Pop Blend," which consists of oldies from the 50s and 60s, performed by the original artists. There may be something to this—a recent study by Loyola University suggests that businesses can increase sales by up to 40 percent simply by playing music that puts people in a good mood.

And Some People Thought He Was Crackers A Presbyterian preacher from West Suffield, Connecticut, named Sylvester Graham might be properly considered the great-granddaddy of the high-fiber movement. In the early 1800s he lectured widely, preaching passionately against the use of condiments (which he said could cause insanity) and proclaiming the virtues of loose clothing, cold showers, hard mattresses and, above all, bran. He campaigned to have bran put back into wheat flour, for the good of the nation, and therein lies his claim to fame. When the bran *was* put back, the result was given the name, reasonably enough, of graham flour. Also, named for him was the Graham cracker, made from graham flour.

Century Of Bounty Pear trees planted over 100 years ago on the banks of the Sacramento River in California still produce abundant crops every year.

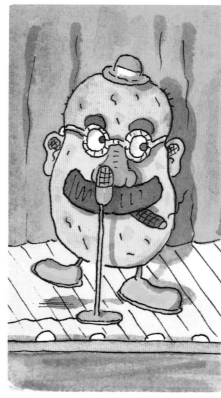

Unloved A recent Gallup survey of 1,540 American adults found that the top ten most unloved foods were: snails, brains, squid, shark, tripe, beef kidneys, beef tongue, oxtail, squab, mussels.

Citymeals On Wheels

In 1981, an article in *The New York Times* about Meals on Wheels—a federally funded program which delivers hot meals to homebound senior citizens in New York City—caught the eye of Gael Greene, restaurant critic for *New York* magazine. Struck by a major limitation of Meals on Wheels—that food is delivered only on weekdays—Greene enlisted the help of some influential food-world colleagues, including James Beard, Barbara Kafka and George Lang, and formed Citymeals on Wheels. Working with the city's Department for the Aging, Citymeals on Wheels was able to raise enough money in its first few months of existence to provide Christmas and Chanukah dinners for some 6,000 elderly people. Since then, thanks to contributions from corporations and individuals, Citymeals on Wheels has managed to feed even more needy souls. In 1985, 6,600 elderly New Yorkers received a hot meal each weekend, and, in addition, 11,000 were served Christmas and Chanukah dinners and 25,800 received emergency food packages.

Potato What?

Without endorsing the author's view of what these are, we pass along the following from a booklet called *Potato Jokes* by Paul McMahon, published by Simon & Schuster:

What holiday is sacred to all potatoes? Mash Wednesday.

Who was the first potato in outer space? Spudnick.

Why are potatoes so afraid of Indians? They don't want to get scalloped.

Why do potatoes vacation on the French Riviera? They like to see the French fry.

What do they do there? Nothing, they just sit and bake. They can't stay out too long, though....They peel easily.

Judge Not, Lest Ye Be Judged Restaurant critic Mimi Sheraton notes: "Restaurants and chefs want to be judged by their goals and not their achievements."

Building Better Bodies...
"Meat and potatoes has taken something of a bad rap in recent years, assaulted on all sides by gourmets who think it too common a meal, by nutritionists who insist that it is too full of cholesterol and fat and by polemicists who believe there would be a lot less macho posturing in the world if people ate less red meat. I usually remind the latter that Sylvester Stallone subsisted on wheat germ and fish while filming his carnage scenes for the Rambo and Rocky sagas."
John Mariani, food and wine writer, *Food & Wine*

The Fizz Has It According to the Food Marketing Institute, people drink more soft drinks than water.

So What If It Is Only Fermented Milk
Yogurt is currently so big on the American scene that there are no fewer than 45 separate brands ringing up over $1 billion in annual retail sales.

Waitpersonality There is a search under way for a new, more appropriate unisex name for a waiter. Laura Brody, author of *Growing Up on the Chocolate Diet*, suggests that anyone who brings you food and looks after you should be called a "mommy."

AQUABUSINESS

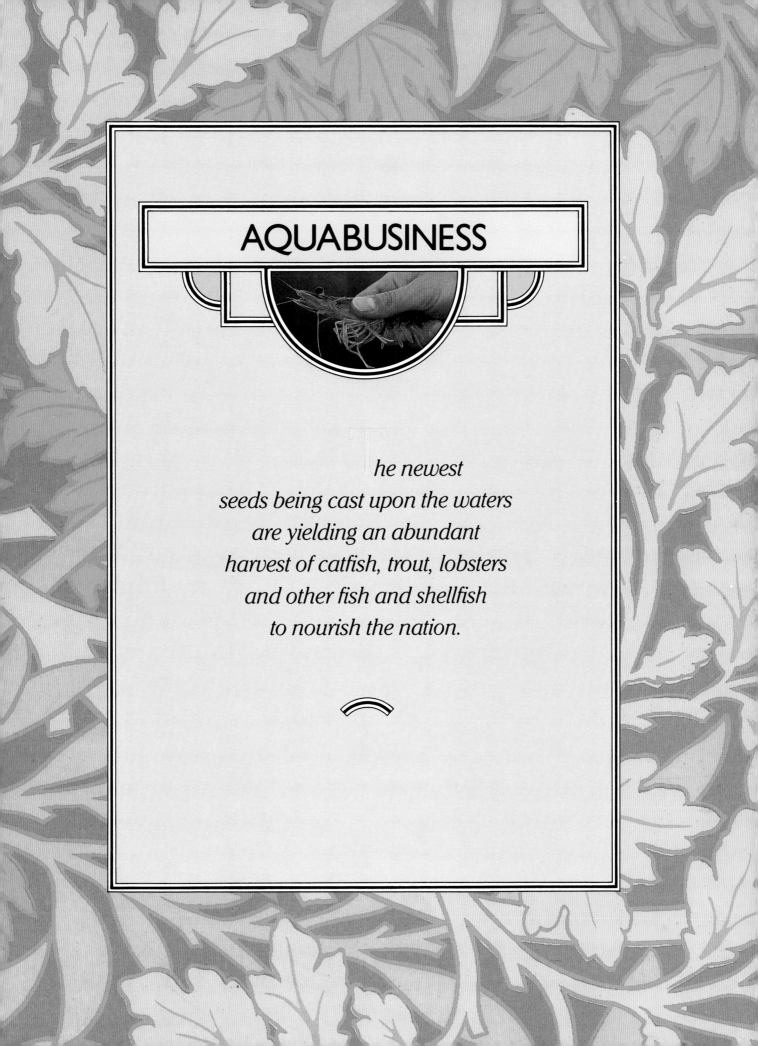

The newest
seeds being cast upon the waters
are yielding an abundant
harvest of catfish, trout, lobsters
and other fish and shellfish
to nourish the nation.

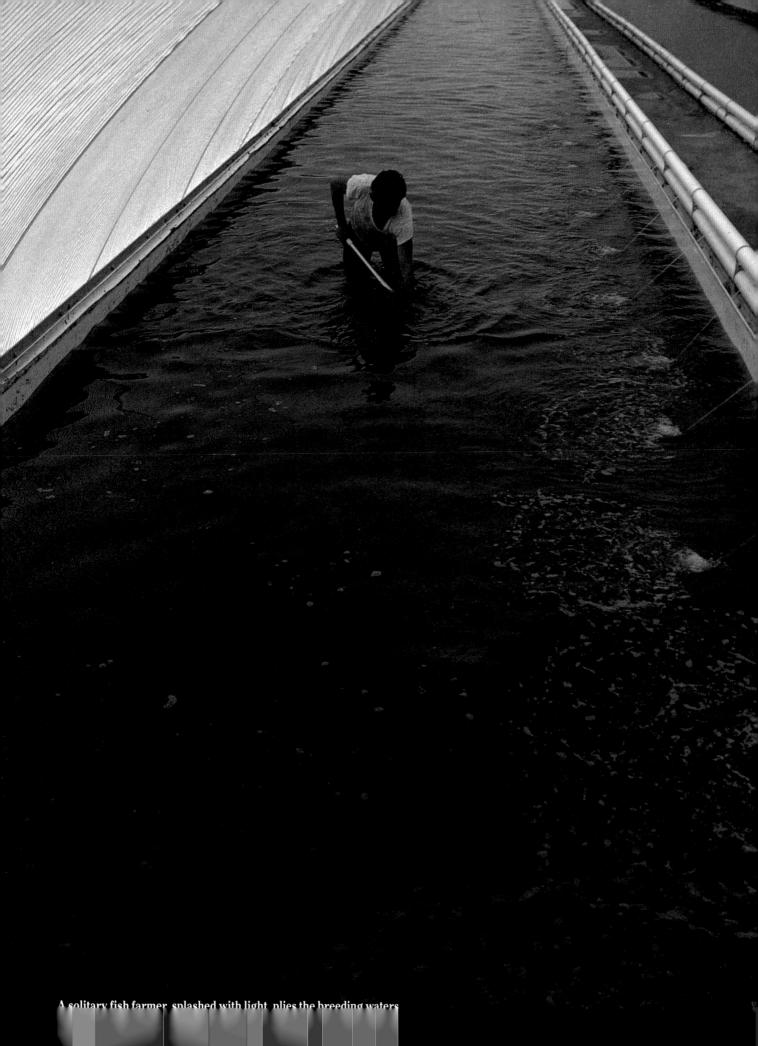

A solitary fish farmer, splashed with light, plies the breeding waters

AQUACULTURE

Bored with beef? Sick of chicken? More and more Americans are turning away from traditional fare toward seafood. According to the National Marine Fisheries Service, U.S. consumption of fish has gone up at least 30 percent over the last two decades to around 13 pounds per capita. But there's just one hitch: The annual seafood catch is going down. To quote *Forbes,* "Seafood is 'in,' just as the oceans are being fished out."

Where is all that fish that Americans are demanding going to come from? Fish farms.

For the past twenty years big companies, such as Coca-Cola, Union Carbide, Ralston Purina and Campbell's, to name just a few, as well as small entrepreneurs have been flocking to this new industry. Its, official title is aquaculture, a moniker that covers just about anything that can be raised in the water—from turtles to trout, from catfish to clams. Even vegetables grown in water hydroponically—or without soil—are considered aquacultural products. Aquaculturists are successfully cultivating over twenty different species, growing such delicacies as prawns, crayfish, lobster, oysters, mussels and clams, much the way a dirt farmer grows corn or wheat.

The first fish farmers in America were the Hawaiians. When Captain Cook landed at Kauai in 1778, he counted 360 fish ponds on the island—covering some 6,000 acres and producing about two million pounds of fish per year.

Last year, U.S. fish farmers raised more than 300 million pounds of seafood. The retail value of their products is over $1 billion a year in the U.S. and worldwide

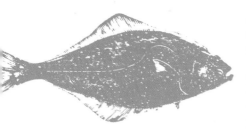

aquaculture provides about nine million tons of seafood, about one-eighth of what's consumed. Already most of the catfish and crayfish, and about 40 percent of the oysters that grace the tables in this country were raised on a farm.

If you imagined that succulent rainbow trout on your plate once cavorted in some sparkling waterfall, think again: Nearly all the rainbow trout consumed in this country comes from farms, most of them in Idaho.

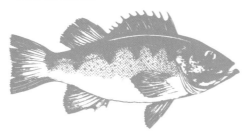

Fish farming probably originated about 4,000 years ago in China, shortly after livestock was domesticated. Carp were kept in ponds, where they were fed grain. The Chinese knew what they were about, since fish, it turns out, convert vegetable matter into protein far more efficiently than other domesticated animals. It takes seven pounds of grain to fatten a steer by one pound; a fish gains a pound on only 1.7 pounds of grain. China and Japan continue to be the world leaders in cultured fish, shellfish and seaweed. Yes, seaweed.

China produces over four million tons of seafood a year.

But aquaculture on a commercial scale in the U.S. has been another kettle of fish. Back in the 1970s, pioneer aquaculturists discovered that they simply didn't know enough about the life cycles, feeding habits and diseases of the species they wanted to raise. Sanders Associates, Inc., for example, a Nashua, N.H. electronics firm spent eight years developing methods to grow lobsters. Nobody knew that it took 8 to 11 years for a lobster to mature to market size, or that young lobsters are so aggressive

they will tear each other apart when kept in a common pen.

The second most abundant farm-raised fish is Tilapia, an African fish with flesh about as exciting as tofu.

With all the unknowns, it's not surprising that the most successful aquaculture ventures have been those producing species whose habits *are* well known. Catfish is the perfect example. Just about every farmer in the south had a pond full of catfish, and turning that backyard hobby into a full-blown commercial operation seemed like a natural to a lot of southern farmers. In fact, it came so easily, southern farmers produced 192 million pounds of the mild, tender fish in 1985. One of the South's catfish giants, Farm Fresh Catfish Company, with its 3,000 acres of man-made ponds had sales in excess of $40 million.

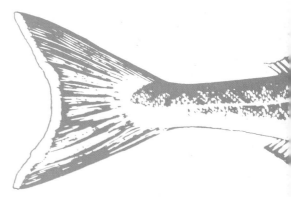

Look for the fast food of the future: catfish burgers.

According to some experts, however, if American aquaculture really takes off, it won't be by raising food as prosaic as catfish. The real future in fish farms lies with the luxury species: lobster, jumbo shrimp, clams, Belon oysters and a real exotic for the American palate—mussels. Steamed with wine and celery as the Belgians do, or stewed in the French manner with garlic and cream, mussels are fast becoming fashionable food.

Some of the most succulent of these

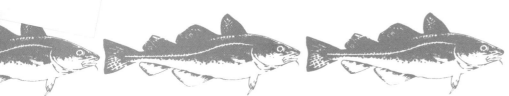

mollusks are being grown in the waters off the coast of Maine. Farmers drag wild mussel beds in the spring to gather "seed mussels," which are no bigger than the head of a pin. These young mussels are then sown in the culturing beds—plots of the ocean floor—about 15 to 20 per square foot. Like most bivalves, they filter seawater to trap and eat the plankton in it, thus benefiting from being given plenty of space.

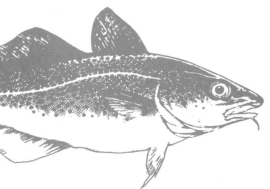

Every week Ecomar, Inc., a California firm, sells about 5,000 pounds of unusually sweet and clean-tasting mussels, which have been harvested from the legs of offshore oil platforms. Out in deep water where the platforms are, there's no pollution or parasites, and most important to mussel-lovers, no sand.

Mussels raised on farms grow to market size, about two inches long, in about two years, more than twice as fast as it takes when they grow in crowded beds in the wild. The mature shellfish are hauled up in huge drags—heavy wire nets—from late August until March. One Maine venture, Great Eastern Mussel Farms, Inc., is one of the largest mussel growers in the U.S., shipping more than 100,000 bushels, $2 million worth annually.

Not everybody has such spectacular success at aquaculture. Take salmon ranching. In concept it's simple: Take a bunch of salmon fry from a fish hatchery, hold them in pens in a stream until they are about two years old, then release them into the ocean to graze and grow fat. When the fish mature, in three to five years, at least a few of them will follow their homing instincts back to the stream where they were born,

foolishly returning to the rancher's waiting corral and processing plant.

Norwegian entrepreneurs growing salmon in fjords have taught their fish to come 'n get it at mealtime when they hear an underwater sound.

Weyerhaeuser Co., the giant forest-products corporation, has poured millions into its salmon rancher subsidiary, Ore-Aqua, but thus far, less than one percent of the fry they have released have returned—and one percent is the break-even point for the ranchers. But Ore-Aqua and other ranchers along the Oregon coast aren't giving up. They've seen a steady, though gradual improvement in their fishy returns even as commercial fishermen catch less and less. If the experts are correct in expecting seafood to replace an increasing percentage of beef, pork and chicken consumed in this country, it's going to have to come from fish farms. Move over, all you cowboys, chicken ranchers and pig farmers. Maybe the song will have to be changed: Home, home on the bay, Where the salmon and shellfish do play.

If cattle ranchers are called cowboys, should salmon ranchers be called fishboys? ●

Good Food—Bad Name

The shark has been around for 350 million years and will probably be here for another 350 million. Ditto cockroaches. The latter *earned* our revulsion; the former *got his* from *Jaws* movies.

The spiny dogfish, three to four feet long, roams up and down the East Coast from Labrador to Florida and is often caught by fishermen seeking more commercial species of fish. Though prized as a delicacy in European markets for hors d'oeuvres, fish 'n chips and so-called belly flaps, our fishermen often consider the dogfish a nuisance. Its sandpaper skin frays nets and its meat requires rapid, special processing to rid it of the chemical urea which causes an unpleasant odor of ammonia. More popular is the 12-foot mako shark, which also roams the Atlantic waters off the U.S. and provides a lot of good protein-rich meat that is appearing in increasing quantities in U.S. fish markets. The best quality is the white or pale pink meat furthest from the skin and it can be poached, baked, broiled or fried like any lean fish. One enterprising New England cookbook author, Hannah Scheets, even suggests curried shark. Shark meat can also be salted, smoked or pickled.

Out of Rumson, New Jersey, William Lane of Universal Marine & Shark Products uses five boats to grab seven tons of shark daily. (That's *tons . . . daily.*) Fins sell in Hong Kong for $50-$75 apiece, for that Chinese delicacy, shark fin soup. The

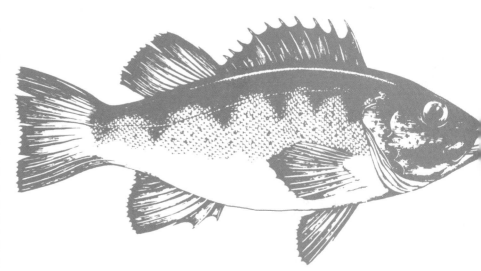

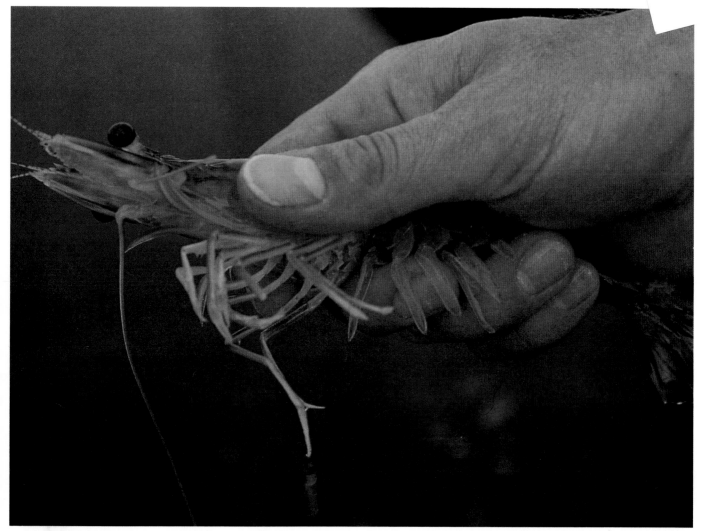

A finger-sized inhabitant of a shrimp farm is held up for inspection. Hawaii is a leader in farming this increasingly popular shellfish.

tanned hides, which are more durable than cowhide, bring $6.50 a square foot for attaché cases, shoes, belts, handbags and wallets.

And scientists, intrigued by the fact that sharks are immune to tumors, diseases and infections (a possible explanation of their long tenure on earth) are probing shark cartilage for the cancer immunity secret. Massachusetts Institute of Technology's Robert Langer told *Forbes*: "What we need to do is purify this molecule out and test it on different animal tumors."

No more *Jaws* movies, please. ●

Please Don't Ice The Oysters Oysters keep for weeks at 40 degrees Fahrenheit. But don't do them a favor and ice them: They'll open their shells, give you a dirty look—and die.

The Undersea World Of Gypsy Rose Crab

Of the 4,400 crab species, the Blue Crab of Chesapeake Bay seems to have the most fun. The growing female does some 20 strip-acts before maturing, pumping herself up like an inflatable woman to break out of her shell during molting. Each time she dons a new and larger shell-costume. During the few hours when she's exposed and squeezable she gets to mate before a new shell forms and hardens. In those same few hours the Bay crabbers grab her—the succulent soft-shell Maryland crab. Her mate also sheds and is also grabbed.

The crabbers watch the maturing decapods in their underwater pens like hawks—waiting for the telltale signs of molting.

First, white lines appear on the shells ten to 14 days before shedding. Two days before the molt, the paddles on the crab's hind legs turn from pink to red. Now the crabs are checked every hour or so, around the clock. When they break free from their shells, out of the water they come and to the market they go. ●

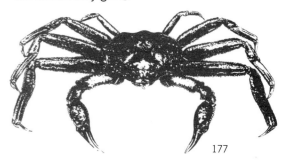

177

Let Them Eat Roe

One hundred fifty years ago, American Indian mothers weaned their babies on caviar. One hundred years ago, we exported caviar to Europe. Seventy-five years ago, saloons put bowls of caviar on their bars to speed up the pace of beer guzzling.

Today we import sturgeon roe—beluga caviar—from the Caspian Sea for $30-$40 per ounce. That's o-u-n-c-e!

What happened to our once plentiful native caviar since the early years of this century? Rivers have been overfished, and, in some areas, polluted; dams have been built, impeding fishes' instinctive urge to return upstream to spawn. That's the bad news.

The good news is that native caviar is making a strong comeback, that sturgeon are again showing up in our rivers from Oregon to Arkansas, from Louisiana to Minnesota, and that the tasty eggs of other freshwater fish—white fish, lumpfish and red salmon, for example—are appearing in our stores and restaurants. The Food and Drug Administration, be it noted, allows *all* domestic roe (not only sturgeon roe) to be called caviar as long as the type is stated.

The renaissance of American caviar began in the late 1970s, sparked by fish processing entrepreneurs like Mats and Daphne Engstrom of San Francisco, who came up with a technique for making caviar from the roe of California sturgeon and turned it into a booming business and Mario Garbarino of New York, a former importer of Russian and Iranian caviar. Garbarino was visiting relatives in Oklahoma in the '70s, when he spotted sturgeon for sale, brimming with roe. Today, his fishermen bring in sturgeon from 12 rivers in the Mississippi system and he has the technique of salting, handling and shipping the roe down pat.

Domestic sturgeon average about 500 pounds in weight compared to the Caspian variety, which can weigh between 1,000 and 2,000 pounds. About 10 percent of the female sturgeon's weight is roe. To get the roe, fishermen intercept the sturgeon on their way upstream to spawn and hit them at a critical spot just below the head so that they experience no trauma when they are killed—otherwise stress releases a chemical in sturgeon that turns its eggs bitter. The Engstroms, however, have developed

a method of giving spawning females a hormone shot and removing the eggs by Caesarian section. The fish are then put back into the water to produce roe for their lifetime—which can be up to 100 years. By whatever method, once the eggs are obtained, they are immediately sorted, washed and salted—a critical process upon which the final taste depends.

Although some purists—shall we say rich purists?—insist that Caspian roe is the

only real caviar and that American roe is ersatz, dozens of respected food critics and chefs give our caviar very high marks. Craig Claiborne, for one, said he'd put the Engstrom caviar "in competition with any import sold in this country." Recently, *The New York Times* reported that U.S. caviar is outselling the imports by six to one.

Price could be a small factor. Beluga: $30 an ounce. U.S. whitefish (golden) caviar: $4.00 for a four-ounce jar. ●

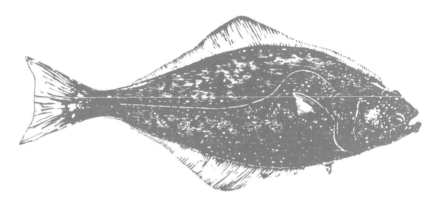

Seaweed For Supper?

Some years ago, I overheard a conversation between Albert Stockli, the brilliant Swiss chef who worked with Joe Baum to create *The Four Seasons*—arguably the greatest restaurant in the country—and his lunch companion. Albert asked her if she was fond of soup. "Thank God," she answered with something of a haughty sniff, "I've never had to eat it." This is the way most of us feel about seaweed. The Japanese people love it; they wrap it around their sushi and think it something really special. We think of seaweed as—well, seaweed.

It's a pity because there is plenty around. For example, there is one variety that grows to an almost unbelievable size off the coast of San Diego—imagine an aquatic tidal wave of brown seaweed 100 feet high and 200 feet wide, undulating from an underwater bed 70-square miles across.

Why should we care that the seaweed is there at all if we don't want to eat it? For one thing, because scientists have discovered that algin, which is derived from seaweed,

is a complex sugar that is thought to reduce the surface tension of seawater. Not very interesting, perhaps, until you realize that algin can do the same thing for ice cream and salad dressings! It prevents crystals from forming in the ice cream as it freezes and stops the vinegar from huddling in the bottom of the bottle of the dressing. Not only that—it makes a bigger froth on a mug of beer. It can also make a gloss on lipstick and a high shiny surface on the kind of paper that is used for upscale magazines.

If you are impressed by this you may be even more surprised to learn that a pellet of this magical algin, when set loose in a waste treatment plant, will separate the components into new forms of fats, proteins and carbohydrates. These can then be used as a nutritious cattle or poultry feed; or they can become a fertilizer for feed grains.

So—while we may not be eating seaweed burgers any time soon—algin will be appearing in our daily lives in all manner of mysterious ways. ●

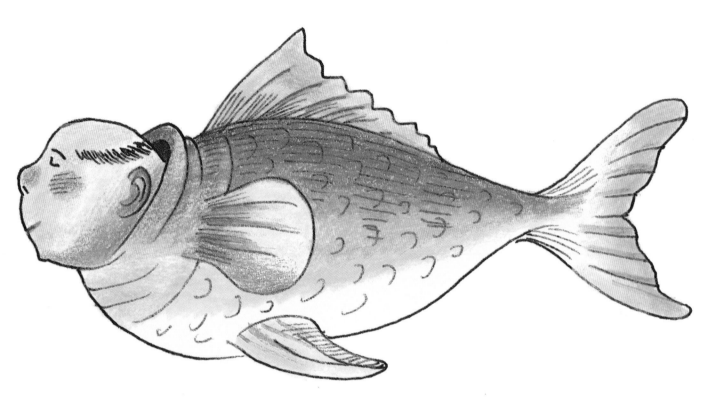

Trash Becomes Flash

Until recently, millions of tons of fish have been discarded each year because people didn't know how to cook them, or the fish were difficult to harvest or lacked the appropriate marketing push. But now that supplies of the more popular species are dwindling, our fishing industry, in a show of American ingenuity, is promoting so-called "trash fish"—fish that were formerly tossed back into the sea if caught by chance. Such fish are often given other, more appealing, names in the market-place—tilefish, for example, becomes "white snapper"—a lesson learned, perhaps, from Madison Avenue, which calls toilet paper "bathroom tissue."

Years ago, believe it or not, lobster was a trash fish. In colonial times, it was planted in corn fields as a fertilizer. And even today, while restaurant-goers in big cities plunk down $16 for a plate of *calamari fritti,* fishermen are using squid for bait. One man's trash, it seems, is another man's treat.

Eel

Once prized by New England's early settlers, but long out of favor here, eel is slowly regaining popularity. It can be used for sushi—brushed with sauce and grilled until crisp, Japanese style. Tiny baby eel that resemble bean sprouts are a delicacy cooked in olive oil and garlic, Mediterranean style.

Monkfish

Beloved by the French, who call it *lotte,* monkfish flesh is firm and succulent and the flavor is so fine that it is known as "poor man's lobster." In fact, restaurants sometimes secretly substitute monkfish for lobster in stews. Monkfish can also be sautéed, grilled, poached or used in chowders.

Mussels

Cheaper than clams, mussels are just as delicious, with a briny, almost smoky flavor. They are also nutritious—high in vitamins and minerals and low in fat.

Sea robin

Small bottom-dwelling fish, abundant in East Coast waters, sea robins have pectoral fins so large that they look like birds' wings. The fins are used for walking along the ocean floor and searching the sand for food—clams, squid, crabs and shrimp.

Sea robins are usually sold as fillets. Use them in bouillabaise but they can also be broiled, sautéed, poached or deep-fried.

Skate

Also known as ray, skate feed on mollusks and, as a result, have a firm, flavorful flesh similar to sea scallops. Only the "wings" are edible and this meat is best poached.

Smelts

Smelts are small (usually about seven inches long, and weighing less than two ounces), silvery, delicate-tasting and very inexpensive. Abundant in the Atlantic and Pacific oceans, the most common species in markets are rainbow and eulachon, or Columbia River smelts. The eulachon are so rich in oil that local Indians would air-dry them, thread a wick through their bodies, and use them as candles—thus their other name: candlefish. Smelts are best prepared simply: lightly coated with flour and sautéed in butter, or grilled with herbs.

Squid

Although there are still plenty of people

who cringe at the idea of eating these homely, ten-armed mollusks, squid have become enormously popular of late, especially in northern California, where they are abundant. Californians prefer to call them by their Italian name, *calamari,* but whatever the nomenclature, this cephalopod is finding its way into scores of restaurants across the country. Squid must be cooked either very quickly or very slowly, or they become rubbery and inedible. When cooked properly, they are sweet and tender.

Tilefish

Large and multi-hued, tilefish are common in the deep waters of the Atlantic, the Pacific and the Gulf of Mexico. They feed on crabs and other crustaceans, which may be the reason for their superb flavor with overtones of shellfish. Tilefish has a firm texture and is therefore generally sold as steaks or fillets. It is best grilled, poached or baked. ●

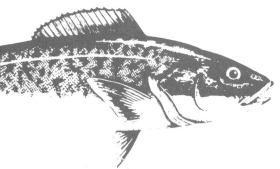

What Is Surimi?

One hundred million pounds of it were consumed in the U.S. last year by people who didn't know what it was. Surimi is really a pig-in-a-poke mystery food from Japan but a big seller in America's take-out shops and restaurants where the notion prevails that if it's Japanese it's good for you—like a Sony Walkman or a Toyota.

The consensus of food technologists is that surimi is mostly pollack, a cousin of cod, found off the coasts of the North Pacific. Pollack swim so close together that "shoals" of them appear on fishing boat sonar screens as vast underwater towers, so Japanese fishermen have no trouble hauling in tons. Taken back to Japan, they

are mixed with the meat of the snow crab and given body by the addition of starches and stiffeners, usually egg white. Dyed a pretty pink, this agglomeration is extruded, formed into the shape of a crab leg and frozen. Presto! Surimi, also known as "Sea Claws." And where is the major export market? Where else but in the U.S.A.

Surimi's main appeal is its price: It's far cheaper than real crabmeat and frequently passes for the real thing! But many food

critics look down their noses at it; one calls it "mock food in a mock shape for a mock dinner, cooked by mock heat." Another calls it "the soybean of the sea."

It is a feeling among some U.S. food processors that since the Japanese are fishing for pollack inside our 200-mile territorial waters—if indeed they are—they should share their surimi technology with us. The Japanese don't agree. It is, as the newsmen say, a breaking story . . . ●

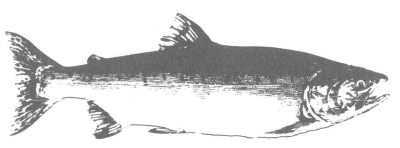

Tinkering With Piscatorial Instincts

In the spring of 1986, biogeneticists from Michigan State University released 100,000 sterile young chinook salmon into Lake Michigan. Sterile fish will not have the urge to seek out their river birthplace to spawn and die at the meager 15-pound weight of their fertile cousins. Instead, they are expected to live to reach weights of 70 pounds before being harvested.

To induce sterility and suppress the spawning instinct, the salmon eggs are exposed briefly to pressures of 6,000-8,000 pounds per square inch in a pressure chamber. This procedure causes chromosomes to multiply, and once there are too many, the fish—like all animals—will become sterile.

Taking an entirely different approach to genetic tinkering, Canadian scientists are exposing baby salmon to growth hormones similar to those used to grow larger livestock and poultry. They hope that greater size will allow more mature fertile salmon to survive the rigors of the sea, and to return to their birthplaces to be harvested. And carrying this approach to a logical conclusion, Johns Hopkins researchers are

injecting fertilized eggs with mammalian growth hormone genes hoping that the salmon will then produce the growth hormones themselves and become a new giant strain.

Salmon fish ranchers would like a higher proportion of females to males: the more females the more eggs. Injecting females with the male sex hormone, testosterone, turns them into "males" with the genetic make-up of females. As a result, when they mate with normal females, only female offspring hatch.

Shellfish are also getting the geneticists' attention. Scientists at the University of California at Santa Barbara have discovered that the addition of very small amounts of hydrogen peroxide to the environment of abalone, oysters, mussels, clams and other shellfish stimulates them to produce the hormone prostaglandin—also present in humans—which in turn stimulates them to spawn. And in yet another experiment to speed the growth rate of abalone, insulin and a growth hormone from livestock have been added to their waters. The result: a 25 percent increase in growth rate. ●

Food Festivals

Food festivals are becoming increasingly popular. Everywhere folk are flocking to rejoice in the first appearance of shad, to taste the crawfish, the strawberries and to indulge in persimmons prepared in a hundred different ways. Alice M. Geffen and Carole Berglie have studied this happy phenomena and written *Food Festival—The Ultimate Guidebook to America's Best Regional Food Celebrations* (published by Pantheon). They invite us to travel around the country to savor the local flavors and for those who cannot journey with them, there are recipes from the Black-eyed Pea Jamboree, the Watermelon Festival and hundreds of other fabulous fresh tastes to savor. Listed below are the authors' choices of the best of the celebrations.

February

Boudin Festival—last weekend
Martin Richard
Broussard, Louisiana 70518

National Date Festival—mid-month
Indio, California
(714) 342-8247

Swamp Cabbage Festival—last weekend
La Belle, Florida
(813) 675-0125

April

Vermont Maple Festival—mid-month
St. Albans, Vermont
(802) 524-5800

World Catfish Festival—every Saturday
Belzoni, Mississippi
(601) 247-2616

May

Cosby Ramp Festival—1st Sunday
Cosby, Tennessee
(800) 438-4404 (out-of-state)
(800) 334-1051 (in-state)

Breaux Bridge Crawfish Festival—1st Saturday
Breaux Bridge, Louisiana
(318) 332-2345

Eastern Shore Seafood Festival—1st Wednesday
Chincoteague, Virginia
(804) 787-2460

National Mushroom Hunting Championship—Mothers Day weekend
Boyne City, Michigan
(616) 582-6222

Harrison Mushroom Festival—early in the month
Harrison, Michigan
(517) 539-6011

Windsor Shad Derby—entire month
P.O. Box 502
Windsor, Connecticut 06095

June

Delmarva Chicken Festival—early in the month
Georgetown, Delaware
(312) 856-2971

Pink Tomato Festival—early in the month
Warren, Arkansas
(501) 226-5225

Jambalaya Festival—2nd weekend
P.O. Box 1243
Gonzales, Louisiana 70737

National Asparagus Festival—2nd weekend
Box 153
Shelby/Hart, Michigan 49455

Ipswich Strawberry Festival—mid-month
Ipswich, Massachusetts
(617) 356-2307

July

National Cherry Festival—early in the month
P.O. Box 141
Traverse City, Michigan 49684

Minnesota Wild Rice Festival—early in the month
Kelliher/Waskish, Minnesota 56650

Black-Eyed Pea Jamboree—mid-month
Athens, Texas
(214) 675-5181

Central Maine Egg Festival—4th weekend
Pittsfield, Maine 04967

Pork, Peanut and Pine Festival—mid-month
Chippokes State Park
Surry, Virginia 23883

Gilroy Garlic Festival—end of month
P.O. Box 2311
Gilroy, California 95020

August

Indian-Style Salmon Bake—1st Sunday
Sequim Chamber of Commerce
P.O. Box 907
Sequim, Washington 98382

Shaker Kitchen Festival—1st week
Hancock, Massachusetts
Hancock Shaker Village
P.O. Box 898
Pittsfield, Massachusetts 01202

Maine Lobster Festival—mid-month
Winter Harbor, Maine
(207) 963-2235

Beefiesta—mid-month
Scott City, Kansas
(316) 872-3525

Strange Seafood Exhibition—3rd Thursday
Beaufort, North Carolina
(919) 728-7317

Watermelon Festival—mid-month
Hope, Arkansas
(501) 777-3640

State of Maine Blueberry Festival—3rd week
Union Fair
Knox Agricultural Society
Union, Maine 04862

International Zucchini Festival—last Saturday
Harrisville, New Hampshire
(603) 827-3033

September

Hatch Chile Festival—Labor Day weekend
Hatch Valley Chamber of Commerce
P.O. Box 38
Hatch, New Mexico 87937

National Hard Crab Derby—Labor Day weekend
P.O. Box 215
Crisfield, Maryland 21817

Feast of San Esteban—September 2
Acoma Pueblo, New Mexico
(505) 552-6606

Castroville Artichoke Festival—2nd weekend
Castroville, California
(408) 633-2465

McClure Bean Soup Festival—mid-month
McClure, Pennsylvania
(717) 658-8425

Sorghum Sopping Days—3rd weekend
Waldo, Alabama
Town of Waldo, Route 3
Talladega, Alabama 35160

Persimmon Festival—last week
Mitchell, Indiana
(812) 849-2151

Marion County Ham Days—last weekend
Lebanon, Kentucky
(512) 692-2661

October

Apple Harvest Festival—last weekend in September, 1st weekend in October
Southington, Connecticut
(203) 628-8036

Cranberry Festival—last weekend in September, 1st weekend in October
P.O. Box 7
South Carver, Massachusetts 02366

Cherokee Fall Festival—early part of month
Cherokee, North Carolina
(704) 497-9195

Okra Strut—1st Saturday
Irmo, South Carolina
(803) 781-7050

Arkansas Rice Festival—2nd weekend
Weiner, Arkansas
(501) 684-2284

Chincoteague Oyster Festival—Saturday of Columbus Day weekend
Chamber of Commerce
Box 258
Chincoteague, Virginia 23336

Gumbo Festival—2nd weekend
P.O. Box 9069
Bridge City, Louisiana 70094

West Virginia Black Walnut Festival—2nd weekend
Spencer, West Virginia
(304) 927-3708

Burgoo Festival—2nd Sunday
Utica, Illinois
(815) 667-4861

National Shrimp Festival—3rd weekend
Chamber of Commerce
Gulf Shores, Alabama 36542

Boggy Bayou Mullet Festival—3rd weekend
Niceville, Florida
(904) 678-3099

Circleville Pumpkin Show—3rd Wednesday
P.O. Box 288
Circleville, Ohio 43113

Usquepaugh Johnnycake Festival—last weekend
Usquepaugh, Rhode Island
(401) 783-4054

Andouille Festival—last weekend
LaPlace, Louisiana
(504) 652-2065

Lexington Barbecue Festival—last weekend
Lexington, North Carolina
(704) 243-2629

Yambilee—end of month
Opelousas, Louisiana
(318) 948-8848

November

Louisiana Pecan Festival—1st weekend
Colfax, Louisiana
(318) 627-3711

Annual Indian Foods Dinner—2nd and 3rd Saturday
Salamanca, New York
(716) 945-1252

Bradford Wild Game Supper—3rd Saturday
Mrs. Raymond Green
Box 356
Bradford, Vermont 05033

December

Bracebridge Dinner—Christmas Eve, Christmas Day and Christmas Night
Yosemite National Park, California
(209) 373-4171

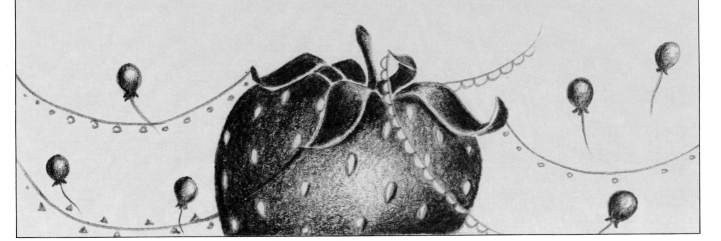

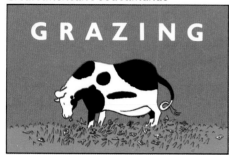

GRAZING

Grunion To The Max

Eating outdoors, whether at a beachside picnic or a backyard barbecue, is a fundamental part of life in Southern California. Therefore, each spring and summer, residents eagerly anticipate the traditional grunion run, which provides them with one more excuse for an outdoor feast.

Grunion are small, silvery fish which are borne onto Southern California beaches by the high tides whenever there is a full moon. The females quickly lay their eggs in the damp sand, and the males fertilize them. Meanwhile, hordes of hungry natives stand poised to grab the hapless little fish before they are spirited back out to sea on the next big wave.

California law states that grunion may be caught only by children under 16 or by adults with state licenses, and only with bare hands. As soon as the fish are caught, they are cleaned and cooked right on the beach, and eaten with—what else—bare hands.

Forty-Eight Minutes Of Jogging That's what you'd have to do to mend the damage done by devouring just one chocolate truffle, according to Judith Olney, author of *The Joy of Chocolate.*

Oh Gosh, Look At The Potato—I've Got To Run E. Thomas Hughes, a teacher at the Potomac School in suburban Virginia, is also the proprietor of the Potato Museum in Washington D.C., which is open by appointment. His wife, Meredith Hughes, is editor of *Peelings*, a newsletter concerned with the same subject. Tom Hughes is the originator of the idea that Washington should be designated the "Hot Potato" as competition to the Big Apple. Among the 350 objects on display at the museum is a potato clock, which is to say a potato with a big hand and a little hand and some zinc and copper wires. It was invented by Bill Borst of North Carolina, who, by using the flow of electrons through the potato, created a primitive battery that could run a clock mechanism. It works.

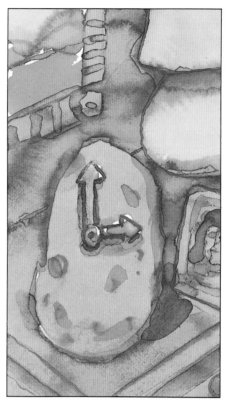

Steak Is Just A By-Product Our four-hooved friends, according to the California Beef Council, whose business it is to know such things, provide the world with the following inedible products: upholstery, clothing, luggage, felt, ointment bases, artists' brushes, rug pads, insulation, powder and rouge, buttons, bone china, dice, crochet needles, glues, bone charcoal, photographic film gelatins, neat's-foot oil, combs and barrettes, jewelry, hand soaps, shampoos, candles, crayons, industrial oils, lipsticks, hand creams, shoe polishes, fertilizers, methane gas, detergents, tires, gloves, boots, shaving creams, polishes, floor waxes, adobe bricks, paints, asphalt.

I Get No Kick From Champagne . . . "Nouvelle bothers me mightily: dainty portions of this and that; entrees and accompaniments plated so exquisitely you are sure the chef spent more time arranging the food than he did preparing it. Don't get me wrong: Nouvelle done well is swell. Unhappily only a handful know swell from swill."

Stephen Michaelides, editor, *Restaurant Hospitality*

(Don't) Think Pink If you order New England boiled dinner in Boston and find that the corned beef is gray, don't send it back. Bostonians, and people living within a 50-mile radius of that city, *like* it that way. The rest of the country prefers pink corned beef, which is cured twice as long as the Boston variety, and contains sodium nitrite to preserve the meat's pink color.

Cold And Big

The ice cream industry is currently worth $3.7 *billion* a year, with the average American eating just over 22 quarts of ice cream, sherbets or ices annually, according to the International Association of Ice Cream Manufacturers. And another source, *Advertising Age*, tells us that the 53 billion scoops of ice cream produced by the industry in this country could supply 12 cones for every inhabitant of the planet. Our ice cream production could also fill enough half-gallon containers to encircle the earth 11 times.

The Kreplach Joke

This is the third-oldest joke in the world. Little Irving has an unreasoning fear, a terror of kreplach, those little Jewish wontons. His mother takes him to the family doctor—not for old Jewish families anything so modern as psychiatry, it's gotta be an M.D. or a rabbi—and the doctor says: "Do this, Mrs. Feinstein. Take him in the kitchen and show him every step in the making of kreplach. When he sees there's nothing to be afraid of, he won't be afraid." Okay? That's the setup; here's the joke.

Mamma: Oiving, come here, dollink. Come into mine kitchen.

Irving: Okay, here I am.

Mamma: And vot is mamma doing?

Irving: You're rolling out dough . . . and now you're cutting out triangles.

Mamma: Right, pussyket. And now vot is mamma doing?

Irving: You're putting in chopped meat with chopped onions, a little in every triangle.

Mamma: Correct, svitthott, and now vot?

Irving: Now you're folding over one corner . . . now the second corner . . .

Mamma: Yes? And now . . .?

Irving: Yiiiiiiiiii! Kreplach!

Leonore Fleischer, contributing editor, *Publishers Weekly*

Take Three Rose Petals Most of us have heard of dandelion wine but how about marigold cheese balls, lavender caviar dip or lime geranium muffins? A few other edible blossoms to enhance your recipies: fuchsia, lily, peony, nasturtium and chrysanthemum.

FOOD SERVICE

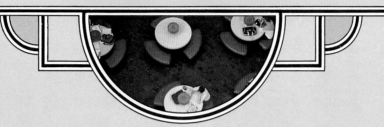

*Whether
you eat on a train or plane,
there is an
increasing chance that
the cook is Marriott or a friendly
face from a fast food chain.*

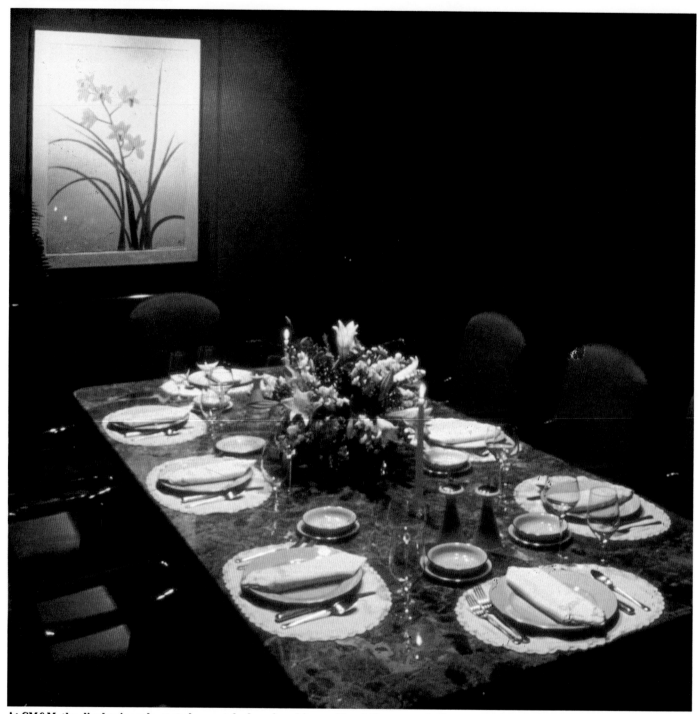

At CM&M, the display is understated—crystal, gleaming china and fresh flowers artfully arranged on polished marble.

EXECUTIVE DINING ROOMS

"What we serve is big, big business," says Stephen Elmont, president of Boston-based Creative Gourmets, Inc. His firm specializes in catering for executive dining rooms and his clients are primarily insurance companies, banks and investment firms.

Discretion is the better part
One of the most pressing reasons for the private dining room, at least to the moguls of the money world, is discretion. Mergers, international transactions and negotiations involving unparalleled sums need secrecy, and if Tycoon A is seen at a restaurant with Oil Minister B or Banker C, tremors might shake the stock market. Even within the executive dining room more caution might be taken: "I've seen men draw their chairs away from the table and confer in whispers," says executive dining room chef Miriam Brickman.

In principle, executive dining rooms are used mainly for lunch, although some are opened for the occasional breakfast or dinner meeting as well as for cocktail parties or receptions. Depending on company policy, the room may be used by one exalted chief executive officer or by 50 partners of a law firm and their guests.

It is difficult to estimate just how many executive dining rooms really exist in the country. Many companies veil the executive dining room from the public eye, fearing complaints of money-wasting from disgruntled stockholders who don't understand that, in most cases, the use is strictly for business. To a client, an invitation to an executive dining room is frequently more coveted than one to the finest restaurant in any city. In addition, these dining rooms often enable executives to make the most efficient use of time—a very elevated form of grabbing lunch at the desk.

Food for thought

Apparently the rich are not all alike, at least when it comes to lunch: "Each corporate culture requires a different form of cuisine," says Mr. Elmont. "A very traditional company will want, figuratively speaking, meat and potatoes, and at a firm that perceives itself as avant-garde, we'll see grilled baby vegetables and breast of duck."

Although Mr. Elmont was speaking figuratively of "meat and potatoes," that is a combination that appears with increasing rarity on the executive table. Red meat is seen as an unhealthful substance that can dull the keen competitive edge or encourage the occupational coronary threatening the strongly driven. Chicken and fish are most frequently served.

"Less red meat, absolutely, in the last five years," says Ivar Christensen, head of Restaurant Marketing Associates which operates a dozen executive dining rooms, "and in some cases we will list calorie and cholesterol information on the menu."

Gerd Johannsen, banquet manager of the United Nations dining rooms (a Restaurant Associates operation), finds that, contrary to the trend, red meat is very much in demand. Curries and other national dishes can be supplied on request, but there is little emphasis on them. Given the dietary restrictions of many delegates, pork is served only when asked for. The menu for a recent luncheon for 15:

**Smoked Trout
with Dill and Mustard Sauce
Medallion of Beef
with Braised Leeks
Chocolate Truffle Gâteau**

The legendary perfection of the old Lehman Brothers, under the direction of the distinguished William Proops (École Hôtelière in Lausanne, Cordon Bleu) continues at Shearson Lehman Brothers Inc. There is a set menu for the day, but partners and guests may choose whatever else they like from a dozen alternatives. Two hundred to 225 lunches are served each weekday in 11 dining rooms.

The lunch menu for a recent Monday:

**Consommé Julienne
Loin of Veal
Braised Leeks and Onions
White Asparagus
Salad of Endive and Arugula
Sorbet de Cassis**

Chef Julien Stuart will serve from 1 to 12 in the *Forbes Magazine* dining room. Although most executive lunches run from 40 to 45 minutes, the formalities at *Forbes* take considerably longer: A lunch given for Princess Lalla Miriem of Morocco took two hours. The menu:

**Spinach Dumplings
with Provençale Tomato Sauce
Veal Scallops with Wild Mushrooms
Fresh Asparagus
Saffron Lemon Rice
Fall Fruit Compote with Custard Sauce**

Another *Forbes* lunch, for the chairman of an important board:

**Galantine of Duck
Paupiettes of Sole
stuffed with Crabmeat
Sautéed Sugar Snap Peas
Glazed Finger Carrots
Raspberry-Mango Sorbet**

Art Wintermyer, general manager of food services at *The Washington Post*, reports that Lobster Tails in Cumberland Sauce is a hot-weather favorite. Veal—prime ribs and roulades—is replacing beef. For working

meetings, an omelette station, with individual omelettes whipped up to order, is popular.

Wall Street chef Rona Moulu cooks lunch for members of the CM&M Group, Inc., primary dealers in government securities. The executives host lunch on different days. "The executive who has the room on Mondays has gastroenteritis, and I know he always wants fish. So today's menu is Grilled Eggplant Slices with Garlic, drizzled with olive oil, Grilled Swordfish with Tarragon Butter, and Carrot Torte. One of the executives is both Italian *and* diabetic, so when he lunches I take both factors into account," she says. "When I came here four years ago there was lots of meat, but now that's out. But there is no holding back on dessert. And for the Monday and Tuesday breakfasts, there are requests for buttery three-egg omelettes and bacon. But red meat—no!"

Rona Moulu adds that some of the top men often *do* eat in their offices, but it's food that she prepares.

Alcohol in the executive dining room? That depends very much on the "corporate culture." Yes, at Shearson-Lehman Brothers (house wines and a wine list) and at the United Nations (both house and list); no, at the Dreyfus Fund and *The Washington Post*, where a bar is set up, but the offerings are sparkling waters, sparkling cider and sodas. At the J. Walter Thompson advertising agency, no hard liquor is served in the dining rooms until after business hours; but at lunch, wine (one board member owns a vineyard) and Miller Beer (Miller is a client) are available. The house wines served at *Forbes* are Mâcon-Lugny white and Château Duhart-Milon Rothschild red.

"I have been in this business since 1960," says Ivar Christensen, "and over the course of the years I have never seen an abundance of wine. And no three-martini lunches."

A setting to match

The rooms in which the carefully prepared food is served vary from the timeless elegance of the World Bank Headquarters to a seventeenth century room, removed from Ipswich, Massachusetts, and installed at the J. Walter Thompson Agency. Typical is the serenely lovely room at CM&M Group, with custom marble table, salmon paneled walls and a sweeping view of the Hudson River and the World Trade Towers.

Prestigious interior decorators are often responsible for the decor, and some food service contractors have their own in-house designers. "We can get in early on new buildings," says Ivar Christensen. "The request may be for an ultra-modern style or an ultra-conservative one, and we decorate accordingly."

Only a dyspeptic curmudgeon would fail to be charmed by the dining room in the New York townhouse of *Forbes Magazine*, designed by top-flight interior decorator Mario Buatta.

It's a small room, not much more than 12-feet-square, but the Waterford crystal chandelier hung from a silver ceiling illuminates a circular English table and Queen Anne chairs covered in needlework. The floor is *faux marbre*, in shades of green, yellow, beige and red. Mahogany-stained poles run around the top of the room, suspending, on brass rings, vibrant orange-red curtains of cotton printed moiré that cover all the walls. Paintings befitting the *Forbes* collection grace the room. A setting made for talk, both serious and convivial, this little room is a veritable Capitalist Power Lunchbox.

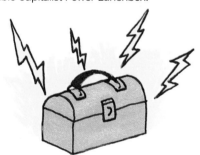

Behind the scenes

The position of executive dining room chef is considered a plum. To begin with, the hours are good—that is, for early risers. Chefs are often on the job between 7 A.M. and 8:15 A.M., and work until 2 P.M. or as late as 3:30 P.M. Dinners, cocktail parties and receptions extend the hours, of course, but there is generally a good bit of notice. More importantly, a chef usually has complete control of the kitchen and does as she or he pleases, within the limits set by the employer. Most chefs have a free hand to select the finest provisions, even when the executive dining room is run by a food service contractor.

Many chefs relish the opportunity to cook

consistently for the same person or persons, as opposed to the anonymous patrons of a restaurant. "I like the challenge of keeping them pleased," said one, "and that in turn pleases me." Whether a meal is simple or complex, the standards are exacting. Service must flow smoothly. "I've finally found a silent buzzer," says Rodney Madden, chef at *New York* magazine. "The host steps on it, and alerts me when the next course is wanted.

Salaries are considered good. "They [chefs] can make $30,000 a year for a Monday-to-Friday, six-hour-a-day job, with no stress," says Stephen Elmont, who employs a number of chefs for the companies he serves. That may be, but a chef expresses another point of view: "To come up to the highest level every day?" says Julien Stuart. "I'd say there's some stress."

In most dining rooms the chef might never see those at table, but others do—the waiting staff. These people must be trusted not to repeat anything they overhear. "Confidentiality is vital," says Ivar Christensen. "We try to screen the waiters and waitresses to see that they are reliable; we impress on them that they are here to serve. They make pretty good money, and we are able to train and keep a pool of trustworthy people wherever we need them—New York, Indianapolis or Phoenix."

Executive dining style depends on the boss. The $4.2 billion Marriott Corporation is perhaps the leader in the executive food service field. "We can put together an executive dining room that will knock your socks off," says a spokesman at the Bethesda, Maryland headquarters, "but that's not Bill Marriott's style. The executive dining room at Marriott is the employees' cafeteria." ●

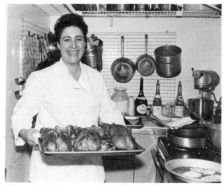

Rona Moulu serves duck to bulls and bears.

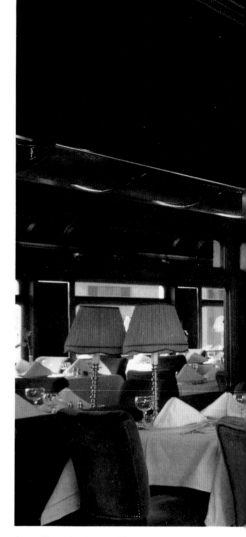

A replica of a luxury French restaurant car

Eating To The Lonesome Whistle

Advocates of *yesteryear* as the *better year* look fondly back to the 1930s and 40s as the time when train dining in America reached its peak of elegance. But nostalgia tends to be selective: Compared to an earlier yesteryear, say the 1830s, today doesn't look too bad. Back then, trains were merely stagecoaches drawn on tracks by mule or horse teams. You brought your own food or went hungry. When the real iron horse emerged, with central aisles, enterprising newsboys hawked not only papers but fruit, cake and water—poured into communal cups.

The next evolution anticipated airline food service. In 1853, the first caterers came on board, serving pre-cooked food on long ta-

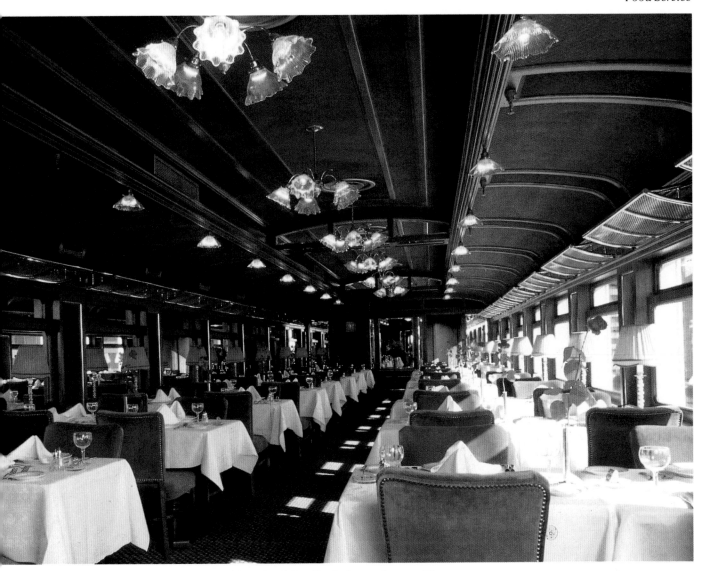

from the fabled *Train Bleu* as re-created for Bloomingdales. No shake, rattle, or roll here.

bles set up in coaches or baggage cars. If this was beyond your means, you made do with "station buffets," where greasy meals were offered during a 20-minute stop.

George Pullman introduced his restaurant car in 1868, making true dining on the move a reality. Suddenly, there was champagne for breakfast and other wonders, like regional specialities—buffalo, elk, mutton chops and grouse, for example, on a Western Territories line. Brand new railroad commissaries supplied trains with delicacies such as Alaska shrimp, California artichokes and Idaho trout. Train kitchens pulled out all the stops: One 1870s railroad menu offered 15 seafood items and 37 meat and game dishes.

Kitchen cars coped ingeniously with the hazards of fire and slithering containers. Thick iron slabs, called "flattops," transmitted heat from fires safely contained below, and brass rails kept the pots aboard when the train took curves at 40 miles per.

Restaurant cars grew more and more ornate throughout the 1890s, boasting stained glass, crystal and oriental carpets. But with the turn of the century, new notions of economy began to tangle with the good old ways.

By World War I, the Pennsylvania Railroad, for example, was losing $1 million a year on its dining car operations and economic realities are tough to ignore. The railroads didn't ignore them and reduced or totally eliminated their dining services. Snack bars, lunch counters and vending machines became the traveler's options and on some trains, the latter provided the only available food, even on overnight runs. To hardly anyone's surprise, "this was found to have a negative effect on ridership," says Barry Williams of the National Association of Railroad Passengers.

Fortunately for train lovers, this dismal dining scene doesn't end the tale. On Amtrak, the quasi-governmental entity that has operated all intercity passenger service in the U.S. since 1977, you'll still get microwaved snacks on short runs, but things are looking up. According to a company spokesman,

"We've recently advised all our cooks that hamburger patties must be heated separately from the buns, to keep them from tasting like cardboard."

On many overnight lines, Amtrak has restored full service dining, so you are likely to find real chefs, waiters and sometimes a maître d' in the dining car. Stainless steel tableware has replaced plastic utensils, and the fake table flower is now a silk rose. But Congress still isn't funding real flowers. ●

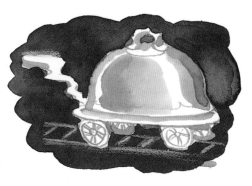

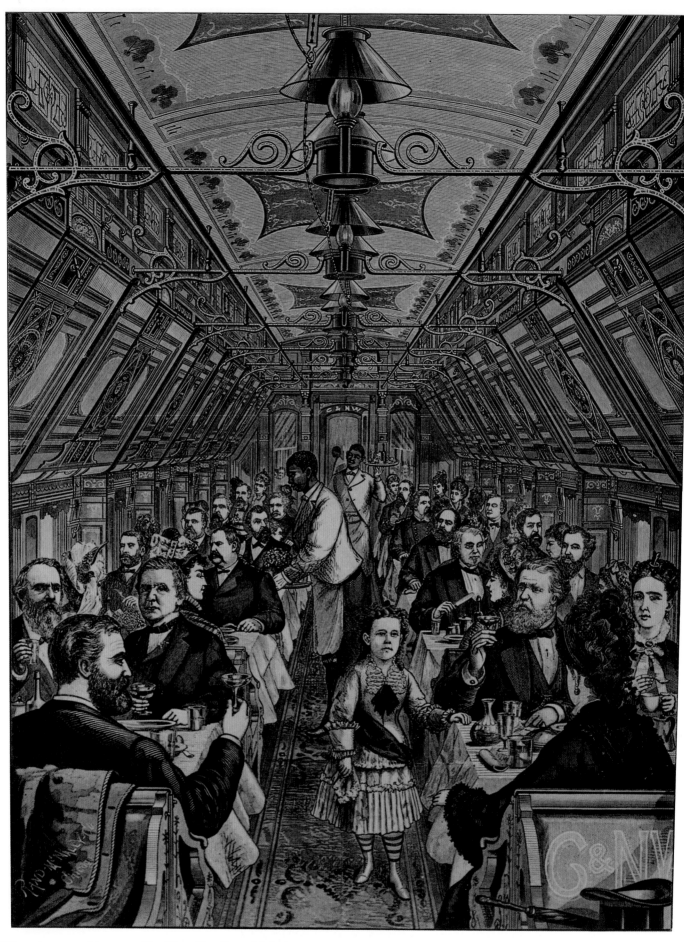

When steam was king, even Tom Thumb's wife couldn't always get a decent table.

High Style On Wheels

You can still eat in high style on an American train—in regal style if your garage shelters one of the nation's hundred or so privately owned railroad cars. It doesn't? Then ride one of the commercial luxury trains that sell the romance of railroad dining:

The Star Clipper

Two dining cars and a kitchen car, pulled by their own engine, make a round trip nightly on the Cedar Valley Railroad line between Osage and Cedar Falls, Iowa.

The three-and-a-half-hour ride allows 144 passengers to forage at a leisurely pace through their $35 classic midwestern dinner: a cream soup, followed by prime ribs, crabmeat in puff pastry or Rock Cornish hen on rice and Mud Pie for dessert. The Star Clipper's speed, a leisurely 12 miles per hour, encourages thorough digestion.

As you eat, you gaze out on a landscape floodlit to a distance of 60 feet. "There are lots of wild animals out there," says Walter Vining, the train's 74-year-old manager. "The countryside is beautiful. You see things you won't see from the highway or at 30,000 feet."

The American Zephyr

It was launched in 1984 by train buff John Hickman and Ken Wilson, a Maryland entrepreneur.

The train is lavish with Art Deco motifs: two cars elegantly dressed in black, silver and maroon fabrics, etched glass and chrome, with stainless steel exteriors. Name your poison, it's there—any brand, any land—in the lounge car's black-topped bar.

Replete with caviar and cocktails, you enter the dining car, with its small islands of pristine linen accented by fresh flowers in silver bud vases. Tonight you're dining on snapper turtle soup, Duck Scallopini Framboise and salad with chèvre cheese and raspberry vinaigrette. The dinner wines are fine Bordeaux. All is luxe.

The American Zephyr is mostly seen on the New York-Washington axis, but it also runs weekend excursions to Colonial Williamsburg, as well as to those opulent watering holes: The Homestead in Virginia and The Greenbrier in White Sulphur Springs, West Virginia.

As for the fare, bring your credit card. New York to Washington will nick you about $200, not exactly Amtrak prices. Passengers, however, don't complain. Some of them compare the American Zephyr favorably to the fabled Orient Express. And one young professional, a frequent Zephyr traveler, says, "All other ways to New York are insane by comparison." ●

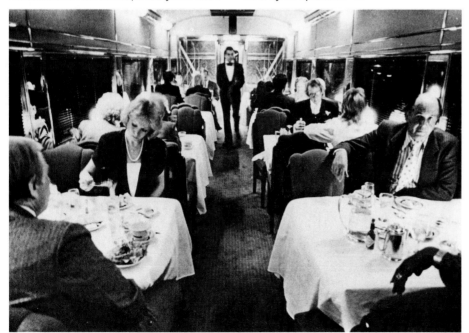

Attentive waiters, impeccable in black tie, recreate railroad romance—Zephyr style.

CAFE BEAUJOLAIS SOUR CREAM WAFFLES

Waffles are on the move in the popularity polls again.

Makes 8 waffles

Ingredients:
Sautéed apples:
2 tablespoons unsalted butter
1 firm, medium-size apple, peeled, cored and sliced
1/8 teaspoon ground cinnamon
1 1/2 teaspoons brown sugar

Waffles:
2 cups flour
2 1/2 teaspoons baking powder
3/4 teaspoon baking soda
1/2 teaspoon salt
1 1/2 tablespoons sugar
4 eggs, separated
1 cup sour cream
1 1/2 cups milk
3/4 cup plus 2 tablespoons melted unsalted butter or corn oil
1/2 cup chopped toasted pecans

Method:
1. To cook the apples, melt the butter in an 8-inch skillet over moderate heat. Add the apples and cook, stirring frequently, for 2 to 3 minutes. Stir in the cinnamon and sugar, reduce the heat to low, and cook, covered, for 2 to 3 minutes, until tender and golden brown. Cool slightly.

2. To make the waffles, sift together the dry ingredients.

3. Beat the egg yolks with the sour cream, milk and melted butter in a separate bowl until blended. Stir into the dry ingredients until blended well. Stir in the apples and the pecans.

4. Beat the egg whites until stiff, moist peaks form. Stir about 3 tablespoons of the beaten whites into the batter, then gently fold in the remaining egg whites until just combined.

5. Pour or ladle the batter over the center two-thirds of a hot waffle iron. Close the lid and cook for about 4 minutes, until the steam is no longer emerging from the crack. Remove the waffle and keep it warm in a warm oven while you cook the rest. Serve with butter and maple syrup.

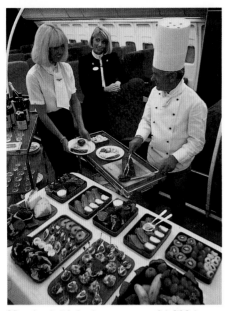

Marriott's high-class eats—at 34,000 feet.

Recipe For Mile High Meals

Airlines are bustling to bolster their food image, but fliers still have reservations.

"I dislike eating at a restaurant that's 30,000 feet in the air," says comedian Alan King. "You can't walk out."

Do passengers really suffer from the fare of flying, or is the whining about dining just a case of snob appeal?

"It's chic to say that airline food is terrible," says Jack Costello, United Airline's president of food services. "People are embarrassed to admit they really like it."

Last year, U.S.A. carriers spent about $1.5 billion on an estimated 150 million meals. Airline cuisine may never soar to the gastronomic heights of a Lutèce or Maxim's, but landlocked chefs aren't faced with the task of serving steak Diane in a metal tube hurtling through the stratosphere.

"It's a bad rap," says Terry Souers, director of corporate relations at Marriott, the nation's biggest airline food caterer. "Given the constraints, it's relatively good food.

"For a lot of people, not necessarily frequent fliers, flying is a big occasion," Souers says. "They expect it to be very special, like going to a really nice restaurant. It's an invalid comparison."

Yet airlines do strive for restaurant quality, even offering dozens of special-order meals including kosher, diabetic, low cholesterol, Hindu, Oriental, lactose-restricted, hypoglycemic, low sodium and children's portions. Specials, which account for less than 2 percent of all meals served, aren't widely advertised, primarily because they cost the airlines—not the passenger—more money.

"At every conference, every trade show, food is a major topic," says Barbara Losman, vice president at *Air and Travel Food Service*, a trade magazine. "Airlines are very aware of their image. Presentation is getting more sophisticated."

Fancy and fussy dinners, once the bane of airline caterers, are flying the trendy skies. First-class passengers are treated to stuffed quail eggs and smoked salmon on American and chicken Wellington on United.

Even People Express, the budget carrier with a no-frills reputation, offers (at extra charge) a gourmet buffet and chocolate-covered macadamia nuts.

Now in vogue: light meals. Delta frequently serves seafood, Eastern leans toward fish and pasta, and United just introduced shrimp in puff pastry and shredded chicken on a bed of spaetzle.

"It's a complex environment," says Jim Jette, Republic's director of food service. "You precook the food, freeze it, transport it to a plane, take it up to 34,000 feet, reheat and reconstitute it and serve it to maybe 150 passengers."

The complications:

Timetable

Because food is not delivered directly from the kitchen to the customer, only items that "hold" well are considered. "The food is put on a food truck one hour before field departure and served maybe another 1½ hours later," says Costello at United, which preps and boards meals at 110 locations. "That's a long delay." Fragile substances, such as poached eggs, don't have the necessary durability.

Turbulence

Obviously, chicken soup won't fly.

Dehydration

Gravy is a vital ingredient "partly for flavor enhancement but also to preserve food in an extremely dehydrated atmosphere," Eastern's Hal Carper says. "Beef with no sauce or maitre d' butter would get completely dried out." Dehydration also alters taste perceptions, perhaps contributing to the notion that airline food "tastes funny."

Cramped quarters

Weight and space limitations preclude the luxuries of onboard cooks. Seating arrangements render a meal of crab legs or barbecue ribs logistically impossible. And foods such as sauerkraut and grouper are nixed for their pungent odors.

Consistency

When a caterer receives airline menu instructions, nothing—from the grade of eggs to the placement of salt packets—is left to the imagination. "There is absolutely no flexibility in an airline menu," Jette says.

Several airlines that experimented with fresh meals are returning to composite meals, or "popouts," prepared by frozen food manufacturers. "The quality is more consistent when food is prepared at a single site instead of 120," Eastern's Carper says. "Trays have to be identical. You look at my plate, I look at yours. Everyone compares."

Menu fatigue

Menus are frequently rotated to assuage easily bored frequent fliers. When passengers grumbled, Eastern replaced its longstanding French toast breakfast with blueberry pancakes.

Expense

Carriers devote up to 4 percent of operating expenses toward meals. But airlines can't afford to be too lavish with food, particularly when fare wars cut profits to the bone. "We're always constrained by the almighty dollar," Jette says. "We carry food dollars to four decimal points. We know the exact yield of a case of leaf lettuce."

Striking a happy mediocrity

Airline meals are bland by design. Not only are fussy and exotic dishes a pain to prepare, but they tend to entice a smaller audience than such sure hits as ham sandwiches. "Spinach is very popular right now," Carper says. "That astounded us. Spinach doesn't look that attractive on the plate. But it's familiar. We hear that people are clamoring for what's innovative and different, but the dramatic dishes get very negative feedback."

United's Costello says, "We avoid extremes. We tried chili once. A chili eater loves it, but other people can't tolerate it." ●

Edna Gundersen, reporter, USA TODAY

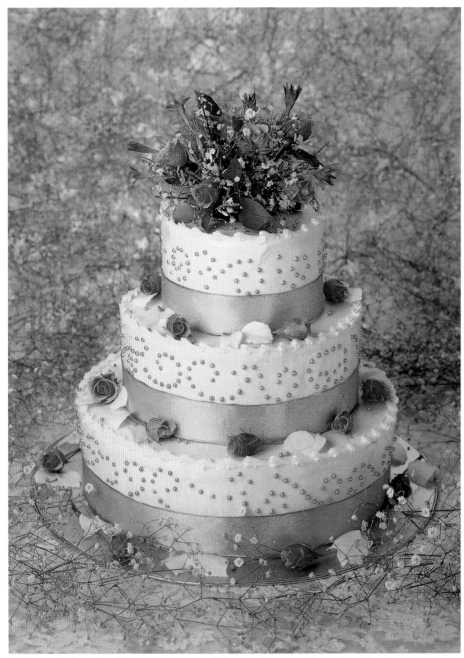

A famous baker of cakes never gets carried away, but sometimes the cake does.

My Brother's Wedding Cake

Rose Levy Beranbaum

Valentine's Day 1983 was the scheduled date for my only and beloved brother's San Francisco wedding. And it was with great joy that several weeks ahead of the event in my New York kitchen, I began to prepare a most spectacular wedding cake as my present to Michael and Suzy, his wife-to-be.

The cake was a triple-tiered fantasy, large enough to feed the 150 invited guests. The tiers consisted of layers of the softest white butter cake, filled with creamy classic buttercream and topped with pistachio marzipan. The frosting

was a Swiss white chocolate buttercream (invented especially for the occasion), and the cake was decorated with gold lamé ribbon from Paris, gold dragées, white chocolate rose leaves and a dozen real pink sweetheart roses. This was a very special cake not only because it was intended for my brother's wedding but also because it was destined to appear in Cook's *magazine,* and subsequently on the cover of and inside thousands of recipe booklets.

My cake's arrival at its most important destination, San Francisco, however, was

thwarted by fate: the great snowstorm of February 1983 which locked in the entire Northeast coast along with me and my cake.

Much planning had gone into the projected transportation of this perishable masterpiece. Because the photography for the magazine had been scheduled a few weeks before the wedding, the cake needed to be frozen during the interim. An ordinary freezer was not large enough, but my butcher, Ottomanelli, upon learning that the cake was for a family wedding, sympathetically offered a safe corner amongst the carcasses in his spacious walk-in freezer. Our father, a cabinetmaker, fashioned a special protective crate to protect the cake from possible falling sides of beef or lamb in the freezer or from unknown hazards in the belly of the airplane. My publicist arranged special red-carpet treatment for me and the cake en route so the airlines consented to store the crated cake in the plane's kitchen. Fresh roses were ordered from the florist. In short, everything was perfectly planned. The plans of mice and men . . . !

The snow started falling early in the morning the day of the flight. My 98-year-old Grandmother and my Aunt Ruth were already on their way to California from their home in Pompano Beach, Florida. My parents had departed from Kennedy airport hours before. The airlines suggested that I board an earlier flight than the one I had booked, as the snow seemed to be coming faster than anticipated, so I picked up the cake from the butcher shop, optimistically leaving all the baggage for my husband (who was unable to leave work earlier than originally planned), and set out for Newark airport.

No seats in "Tourist" were available on the earlier flight so the airline offered me a First Class seat which I enthusiastically accepted. Having made sure that the cake was safely stored in the kitchen below, I sat looking out the window, watching the snow steadily falling, feeling relieved to have obtained a seat on what was purported to be the last flight to leave Newark airport that day. "Let's go! Let's go!" I thought as the snow fell thicker and thicker. Then the inevitable announcement: "We are now below minimal clearance . . . but this flight has not officially been cancelled." A fellow passenger snickered at the word officially. The key words of doom, "below minimal" and "cancelled," sank in as part of my brain desperately clung to the "not officially" part. Gradually the horrible truth hit me with full impact. Not only was my brother not to have this much-planned and most extraordinary wedding cake, worse yet: He was not going to have me at his wedding!

When it was officially decided that the passengers were to disembark, I obtained permission to store my cake in the terminal's refrigerator. I then called my husband to ask him to pick me up only to hear that the storm had become so severe that the streets in Manhattan were impassable. He suggested that I take the airport bus to the Port Authority.

With some indignation, I got in line for the bus to New York and soon considered myself lucky to have been the last person to get a seat on the last departing bus. Four hours later I began to think I would have been luckier to have missed that bus and luckier still to manage to get back to the airport terminal! All traffic had stopped. The bus had no facilities (the bathroom was locked) and no gas gauge. The driver was forced to open the door for ventilation, thus also admitting the exhaust fumes from countless other vehicles. The situation seemed unbelievable. Could this familiar city terrain have become a wilderness over which we had no control?

Could we all freeze to death, stranded between Newark airport and the Lincoln Tunnel? Would people from the nearby houses take us in or would they panic like those in lifeboats fleeing the sinking Titanic and bar their doors?

Passengers started to take sides. The majority wanted to attempt a turnaround and go back to the terminal. The few who kept insisting that they wanted to go to New York (they simply would not accept the reality that getting to New York was now impossible) were transferred to a bus behind us and several young male passengers forged onto the snow-filled highway to direct traffic to back up or move forward a few feet to give us space to turn. Despite my distress, I could not help but notice what a splendid study of human nature this emergency was presenting. Already our small bus had become a mini-community with its different personality types.

With all remaining passengers in full agreement, we headed back to the airport but got stuck in a drift at the foot of the hill four miles from the first terminal. The snow was already several feet high and I started to wonder how long it takes to get frostbitten without boots. Luckily a nearby taxi offered (after much arm-twisting and demands for fare) to take six of us up to the main terminal. The rest would have to walk.

The first terminal (where my cake was stored) was dark and locked for the night, but the second terminal a quarter mile down the road was filled with people who had already commandeered sleeping areas for themselves and their families. Hordes of people were stretched out on every available chair and all over the floor. Any food in the canteens had long since been consumed. I found a relatively cozy spot on the red-carpeted, snail-shaped section of the baggage unloading area and curled up to sleep. (Here at last was my red-carpet treatment!) I slept fitfully all night, wakened occasionally by the surrounding noise and the empty feeling in my stomach from not having eaten since the night before; remembering that I was going to miss the wedding, trying to swallow the disappointment, then going back to sleep. There was nothing to do.

When dawn broke we were informed that no planes would be able to take off until perhaps one or two days later. I managed to locate one of the managers and asked if the airlines would hold my cake until I could come back by car to reclaim it. He looked at me in a kind of puzzled way and said: "There is no more cake." Then he smiled. So I thought he was teasing me. "Well, what happened to the cake?" I asked, pretending to go along with the joke. "Oh, we ate the cake," he said with imperturbable Oriental calm. "You what?" I practically screamed, starting to believe him. He then explained, with total confidence that I would see the logic of his decision, that there had been no room in the terminal refrigerators for the food from the stranded planes so the crew had removed my cake to make room for those incomparable airline delicacies. Then, evidently, assuming (incorrectly) that the cake would spoil unrefrigerated, they proceeded to consume it so that it would not go to waste. Not even the special crate remained. ●

Rose Levy Beranbaum is a teacher, journalist and author of the forthcoming *Cordon Rose Cake Book* (William Morrow and Company, Inc.).

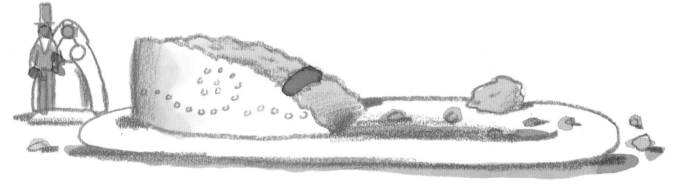

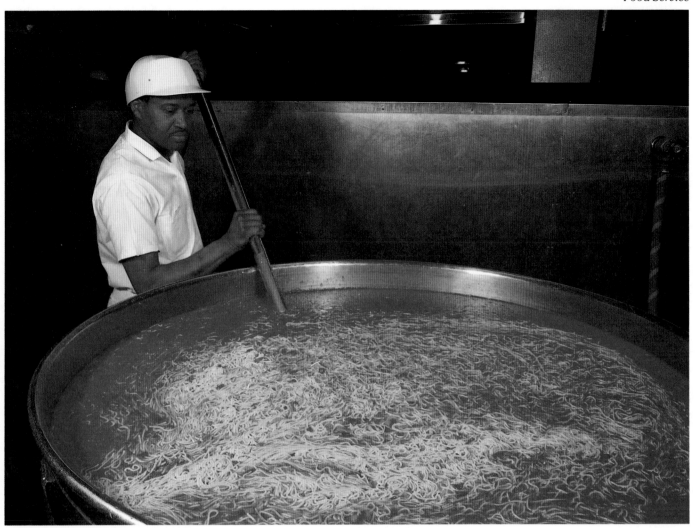

Standing tall among the Mexican, Chinese and even Greek foods on school menus today is that great and nourishing favorite—pasta.

Bringing Up Eaters

Taking the cue from their elders, no doubt, our kids are becoming connoisseurs of tacos, nachos and burritos; of yam threads, sesame noodles and oriental vegetables. They're also into Greek gyros and practically anything that can be stuffed into a pita.

Indeed, we have trained them so well—if our example of eating widely qualifies as "training"—that they are even showing an interest in healthy foods, a truly radical development in children's eating behavior. Radical squared, when you consider that the scene of this exemplary conduct is your public elementary and high school cafeteria.

Not to be believed? Believe.

You have it on the word of Bill Mulcrone, an official at the American School Food Service Association (ASFSA). "The only vegetable kids used to eat voluntarily was corn," he says. "Now they actually ask for broccoli."

A little history is in order here. At one time, schools were obliged to serve the so-called Type A lunch: five boring portions of protein, bread, two vegetables or fruit and milk. Children had to eat every bit of it (well, let's be

honest, *accept* the obligatory menu; after all, the trash bin was always nearby) for the school to get its expenses back.

Some wise regulator, no doubt having seen the rampant opportunities for deception,changed rules in 1976. The government agreed it was OK if a child selected only three approved items. The result was what you usually get when you give people options, not directives.

To compress a lot of history, the new menus made it possible for food service directors to compete successfully with Burger King, bag lunches and school vending machines. And kids can now put together a well-balanced meal—say, an orange plus a slice of pizza and a carton of milk—without having the tiresome message hammered home that "it's good for you."

Choice is wonderful.

Food companies also saw the opportunities in the fast-growing, $10.4 billion school food service market. La Choy, an oriental food company that was rapidly domesticated after its acquisition by the giant Beatrice,

succeeded in spreading its noodles throughout California's public high school system. La Choy egg rolls now come in Italian and Mexican varieties as well as Chinese.

It seems one can't be too young to join this latest consumer surge. The schools in Nashville, Tennessee have installed buffet counters only 27 inches from the floor so that tots short enough to ride public transport for half-fare can practice putting their own meals together. ●

The Great Public Schools Food Lottery	
Currently Favored	Yesterday's Winners
1. Pizza	1. Hamburgers
2. Hamburgers	2. Pizza
3. Tacos	3. Hot dogs
4. Burritos	4. Spaghetti
5. Fried chicken	5. Fried chicken

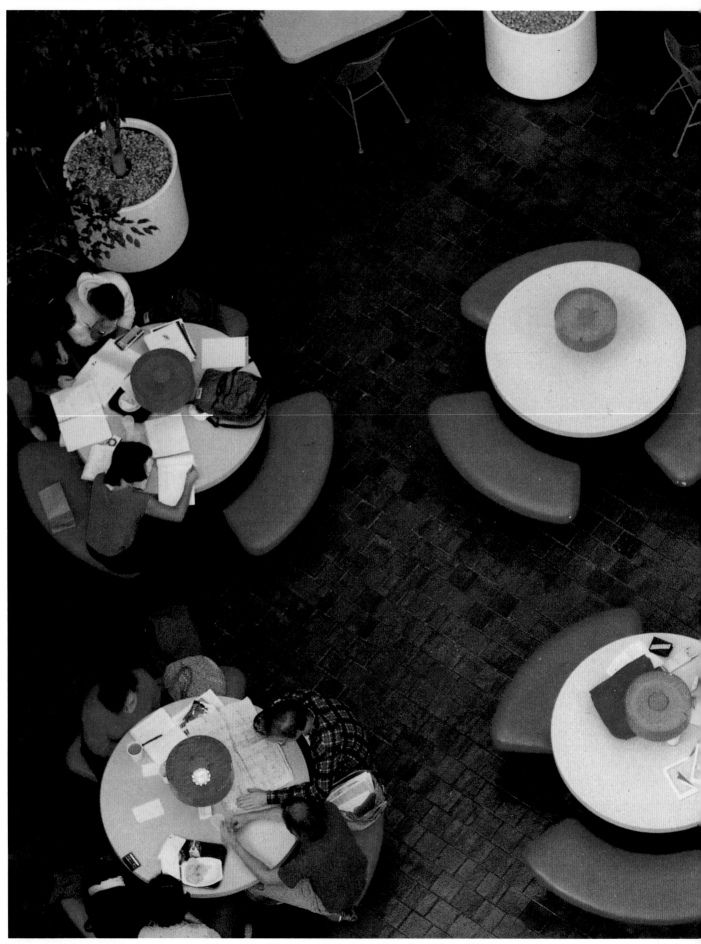

Students eat in colorful splendor at the University of Rochester's dining hall designed by I. M. Pei.

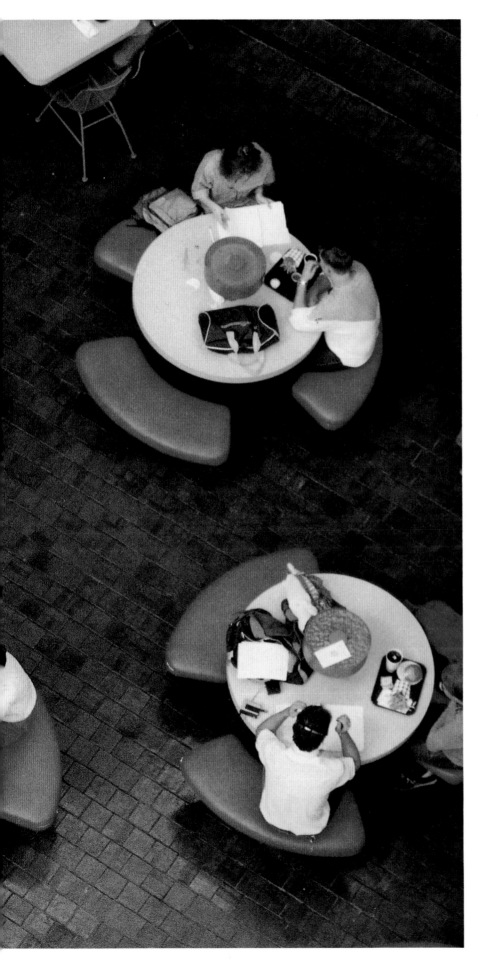

The High End Of Student Eaters

"We're not just selling food, we're selling service and sociability," says Don Jacobs, president of the National Association of College and University Food Services and director of dining services, University of Pennsylvania.

At best, it's an uphill struggle for the $4.4 billion college food service industry, $3 billion of which is handled in-house by colleges and universities without the aid of professional food service contractors. Students aren't playing the old standard game. They're staying home and preparing their own vittles instead of eating in the available institutional establishments. They prefer living in apartments or apartment-style quarters with kitchens (for obvious reasons) rather than in dorms. And even the dormies have discovered the practical utility of hot plates, toaster ovens and microwaves.

One recent study reported that probably 30 percent of college students regularly do their own cooking. As for some-time cooking, about 68 percent of the men and 76 percent of the women polled admitted they cooked at least "occasionally."

This is not heartening news for college food service divisions, but a golden opportunity for convenience food companies, the main suppliers of the foods that students are likely to cook (read "heat"). Students, it turns out, are loyal to brands they first tried while in college. What a bonanza for all those stars in the processed foods firmament—Campbell, General Foods, Beatrice, Carnation, General Mills and the rest—who offer heat-and-eat quality and convenience to the lazy cook.

The battle lines are drawn, with college food service directors right in the line of fire. Many of them are scrambling for aggressive marketing strategies that will not only keep them in a precarious business but, better yet, might even provide them with a return on their investment.

Among the wily players are organizations like SAGA, an experienced supplier of institutional food services that has been the leading off-campus feeder of collegians since 1978. SAGA is meeting the competition of McDonald's et al and campus home cooking head on. It's now delivering pizza, the number one favorite, to dormitories, and is considering an end run around the campus home cookers by opening campus stores where students can shop for staples—SAGA staples, of course. ●

The Restaurant That Aims To Keep You Healthy

"Nobody comes to the hospital to eat," says Ross Bell, Director of Food Services at The Mount Sinai Hospital in Manhattan. "Yet it's amazing how much better some people eat in a hospital than they do at home."

They eat pretty well at Mount Sinai, where the hospital's food operations have been managed in association with the Marriott Corporation's Health Care Division for the past four years. Fresh fruits and salads are always available and patients can choose from over 20 dinner entrées on their restaurant-style menus. There are special alternate food items available for patients who cannot order off the regular menu. Strictly kosher patients have a kosher selection similar to that listed on the restaurant menu.

Moreover, the majority of the food is made from scratch in Mount Sinai's own kitchen, where a staff of 253 prepares around 2,400 meals daily for 900 patients and another 2,500 meals for employees and visitors.

At over $2 million for 1986, the food bud-get is no small potatoes. Mount Sinai goes through 20 cases of 50-pound bags of the tubers per week, in addition to 600 other food items. Heading the list is chicken, at $1,575 spent weekly for 2,500 pounds served in ten-ounce portions. Other big weekly buys include 90 cases of four-ounce orange juice packs, 30 cases of head lettuce and 20 cases of apples. The kitchen computer keeps waste down to a level of two percent. "Five percent is doing good," says Bell.

The bulk of the food is delivered three times a week by a 36-foot Marriott truck that leaves a Maryland distribution center at midnight, reaches a regional warehouse in New Jersey by 4 A.M. and Mount Sinai by 6 A.M. Produce arrives six days a week from the New Jersey warehouse. Other perishables are bought locally: 2,800 half-pints of milk a day from Queens and about 1,200 slices of pre-packaged bread from Brooklyn. And, says Bell, "We'll go out for special requests like white seedless grapes." ●

Happy As We Are, Thanks The indigent patients at Parkland Hospital, a tax-supported county hospital in Dallas, Texas—where John F. Kennedy was taken—couldn't care less about having raw sliced mushrooms on their salads. Or about asparagus.

"We tried them," says Celia Krazit, food services director, "and they bombed." Though questioned monthly, the patients stick to the tried and true items on their two-week, no-choice menu: chicken-fried steak and turnip greens; turkey and cornbread dressing; sweet potato pie, raisin bread pudding and pineapple upside-down cake.

Last year the 750-bed hospital served 1,300,000 meals at a daily raw food cost of $3.35 for each patient. Six years ago, that cost was 40¢ a day for "a hundred versions of ground beef, macaroni and tomato casserole," remembers Krazit. Currently, the state's depressed oil and gas industries are contributing fewer taxes to social programs, and Parkland may have to cut back on next year's food budget by 5 percent. ●

Menu DOs and DON'Ts It can take 20 minutes for food to travel from the hospital kitchen to your bedside. Food with large flat surface areas cools fastest. Therefore, toast may be out, unless there is a toaster on your floor and a willing nurse. Casseroles and meats with gravies will be in.

One enterprising administrator reports, "The dietitians complained that the fish was arriving cold. Now we roll it up instead of serving it flat." ●

They Might Also Starve You

You might be eating better than ever in your hospital luxury suite, but starving in intensive care. "Malnutrition is said to cause 50,000 preventable hospital deaths per year in the U.S. alone, while affecting another half million patients' recoveries," says Pieter Halter, executive editor of *Biomedical Business International*.

Dr. Stanley J. Dudrick, a clinical professor of surgery at the University of Texas at Houston, says that over 30 percent of U.S. hospi-

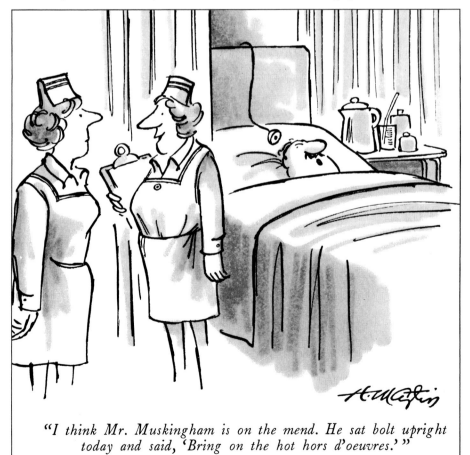

"I think Mr. Muskingham is on the mend. He sat bolt upright today and said, 'Bring on the hot hors d'oeuvres.'"

tal patients are malnourished. And a third of them have lost 30 percent of their ideal body weight, leaving [them] only a 5 percent chance of surviving an operation.

Unlike the need for open heart surgery, malnutrition is hard to spot. Some hospitals ignore basic nutritional support, a costly endeavor that can easily come under pressure from price cutters. And of the 470 categories spelled out by the new Medicare reimbursement policies, not one applies specifically to nutrition.

In 1968, Dudrick invented a new technology to cure the malnutrition problem. Unlike previous methods of intravenous feeding, his Total Parenteral (in a manner other than through the digestive canal) Nutrition system can deliver all necessary nutrients. But neither his invention nor the basic research it inspired have been adequately used.

"However," says Dr. George Blackburn of the Harvard Medical School, "recognition of the problem has been growing, and most medical schools now offer at least one course in nutrition." ●

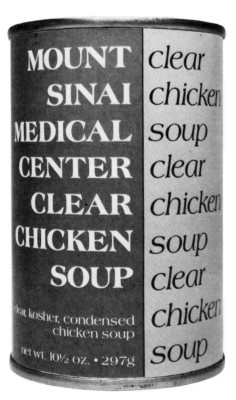

Mt. Sinai (Miami) packages the best treatment your sniffles can expect.

CHICKEN SOUP WITH RICE

Here is a chicken soup that combines all the elements of our most favorite and comforting foods: a pure, homemade, slow-simmered chicken broth with health-giving rice and sparkling fresh vegetables.

Serves 6

Ingredients:
3 1/2 pounds chicken, cut into pieces, with giblets
2 medium-size onions, peeled and coarsely chopped
2 medium-size leeks, coarsely chopped
1 carrot, peeled and sliced
2 stalks celery, sliced
1 bay leaf
1/2 teaspoon thyme
1 teaspoon peppercorns
4 sprigs parsley
8 cups water
1/2 cup uncooked rice
2 carrots, peeled and cut into strips 2 inches long and 1/8 inch wide
2 stalks celery, cut into strips 2 inches long and 1/8 inch wide
1/2 small turnip, peeled and cut into strips 2 inches long and 1/8 inch wide
1 cup freshly shelled peas
1 very ripe tomato, peeled, seeded and chopped
1 teaspoon sage
1 teaspoon salt
Freshly ground black pepper to taste
3 tablespoons finely chopped parsley

Method:
1. Put the chicken and the giblets (except the liver) in a large saucepan. (Note: Do not add the liver because it will make the broth cloudy; reserve for another use.)

2. Add the onions, leeks, carrot, celery, bay leaf, thyme, peppercorns, parsley and water. Adjust the lid so the saucepan is 3/4 covered. Simmer for 45 minutes over low heat.

3. Remove the chicken from the broth and set it aside until it is cool enough to handle. Separate the chicken from the skin and bones. Cut the chicken into bite-size pieces and reserve. Return the skin and bones to the saucepan. Partially cover the saucepan and simmer for 1 1/2 hours.

4. Strain the broth and discard the solids. Cool the broth, pour it into a large jar or bowl and chill it in the refrigerator for 8 hours. Discard the fat which will have risen to the surface.

5. Pour the broth into a clean, large saucepan and bring to the boiling point. Add the rice and cook for 15 minutes. Add the carrots, celery and turnip and continue cooking for 5 minutes. Add the peas, tomato, sage, salt and the reserved chicken and simmer for 5 minutes. Season with pepper, taste and adjust seasoning as needed. Garnish with parsley.

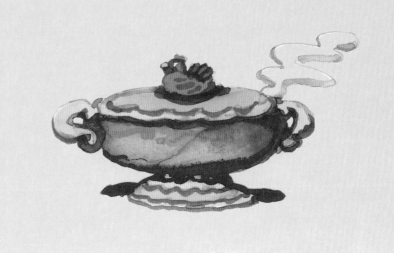

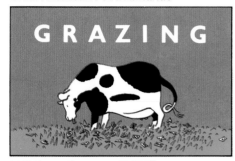

GRAZING

We Are Where We Eat

More ketchup is consumed in New Orleans than in any other city. More popcorn is sold in Dallas than elsewhere, and more candy bars and marshmallows in Salt Lake City. The reasons, as theorized by local residents of these cities quoted by the Associated Press, were: because so much fried seafood is served in New Orleans restaurants to patrons who douse it all with ketchup; because Dallas is still a place where lots of people go out to the movies; and because Mormons, who make up much of the population of Salt Lake City, consume less alcohol than other groups, and therefore make up for it in sugar intake.

One-Tree Orchard If for some reason you longed to raise five varieties of apples but only had a few square feet of earth, you could do it. Due to ingenious grafting, dwarf apple trees can now be obtained from specialist nurseries that grow as many as five varieties on one tree.

Sweet Soup Campbell is now making its chicken soup in five different qualities at five different prices, from 29 cents to $1.99. Because taste tests have shown that people with the least to spend on food have the biggest sweet tooth, the lowest-priced cans will contain the largest amounts of sugar.

Temptation, Thy Name Is Saffron The thrifty Pennsylvania Dutch, who usually deny themselves material pleasures, are major consumers of the world's most expensive spice, saffron. They use it to flavor chicken dishes, such as chicken-corn soup, sauces, noodles, even Schwenkfelder, their traditional wedding cake. This seeming anomaly may be explained by the fact that their ancestors had cultivated saffron in Germany centuries ago, and in 1734, when the Schwenkfelders, a group of Silesian immigrants, settled in Pennsylvania, they brought a supply of the costly spice with them.

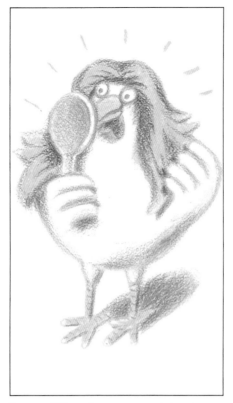

Patented Pies Sugar cream pie has been a specialty of Indiana home cooks for many years. Similar to the transparent pie eaten in the South, sugar cream pie has a flaky lard crust, with a filling made of high-butterfat cream, sugar, vanilla, nutmeg and shortening, and thickened with a little flour.

Duane Wickersham, whose company, Wick's Pies, is the only commercial producer of this regional specialty, believed the pie was so unique that it deserved a patent. The United States Patent Office agreed, and in 1962, Wick's Sugar Cream Pie became the first pie to be so honored.

If Only I'd Been Told Sooner I Could Have Been Doing This All My Life Six paragraphs of detailed instructions on how to wash your hands were recently reprinted in *Restaurant Business* magazine, in their entirety, from a publication called "Safe Food Preparation: It's In Your Hands." The instructions, summarized, were:
1. Wet hands thoroughly.
2. Apply soap to the hands.
3. Wash hands by rubbing one against the other.
4. Rinse off.
5. Dry hands thoroughly.

Nonconformist Fruit It may be perfectly obvious once we point it out, but you probably never gave it a thought: Strawberries, raspberries and blackberries have their seeds on the outside whereas other fruits and vegetables have them within.

Another Unsung Hero Edwin E. Perkins, of Hendley, Nebraska, first offered a flavored syrup called Fruit Smack as a mail-order item in 1922. You may recognize today's name for the product: Kool-Aid.

Egg-Alitarianism

If you encounter slices of hard-boiled egg on an airplane, perhaps, or in a hospital or school cafeteria, each slice is probably not cut from a single egg. It is more likely a slice from a very long egg roll. This is not the sort of egg roll served in Chinese restaurants and not the sort staged on the White House lawn every Easter, but the kind that is created these days by food processors to give "perfect" slices every time keeping the yolk dead center. To accomplish this, an elongated roll of cooked yolks is created and then encased in an elongated ring of cooked whites. This means your slice is actually a single slice of a great many eggs, paradoxical as that may seem.

There's A New Bleached Blonde In Town The preference for white meat over dark among chicken and turkey eaters is so prevalent in America that the food industry has been looking for a way to turn dark meat into light. The answer, which might seem obvious to any hairdresser, has now been found by researchers at Clemson University, who bleach the dark meat with peroxide. They have also found a way to perforate the dark meat in such a way that the result, it is claimed, "has the texture and color of breast meat."

As the customer might have said to the hairdresser: No thanks. I prefer it natural.

1-800-4-Caviar A company called Caviarteria Inc., which also bills itself as "The Caviar Center of the U.S.A.," can be called at this number any hour of the day or night (just in case it's an emergency) to order the precious fish eggs. However, if you're in New York State dial, 212-759-7410.

THE PRINTED WORD

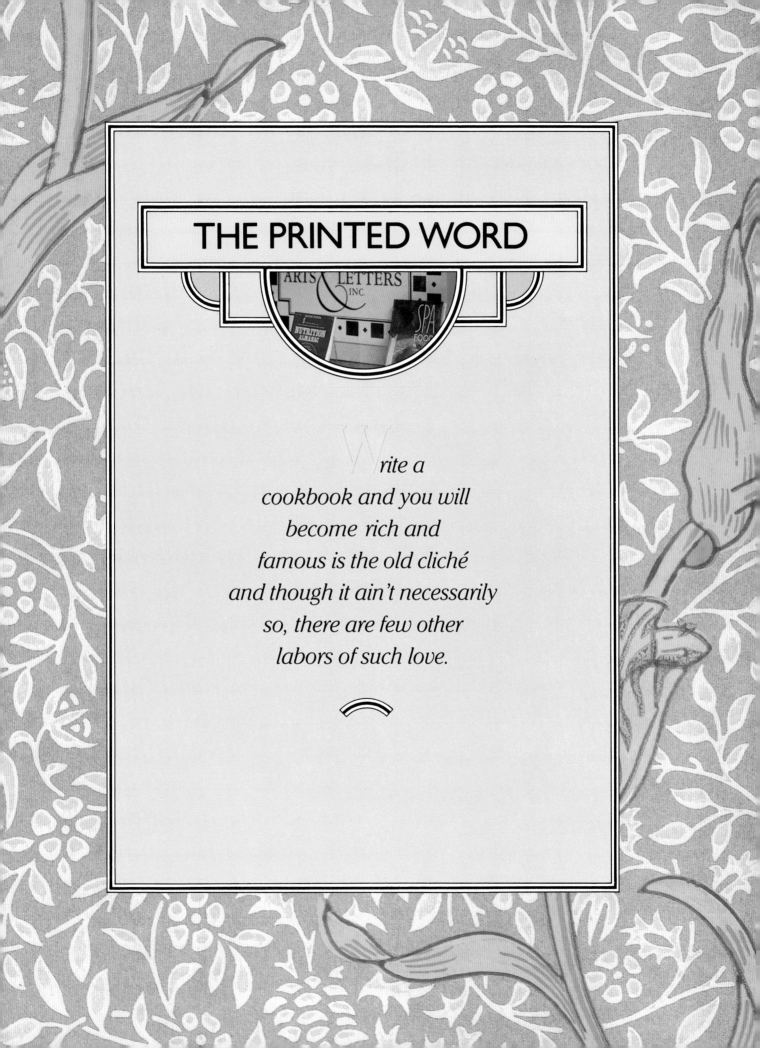

Write a
cookbook and you will
become rich and
famous is the old cliché
and though it ain't necessarily
so, there are few other
labors of such love.

COOKBOOKS: WHO WRITES THEM? WHAT SELLS THEM?

The odd thing about cookbooks is that everyone who was ever praised for kitchen competence thinks he or she could write one, innocently supposing that all it takes to produce a bestseller is a handful of recipes and enough time to type them onto the page.

At the same time, few of us, I think, would take so casual an approach to some other field. Who would suppose that to be a concert pianist, all you need is a bunch of black and white keys, a conductor waving wildly, and there you are taking bows on the stage at Carnegie Hall. To play Wimbledon's Centre Court? Nothing simpler: Just buy a tennis racket and a can of balls. Right!

Yet this assumption is true of cookbooks. If you haven't thought of writing one yourself, I'll bet you can come up quickly with the name of someone you know who either has been involved with a cookbook project, or would like to be.

The commonly-held underlying notion, of course, is that all cookbooks *sell,* but, alas, that is not so. According to statistics gathered by R.R. Bowker for *Subject Guide to Books in Print,* 1,137 books on food and wine were published in 1985, and most of those, according to one industry source, "have a shelf life somewhere between milk and yogurt."

Nothing succeeds like success

This is the way it works. The cookbook industry is not unlike the fashion industry, in that when an idea appears to be successful for one, others rush into imitate. For example, Mrs. Irma Rombauer published *Joy of Cooking* in 1931. It has since sold ten million copies in hardcover alone, and three other editions have, together, sold yet another ten million. That amounts to 20 million in round words. And it is impossible to guess the number of cooks who have referred to it by begging, borrowing or stealing; this classic is to be found in an astoundingly large number of kitchens in America.

The result: Clones of *The Joy* (and any other successful cookbook) abound, hoping for coattail glory. Sometimes it even happens that a subsequent refinement of someone's original idea will do better in sales, especially if the publisher nourishes the clone with infusions of advertising and

publicity. Particularly successful in recent years are the clones that promise to deliver "Everything you ever wanted to know about . . ."

On being definitive

One peculiarly American contribution to the literature of cooking is the establishment of these so-called definitive works. These are books written by authors living in America who make profoundly serious, scholarly studies of the cuisine of another country—somewhat on the order of edible Ph.D. theses. The American food world anointed the late James Beard *President of the U.S.A.* when it was recognized that he was the first author of stature to write admiringly about American food. He had in fact been passionate on the subject for a very long time before it became fashionable to think American Cooking worth discussing.

After Julia Child published *Mastering the Art of French Cooking* (Knopf), food professionals dubbed her *The Queen of France.* Marcella Hazan (*The Classic Italian Cookbook,* Knopf) and Giuliano Bugialli (*The Fine Art of Italian Cooking,* Times Books) are both of Italian origin, and both have produced solidly researched works in their special field. Thus wags have it that Bugialli is *Il Duce,* while Hazan more than shares primacy with him as the *Sophia Loren* of Italian cooking.

Because of the excellence of *The Cuisines of Mexico* (Harper & Row), Diana Kennedy is said to "own" Mexico, while Elizabeth Andoh (*An American Taste of Japan,* William Morrow) is acknowledged *Empress of Japan.* Grace Chu's solid work on Chinese Cooking has won her widespread respect, though—in keeping with the egalitarianism of China today—no imperial title. Paula Wolfert has gone one better than everybody else by standing astride the Mediterranean, one foot in Morocco (*Couscous and Other Good Food,* Harper & Row) and the other in Southwest France (*The Cooking of South-West France,* Dial Press, Doubleday). This makes her a colossus, at least.

Similarly, other authors claim specific segments of the food world. These days we are seeing Sheila Lukins and Julee Rosso, manufacturers of specialty foods, as the

Golden Girls of the Silver Palate. Their two books together have passed the magical 1.5 million-copy mark. Jeff Smith (*The Frugal Gourmet,* William Morrow) has lived on the bestseller list for more than a year; Martha Stewart has seduced and entertained us with her glamorous food; Pierre Franey seems to be able to make anything in 60 minutes; and Jane Brody instructs us firmly on how to eat properly. Reigning over all, M.F.K. Fisher is the undisputed bard of all things culinary.

There is yet another type of definitive work engulfing the food world: Celebrity chefs are now taking up their pens to share their secrets. Alice Waters, Paul Prudhomme (whose *Chef Paul Prudhomme's Louisiana Kitchen,* William Morrow, was a staple on the bestseller list for eight months), Larry Forgione, Bradley Ogden, Christopher Idone, Wolfgang Puck and Jeremiah Tower are among the new stars in our cookbook firmament . . . and, of course, we must have every new book that comes along, to add to our collection. Even if we cook meatloaf—a phenomenon that has lately acquired undreamed-of cachet—every Friday, and eat Lean Cuisine three other nights, there is always the lingering good resolution to do better, to cook Michael Foley's superb Cassoulet of Mussels so that we will be loved by all and acclaimed a *good cook.*

Tying up the package

A very significant segment of the eating community really is passionate about wanting to own every cookbook that comes along. If the subject is really appealing, there's a good chance that the book will be snapped up and carried home by a buyer with high hopes and noble aspirations. Price does not always seem to be the deciding factor. Of far greater significance today is the number of color pictures included; it is also crucial that the recipes appear to be do-able. Most readers are put off by incoherent instructions and the solemnity of black words stacked thick.

The cover alone can make or break a cookbook. If the food on the cover of the book is too beautiful, then the reader will think that he or she can't cook like that, and will simply walk away. If the food is not beautiful enough, the prospective buyer

The Future Of Cookbooks May Be Past

Jason Epstein, vice-president and editorial director of Random House, speaks of the guarded optimism of publishers regarding cookbooks: "People in this country have been irrevocably exposed to good food. The process will slowly be democratized and will eventually translate into the sale of more and more cookbooks—unless something goes drastically wrong with the economy."

Others disagree, and think that the sales of cookbooks will stabilize at a lower plateau. With 49 million women now working, such cooking as can be done must be on the weekend or for entertaining. As *Vogue* contributing editor Barbara Kafka has noted, this is very different from cooking for a family. Some think that the cookbooks of the future will be strongly oriented to fast preparation of fresh ingredients. There will always be room for the deeply researched, 20-times tested recipes from the best of authors. But the days of hoping to sell Aunt Prudence's Favorite Recipes from Cat Hollow, or 365 Exciting New Ways to Cook Leftover Okra, are long gone. ●

The First Real American Cookbook Written By Amelia Simmonds In 1796: *American Cookery: The Art Of Dressing Viands, Fish, Poultry And Vegetables And The Best Modes Of Making Pastes, Puffs, Pies, Tarts, Puddings, Custards And Preserves And All Kinds Of Cakes From The Imperial Plum To The Plain Cake Adapted To This Country And All Grades Of Life.*

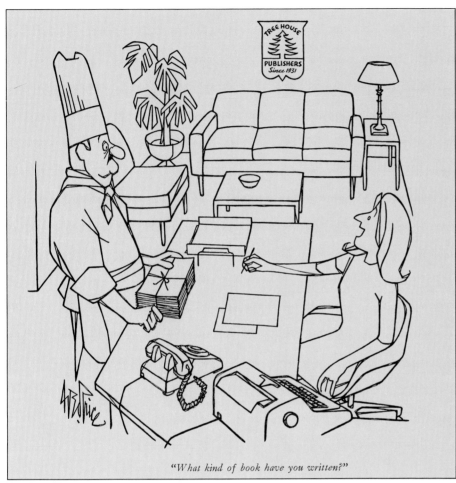

"What kind of book have you written?"

will walk away for a different reason, saying, "Ick! Who wants to cook *that*?" Some think that it is a terrible mistake to put a chef on the cover, dolled up in his *toque* and grinning smugly. The prospective buyer will think that the book is full of impossibly difficult recipes. A picture of an empty kitchen and an empty mixing bowl is no more acceptable than a picture of two eggs, a whisk, a wedge of cheese and one chicken ready for autopsy. Thus, cookbook covers present what book designers call *a challenge.*

Cookbooks are chancy for publishers. They can find a very attractive cookbook author who seems perfect for wowing TV audiences with wit and charm, and the next thing you know, he or she has evoked from the audience not the warm feelings anticipated, but a deep loathing. Shelf life of the new book: zero. Cooking is one of the most competitive indoor sports, and no one likes

to roll up sleeves in the kitchen with a teacher who is too witty, too glamorous, too intimidating. (Martha Stewart, witty, glamorous *and* successful, is one exception to this argument.)

So—you want to write a cookbook

First go to a large bookstore and stand for an hour in the cookbook section, thumbing through the books there. Each represents hundreds and hundreds of hours of author time—thinking and planning, shopping and shopping, unpacking the shopping, putting the food in the refrigerator, cooking four or five or more versions of each dish, washing all those hundreds of pots and pans, and then writing and writing, revising and rewriting, polishing . . . and *worrying to death* . . . Then—say a prayer for the author who has so many hopes pinned on *your* next whim, and wonder whether it's a fix you really want to be in too. ●

Proposed Cookbook Title

A Guarantee To Success: The Best New Instant American Recipes For Calorie-Free, Lite, Fast-Food Using No Salt, No Fat, No Sugar, Grilled Over Mesquite And Then Baked In A Microwave Brick Oven For Spicy, Ethnic Treats From The Napa Valley by Alice Waters with Paul Prudhomme and Martha Stewart. Workman. Paperback, 650 pages. Full color throughout. $2.95.

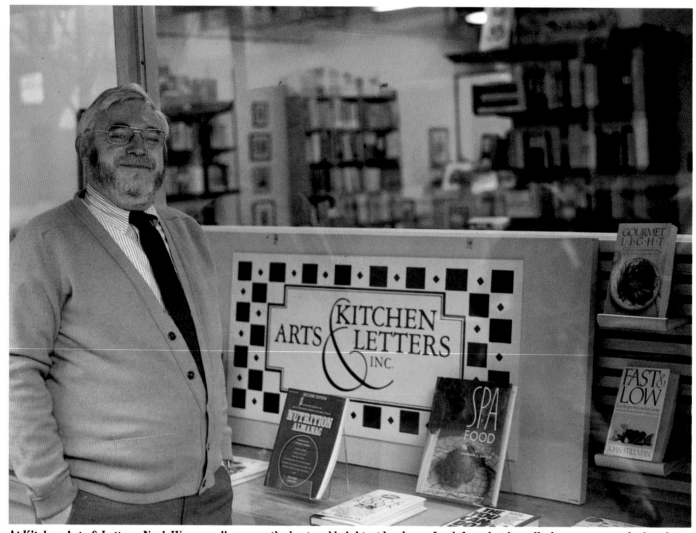

At Kitchen Arts & Letters, Nach Waxman dispenses the best and brightest books on food; for what he calls dopey ones, seek elsewhere.

Conversation With A Bookseller

Nach Waxman is the proprietor of a small retail bookstore called Kitchen Arts & Letters, located in a fashionable residential section of Manhattan, on upper Lexington Avenue. There are plenty of booksellers in New York who sell cookbooks, but Waxman is different; he sells *only* cookbooks, (and other food-related books, for example, those that have to do with the anthropology of food). Waxman opened his shop in September of 1983, but he was no stranger to the cookbook business. Formerly, for 19 years, he was a nonfiction editor for Harper & Row among other publishers, and many a cookbook manuscript became a superior cookbook after passing through his hands.

Isn't retail bookselling a pretty scary business?

If you've got the right thing, and I think we do, retail sales is not a problem. This store corresponds to a felt need in the food community. Seventy percent of our dollar volume comes from people in the food business—chefs, restaurant owners, caterers, food writers, wine importers and food trade organizations. I keep company accounts for several large food companies, such as General Foods. That's how I conceived the business in the first place. For a small business in a neighborhood like this, I need to depend on more than local traffic. My regular customers are people who are buying the tools of their trade here.

Does that situation affect the kind of business you're able to do?

Absolutely. These people are financially valuable, and their business allows the store to run on a higher level than if we were dependent on the general public. I can put in a lot more scholarly, thoughtful and really adventurous books.

Are there other cookbook stores operating as you do?

Not in New York. And nowhere in the U.S. and Canada can such stores as there are operate in this way. There are some five stores I could name on this continent. Toronto and Denver have the best. But they are forced to carry some dopey books along with the good.

Is it true that cookbooks without color pictures or illustrations won't sell anymore?

I wouldn't say that at all. There are some subjects that call for illustration, and plenty more that don't. We have serious people coming here who are not won over by pretty pictures, particularly when the pictures are irrelevant and useless. If the publishers would give as much attention to creating a decent index as they give to silly illustrations, we'd be better off.

It's curious that some books have more than half their value in the illustrations. Chefs, for example, may want them for the sheer presentation value. They'll say, "I *have* the recipe. I just want to know what it *looks* like."

How do you view the cookbook scene today?
Food is the object of popular, faddish attention right now, and this prompts excesses. Happily, natural selection is at work, and the fat and the folly will fall by the way. Thanks to good critics, cookbooks that really don't fill a need are given short shrift today. I'm upbeat on the general quality in the market now, as compared with 20 years ago. Authors are more knowledgeable and better prepared. There are still plenty of bad, silly books being published, but there are also fine, serious books coming out now that wouldn't have seen the light of day two decades ago. And the preposterousness is going to fall off.

Do you think that cooking school video-cassettes are going to make any inroads in the cookbook market?
Not a chance. I personally would be happy to watch Julia Child put her groceries away, because she's so entertaining. But I wouldn't expect to *learn* anything from it. The cassettes will have to get much more seriously instructive before I change my view.

Are you a serious cook yourself?
Well . . . yes, I cook. I do *some* of my cooking to dip into new cookbooks, so I can genuinely recommend a certain book to a customer. And my personal passion is for Indian cooking. I do it all the time.

Why?
Oh . . . long ago my passion was East Asian studies. And I lived out there. I got involved.

Any books you particularly admire?
Yes! *Classic Indian Cooking* and *Classic Indian Vegetarian and Grain Cooking,* both by Julie Sahni, from Morrow.

In your judgment, what are the best cookbooks recently out?
Unquestionably, *The Italian Baker,* by Carol Field, from Harper & Row last fall. This woman knows her stuff! And something else, from Harper & Row this May: *Uncommon Fruits and Vegetables,* by Elizabeth

Schneider. They're calling it a common-sense guide, and it is. This is going to be one of the really important books, and it will have major standing for years and years.

Do you think there ought to be more books of this quality?
I certainly do! And you can quote me on that. ●

Worth A Thousand Words The Benjamin Company reports that 48 percent of all buyers consider that color pictures are essential in a cookbook. This also holds true for catalogs. When products are illustrated with line drawings, buyers tend to think that the product does not yet exist. ●
Lorna Sass, food historian

Cookbook Looks The Vance Research Service reports that American households own an average of 15 cookbooks, try one or two new recipes each month, and look through cookbooks for ideas about 12 times a year. ●
Lorna Sass, food historian

Cookbook Biz

The most recent sales figures for cookbooks date from 1984 and are only estimates. Jonathan Latimer, publisher of adult books at Western, gives a figure of $286 million; a more conservative estimate comes from an industry-wide survey conducted by HP Books: $208 million.

Shelley Hurley, buyer at B. Dalton Bookstore, reports that cookbook sales have increased by 10 to 18 percent annually over the past four years. And Dara Tyson, manager of public relations at Waldenbooks, reports that cookbooks ranked seventh among the 50 bestselling categories in 1984.

According to Andrew Grabois, senior editor of R.R. Bowker's *Subject Guide to Books in Print,* cookbook sales lag only slightly behind those in the very fast-growing field of books on personal computers. ●
Lorna Sass, food historian

Winning By Losing

Diet cookbooks are as popular as ever—we never give up the fond hope that more of them will result in less of us.

Unfortunately, however, no passion for precision has found its way into most of these books that appear with remarkable frequency and startling inventiveness. Few diet books concern themselves with nutrition, a subject that for most doctors, lacks the charisma of open-heart surgery or the drama of life-and-death decisions. Doctors do not necessarily totally reject the idea that there may be a direct link between diet and health, rather they feign boredom with the entire subject. And many of the most esteemed hospitals in the land continue to serve lamentable breakfasts, lunches and dinners that are lacking in any health-giving properties whatsoever. Doctor-authors (and, of course, not all of them have doctorates in medicine) who write diet books seem to be rather more interested in becoming media stars than medical missionaries.

But doctors all seem to be in general agreement about the need for exercise and for the avoidance of all those foods that in the past have given us such infinite pleasure: chocolate, cheese, cholesterol-laden goodies and—alcohol. It is a pity about alcohol, because you may have noticed that most of the really serious and successful cookbook authors have lived to a goodly, ripe old age, partly because they have taken great pains to preserve themselves in alcohol en route. ●

Is There PhD In This? A sampling of articles to appear in *Food & Foodways,* a scholarly journal founded by Steven L. Kaplan, a Cornell University historian:
Hospitality, Women and the Efficacy of Beer.
Feeding Their Faith: Recipe Knowledge Among Thai Buddhist Women.
The American Response to Italian Food, 1880-1930.
Sociology of Taste in the Realist Novel: Representations of Popular Eating in E. Zola.
State-making, Political Legitimation and Food in Early Modern Europe.
Ideology, Power and Nutrition: Soldier's Soup, Prisoner's Soup and Charity Soup. ●
Harper's

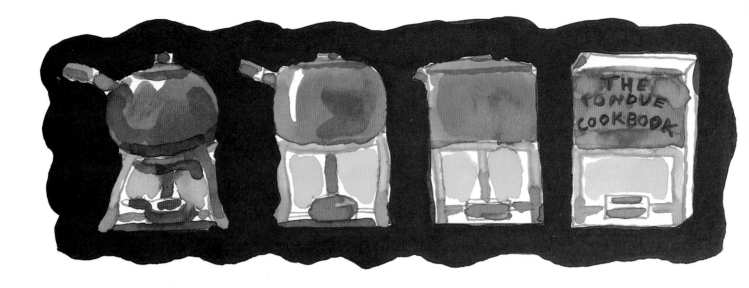

Six Fondue Pots Or How I Became A Publisher

Irena Chalmers

F ads erupt in tumbling profusion. Suddenly hair is long, clothes are short, blue jeans are In and then Out. *All the neighbors are jogging and Having a Good Day, eating Lean Cuisine and gobbling designer chocolates. Perhaps all conditions have to be just right and come together at a precise moment for a new fad to be created, or maybe it is all just chance . . .*

Way back in the late 60s it seemed that, overnight, fondue pots appeared everywhere—in gift shops, in department stores—evoking visions of snow-clad Swiss mountains, lithe fur-fringed skiers and hot, bubbling creamy cheese. Every bride received at least one and some, more than one, fondue pot as a wedding gift. It began to look as though a movement were afoot. So I, too, bought six fondue pots for my small cookware store/ cooking school in North Carolina. Smug, I was pleased to be part of the scene.

There I was, smiling and ready with my gleaming pots, for the next person to walk through the door and say briskly, "One fondue pot, please." I waited, and I waited and no one came; five months later I was still waiting. The smile grew a trifle wan as the six gleaming fondue pots started gathering dust. It is hard to know what to do when you are in the midst of a movement and nothing is moving.

A friend in town had also latched onto the smart new trend. He bought 12 fondue pots for his much larger store in a busy shopping mall. He too was waiting. So, together, we decided to launch an all-

out consumer fondue pot education program. An ad was placed in the local newspaper inviting the entire circulation to come and taste our fondue, to touch the pots—and perhaps even buy them. They came all right and they pronounced the fondue as being "the best thing they ever put in their collective mouth." But no one bought a fondue pot.

All we had done was to compound the problem. We had spent the money for the ad and, between us, we had 17 fondue pots (the one we had cooked in was slightly used and therefore unsaleable). So, we put our heads together and puzzled and worried and decided that the reason that none of the pots had been sold was because we had failed to provide a recipe. You don't exactly need a recipe for melted cheese—nonetheless, we thought that we would put together a poster telling people how to melt cheese. Posters were all the rage at that time.

The local printer was consulted. Not having the right kind of printing press to make up a poster, he warned us sternly of the folly of this approach and instead recommended that we write a small book. The only drawback with this solution was that it created yet another problem. It seems that you can't print 17 copies of a book, or you can if you want to, but it costs just about the same amount to print 2,500 copies.

So that's what we did!

Reasoning that other small stores might, perhaps, have fallen heir to fondue pots that refused to be sold—and could hardly be given away—sample

copies of the book were sent to several small gourmet stores and one large one— Bloomingdale's.

Now if ever there was a store on the cutting edge of knowing what is In, it is Bloomingdale's. An order was received for two dozen copies of the new Fondue Book almost immediately. More orders followed and more and yet more until the entire printing was sold out. What to do? Why, print some more books, of course. So the order was placed for 2,500 more copies. The next print order was for 5,000 and the one after that for 10,000 copies. Pretty close to a million books were sold that first year alone and that book was followed by one on the subject of Chocolate that I thought would be the next big fad. The trouble was that was 20 years ago and the timing was a bit off; nevertheless other little books followed at a rapid pace, published under the banner of Potpourri Press. More than a 100 titles were completed, each one written in response to what was perceived as a definite gap in the marketplace. The books were, and still are, tied to a trend or to a cooking utensil.

The book business thrived and prospered though both my friend's store and mine are long gone. David Grimes, my friend, is no longer in the book business but I am still looking for the next big cheese *to come along.* ●

Irena Chalmers has written and published more than 100 minibooks with sales exceeding 20 million copies. She believes firmly in excess in all things.

Why You Order Crawfish And I Order Crayfish

Stanley Dry

Do you know how a cobbler *differs from a* pandowdy, *a* cob pie *from a* country pie *or a* bungler *from a* bald-headed pie? *If you're confused, it's no wonder—because the principal differences have more to do with geography than method of preparation. All of the examples above refer to the same dessert—a deep-dish fruit pie made with a crust, often of biscuit dough—but it goes by different names in different parts of the country. The same dish is also called a* gobbler, dowdy, grunt, pot pie, slump, deep-dish pie, stew pie *and* clobber.

Those regional and folk expressions and some 12,000 unusual others—words and phrases not found in standard dictionaries, as well as out-of-the-way meanings for common terms—are contained in Volume One of the Dictionary of American Regional English *(Frederick G. Cassidy, chief editor; Belknap/Harvard University Press; $60), a monumental work that has been over 20 years in the making. The first volume contains entries from "A" to "C." Another four volumes, to be published periodically during the next decade, will complete the alphabet.*

If the word "dictionary" in the title makes you think of a dry and tedious tome, think again. Although it is primarily a reference work that undoubtedly will be consulted to settle many a linguistic dispute, it's also a timely diversion for anyone who travels, shops for food or eats out, as its publication coincides with the great revival of interest in American regional cooking.

Regional differences in terminology and usage are far more pronounced and complex than one might assume. For starters, forget about any simplified scheme that divides the country into north, south, east and west. The dictionary uses 37 basic regional labels— so we're talking about regions that most of us aren't even aware of.

Take that word cobbler, *for example, forgetting for the moment all the other regional expressions for the same dish. The term cobbler is used chiefly in the South and South Midland regions, an area that includes parts of Texas, Oklahoma, Missouri, Illinois, Indiana, Ohio,*

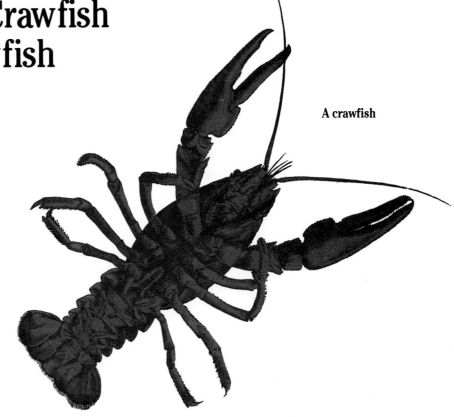

A crawfish

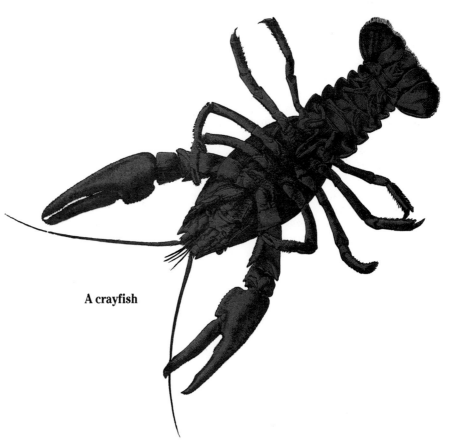

A crayfish

West Virginia, Maryland, Delaware and all the southern states. But even within the South and South Midland regions, cobblers vary considerably from place to place. In some areas they're made with only a top crust; in others they have both a top crust and a bottom crust.

The latter is what I remember having as a child in West Texas, and I'm always disappointed by a cobbler that has only a top crust. In fact, it's been years since I've tasted what I consider the real McCoy, and I had actually begun to suspect that my memory of a cobbler with a bottom crust was more imagined than real. But, lo and behold, under the heading cobbler is a shorthand recipe from a woman in Walker, Kentucky, one of the 2,777 "informants" (natives of 1,002 representative communities in all 50 states) who were interviewed by field workers for the dictionary. She calls it a cobbler pie and gives this description of how it's made: "A biscuit-like dough is put into the bottom of a large square pan and baked. Fruit is put on this and another layer of dough on top. This is baked; the results are superb, especially with wild blackberries or fresh peaches." I get hungry just thinking about it.

When is a turkey not a turkey?
Regional American cooking has always been based on local ingredients, which has given rise to a myriad of colorful expressions. For example, an Alaska turkey *is a salmon, as is a* Columbia River turkey. *But in Massachusetts, if you're offered either a* Cape Cod turkey *or a* Cape Ann turkey, *you'll get a codfish dinner. When sturgeon were plentiful in the Hudson River, they were called* Albany beef. *Similarly, the term* Connecticut River pork *for shad referred to the abundance of the fish in that river. Cincinnati, when it was a center of the pork-packing industry, gave rise to a number of euphemisms. Among them:* Cincinnati oysters *for pigs' feet,* Cincinnati turkey *for salt pork and* Cincinnati chicken, *which was made from pork tenderloin. A* Boston woodcock *is a dish of pork and beans,* Arkansas chicken *is salt pork,* Arkansas T-bone *is bacon and* Arkansas wedding cake *is corn bread.*

There are listings for both Arizona strawberry *and* Boston strawberry, *but both are cross-referenced to* strawberry, *which will be included in a later volume. So we'll just have to wait. But there is an entry for* Alabama egg, *which is also called a* hobo egg *or a* Rocky Mountain egg, *and it sounds delicious—"an egg fried in the hollow center of a piece of bread."*

Some terms change meanings over time as well as from one section of the country to another. In the 1870s and 80s, for example, a Coney Island *meant fried clams. Now it's understood to be "a hot dog, usually served in a bun with condiments." But informants in Ohio, Missouri and Oklahoma used the term to designate a hamburger. And other informants in Nebraska, Washington, Indiana and Oklahoma called a submarine sandwich a* Coney Island. *There is, however, only one translation offered for* Coney Island butter: *mustard.*

The crayfish, a freshwater crustacean that is in great vogue these days, goes by a variety of names. Crawfish *is in widespread usage in the South and the Midland.* Crayfish *is in scattered usage throughout the country. Other terms include* clawfish, crab *(especially around the Great Lakes),* water crab, crabfish, crawdad, crawdaddy, crawldaddy, crowdad, crawcrab, crawdab, crawdabber, crawjinny, crawpappy *and* craydad, *not to mention* mud bug, *which presumably will appear in a later volume. The variety of names is a blessing for menu writers, although I'm not sure that they've taken full advantage of their many colorful options.*

So, the language is sometimes enormously complicated—but always fascinating, in flux and generating new expressions. I was reminded of that by a sign posted outside a café on Ellis Street in San Francisco. It listed the house specials as French coffee, French Submarine, Vietnamese Fast Food.

Personally, I hope that the next volume of the dictionary includes an entry on French Submarine. ●

Stanley Dry is associate editor, *Food and Wine* magazine.

ARCADIA'S LOBSTER CLUB SANDWICH
Another Arcadia triumph to haunt you in the night.

Serves 2

Ingredients:
Lemon mayonnaise:
1 egg yolk
3/4 teaspoon Dijon mustard
2 tablespoons fresh lemon juice
3/4 cup soy oil
2 teaspoons grated lemon zest
Salt and freshly ground pepper

Sandwich:
6 slices toasted brioche
1 1/2 cups cooked lobster meat
Butter lettuce leaves
8 slices cooked bacon
8–12 slices ripe tomato

Method:
1. To prepare the lemon mayonnaise, first have all the ingredients at room temperature.
2. Whisk together the egg yolk, mustard and lemon juice in a small bowl until thick.
3. Add the oil by droplets, whisking constantly, until the mayonnaise begins to emulsify. At that point, the remaining oil may be added slowly, in a thin stream, until the mayonnaise is thick.
4. Fold in the lemon zest and season to taste with salt and pepper. Refrigerate, covered, for at least an hour, until you are ready to make the sandwich.
5. To construct the sandwich, follow illustration.

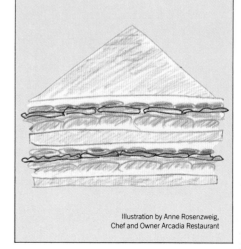

Illustration by Anne Rosenzweig, Chef and Owner Arcadia Restaurant

Cookbook Bestsellers

It appears there are three factors to make a book into a bestseller: We trust books that come from *An Institution* such as *Better Homes and Gardens, Family Circle* or *The New York Times* for example. A second category of potential winners is written by the so-called *Big Name Author* whose strong voice rings forth with authority and the third is the *Diet* or other focused *Single Subject* genre.

1985 Bestsellers

The Frugal Gourmet by Jeff Smith (Morrow, 1984)

The Silver Palate Good Times Cookbook by Julee Rosso and Sheila Lukins (Workman, 1985)

Weight Watchers New International Cookbook by Jean Nidetch (NAL Books, 1985)

Paul Prudhomme's Louisiana Kitchen (Morrow, 1984)

Jane Brody's Good Food Book: Living the High Carbohydrate Way (Norton, 1985)

The New York Times

All-time Bestsellers

HARDCOVERS
The Betty Crocker Cookbook (Gol. Books, 1950) 22,000,000

Better Homes & Gardens New Cook Book—Ringbound Version (Meredith, 1930) 20,685,435

The Joy of Cooking by Irma S. Rombauer and Marion Rombauer Becker (Bobbs-Merrill, 1931) 10,000,000

Mr. Boston Bartender's Guide edited by Leo Cotton (Warner Books, 1935) 8,659,686

Better Homes and Gardens New Garden Book (Meredith, 1959) 2,526,953 (OP)

Better Homes and Gardens New Junior Cook Book (Meredith, 1975) 1,652,417

Better Homes and Gardens Cooking for Two (Meredith, 1968) 1,585,418

Better Homes and Gardens Fondue Book (Meredith, 1970) 1,484,278 (OP)

Weight Watchers® International Cookbook by Weight Watchers International (NAL Books, 1980) 1,245,000

Better Homes and Gardens Eat and Stay Slim (Meredith, 1968) 1,158,247

Better Homes and Gardens Home Canning and Freezing (Meredith, 1973) 1,152,372

Better Homes and Gardens Barbecue Cook Book (Meredith, 1956) 1,148,612 (OP)

Fannie Farmer Cookbook by Fannie Farmer (Little, Brown, 1896) 1,009,849 (OP)

Better Homes and Gardens Meat Cook Book (Meredith, 1959) 956,587 (OP)

Better Homes and Gardens Salad Book (Meredith, 1957) 954,012 (OP)

Better Homes and Gardens Meals in Minutes (Meredith, 1963) 921,499 (OP)

Weight Watchers® New Program Cookbook by Jean Nidetch (NAL Books, 1980) 900,000

Better Homes and Gardens Casserole Cook Book (Meredith, 1961) 896,053 (OP)

Better Homes and Gardens Crockery Cook Book (Meredith, 1976) 836,463

Better Homes and Gardens Calorie Counters (Meredith, 1970) 803,230

Better Homes and Gardens Best Buffets (Meredith, 1963) 775,704 (OP)

Better Homes and Gardens Blender Cook Book (Meredith, 1971) 766,440

TRADE PAPERBACKS
Crockery Cookery by Mable Hoffman (HP Books, 1975) 2,307,253

The Nutrition Almanac by John Kirschmann (McGraw-Hill, 1979) 2,150,000

Joy of Cooking by Irma Rombauer and Marion Rombauer Becker (NAL, 1973) 1,920,000

Mexican Cook Book by Editors of Sunset Books (Sunset Books/Lane Publishing Co., 1969) 1,796,464

Barbecue Cook Book by Editors of Sunset Books (Sunset Books/Lane Publishing Co., 1938) 1,759,269

Breads by Editors of Sunset Books (Sunset Books/Lane Publishing Co., 1963) 1,285,289

Wok Cookery by Ceil Dyer (HP Books, 1977) 1,239,267

Crepe Cookery by Mable Hoffman (HP Books, 1976) 1,219,000

Favorite Recipes I by Editors of Sunset Books (Sunset Books/Lane Publishing Co., 1949) 1,182,777

Canning by Editors of Sunset Books (Sunset Books/Lane Publishing Co., 1975) 1,117,498

Oriental Cook Book by Editors of Sunset Books (Sunset Books/Lane Publishing Co., 1970) 1,108,108

Hors D'Oeuvres by Editors of Sunset Books (Sunset Books/Lane Publishing Co., 1976) 1,074,760

Make-a-Mix Cookery by Karine Eliason and others (HP Books, 1978) 1,012,754

Publishers Weekly

Newsletters of Interest

Foodtalk San Francisco CA

Shrimp Notes New Orleans LA

The Microwave Times Burnsville MN

Macaroni Journal Arlington VA

Food Chemical News Washington DC

Meat Sheet Elmhurst IL

Picklepak (Pickles) St. Charles IL

Dietetic Foods Industry Carlsbad CA

Shellfish Soundings Washington DC

Management Letter (Food Service) Biloxi MS

Vinegar Institute News Atlanta GA

Shop Talks (Food Stores) Lumberton NC

The Pennsylvania Baker Harrisburg PA

American Bee Journal (Honey) Hamilton IL

Aquaculture Digest San Diego CA

Chipper Snacker (Potato Chips) Alexandria VA

Seafood America Rockville MD

Great Taste (Connoisseur Food) New York NY

Briefing (Restaurants) New York NY

The Concessionaire (Snack Bars) Chicago IL

Panacea (Macrobiotics) Brookline MA

Soyfoods (Soy Beans) Encintas CA

Quick Topics (Candy) Washington DC

Sproutletter (Beansprouts) Ashland OR

Cereal Industry Newsletter St. Paul MN

Mountain Muse Herbal Journal Philadelphia PA

Information Letter (Food Processing) Washington DC

Cornucopia Project Newsletter Emmaus PA

Food Conspiracy Newsletter Tucson AZ

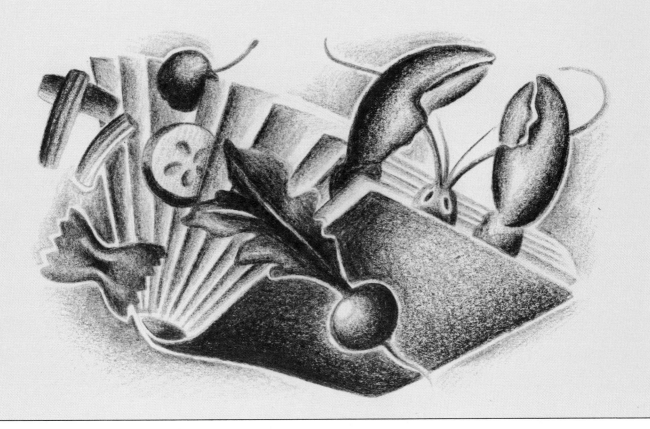

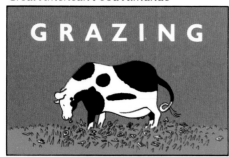

GRAZING

The Great Tomato Debate

The Florida Tomato Exchange had a problem to solve in marketing the states crop of winter tomatoes. According to *The Wall Street Journal*, even it had acknowledged that the tomatoes were so hard when freshly picked that you could easily smash a window with one. But after spending $2.3 million on an advertising campaign, the Exchange thought it had the battle won by convincing consumers to keep those hard tomatoes out of America's refrigerators. Tomatoes, said the Exchange, need time to ripen at room temperature.

Then along came an issue of *Consumer Reports* with word that their tomato judge had likened these tomatoes to "tie-dye baseballs." In addition, they alleged that no amount of patience would allow them to ripen and taste like vine-ripened tomatoes. The Tomato Exchange called the report "irresponsible," but the final judge will, of course, be you, the consumer.

There's One Born Every Minute In the fall of 1985, La Récolte, a toney restaurant in New York City, announced that for $300, anyone who desired could work in the kitchen for a night with chef Christian Levèque. Over 300 people responded.

Saving The Good Stuff A U.S. Department of Agriculture publication called "Conserving the Nutritive Value in Foods" has some valuable tips on getting the best nutrition out of our foods.

- Canned foods should be stored at about a 65-degree temperature; at 15 degrees higher they can lose a quarter of their food value over a year.
- Vine-ripened summer tomatoes are likely to have twice the vitamin C of those grown in a greenhouse or treated with ethylene gas to redden them.
- Oranges in segments are more nutritious than in juice.
- Beef served rare has more of the B vitamins than if it is well done.

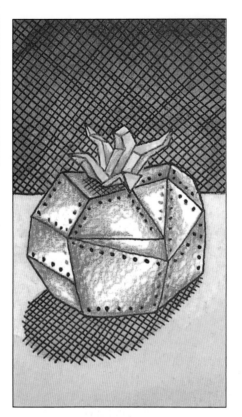

All God's Chillun Got Shoes The International Banana Association must be onto a winner this time. Banana skins were formerly considered useful only for sliding to a pratfall—and how many slapstick comedians can there be? Not enough to comprise a major market segment, surely. Now the Association announces that banana skins are just the thing for polishing shoes.

Is There A Conspiracy Here? Or, On The Other Hand, Why Isn't There One? If you buy a standard package of hot dogs why can't you find a standard package of hot dog rolls to match?

Powerful Bites

In the book *Power Lunching: How You Can Profit From More Effective Business Lunch Strategy*, the authors, Ligita Dienhart and E. Melvin Pinsel, characterize certain foods as either P (Power) or W (Wimp) choices to make when ordering at lunch with business associates. Perhaps predictably, steak is P, as is smoked salmon (but not with a bagel), while banana bread is W. But at least one reviewer, Adam Hochschild of *Mother Jones* magazine, takes issue with some of their choices: He is "shocked" that they gave a W to Perrier, and that's not all. "I would disagree with their characterization of shish kebab as W," he writes, "especially when we consider that it was originally supposed to be grilled on a sword."

Dream Food

In *The Dream and the Underworld*, psychologist James Hillman asserts that food is "so fundamental," even more so than sex, that "examining what and how you eat in the underworld of your dreams can reveal much about your psychic hungers and thirst." One food editor we know was so impressed with this idea that she began recording her dreams. "I did visit the underworld in a dream," she reports, "and found it to be a rather good Italian restaurant. But only the apprentice chefs were eating, in a shadowy back room. The restaurant *wasn't serving!*" She is still pondering what this reveals and hopes it doesn't mean that her psyche is out to lunch.

Merlins Of Flavor

Food flavoring is now a $1.5 billion industry in the U.S. Choosing from bottles of the 2,000 government-approved ingredients which line a laboratory wall, flavorists can create flavors to order—from kiwi, guava, watermelon and papaya to mesquite and clams. One bite of a food will guide the flavorist's hand toward the 20 or more bottles needed to re-create that flavor. Five years ago, 75 percent of all food flavors were made from artificial ingredients and the rest from natural sources. Today, the natural food craze has reversed that percentage and three quarters of the flavors are derived from natural foodstuffs. Often, "better" flavors can be derived from the esters, aldehydes, alcohols, ketones and ethyl acetates in the laboratory bottles. But if the label says "natural flavors" they *must* come from fruits, berries, herbs, botanicals, grains and roots. One seemingly "natural flavor"—peach—isn't. Oddly enough, you can't get peach flavor from a peach—it gets pruney and loses its freshness. Artificial peach flavor seems more "peachy."

Where Did The Name Gumbo Come From? Gumbo is a Bantu word for okra, an ingredient which is often, but not always, included in the dish.

FOOD ON VIDEO

In California
you can order your food via
your personal computer,
get a nutritional printout and
ask for a lite meal
in a restaurant using a
beam of light.

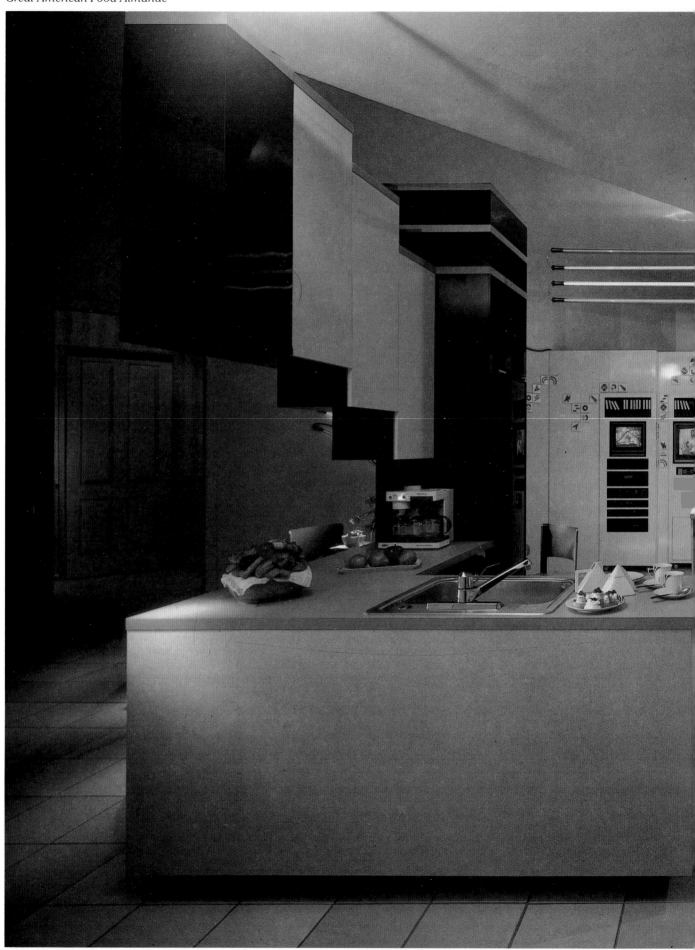

Betty Crocker meets high-tech in this kitchen, where one can cook along with Julia Child, access a recipe and work out to Jane Fonda.

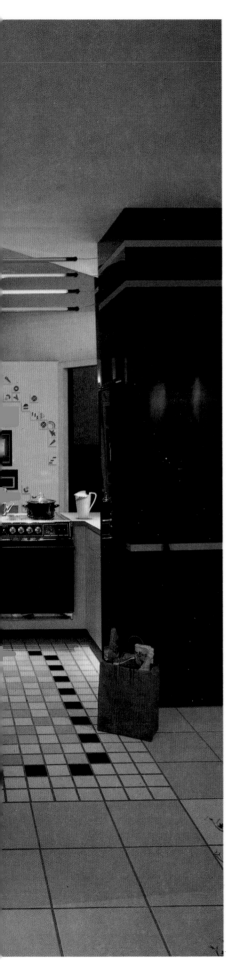

JUST YOU AND YOUR SCREEN

"I wish the heck they sold food. I'd never go out."—Mrs. Ron Birkner, to a *New York Times* reporter, discussing *Home Shopping Network*, a national TV show that allows consumers to shop by TV up to 24 hours a day, seven days a week.

You can now shop at home on your TV; you can watch TV shows on your VCR; you can see people when they're not there on video-telephones. Will the small screen replace all other forms of communication, including the printed page?

If your gut reaction is "not likely," most experts would agree with you. For all the vaunted computer revolutions and communications explosions, computers have not yet made drastic inroads into everyday life. And historians can tell you that new forms of communication have a tendency not to replace earlier forms, but rather to add to them.

Television did not outmode radio; people still write letters; newspapers are still considered *de rigueur* for a community. But screen information presentation is fast finding a niche in our homes—how big a niche is still to be explored.

Videocassettes are certainly familiar by now: 30 percent of all U.S. households have VCRs. Software for computers is also something many of us can discuss—if not with first-hand knowledge, at least second- or third-hand. Less well-known, but perhaps much more exciting, are some new video information systems being tried: videotex and teletext.

Both videotex and teletext are forms of electronic communication whereby people can receive information in either of two ways: on their computer or on their home TV screen. Reception on a TV screen requires a decoder (like the box the cable company gives you) and a keyboard on which to request information from the system; both TV and computer require a modem to make a communications link.

Teletext and videotex "frames" (information on screens like the free-standing ones you can see at airports announcing flight arrivals and departures) can either be stored on a computer and retrieved from there, or transmitted on the "vertical blanking interval"—the high-tech name for the space between channels or the black lines that you see above or below your TV picture if your reception sometimes rolls the image.

Frames can be either all-text, like the airport ones, or have hand-drawn pictures in up to 16 colors, with some animation—enough to illustrate a knife going up and down, or a storm coming closer on a weather map.

Teletext is a one-way system. It offers a bank of information of up to 100,000 frames. You can call up any of those frames and have them appear on your TV screen but you cannot change anything on the frames with your keyboard.

Videotex, on the other hand, is "interactive"—a very important word in today's communication technologies. It means that the computer can respond to your requests by changing—permanently—files to which it has access. Cash machines are videotex: If you want $50, the computer will have its mechanical cashier count out $50, which you can walk away with, and the computer will change the balance of your account just as accurately as any teller could. The cash machine may seem as if it is doing the same thing for everybody, but every transaction is handled in a separate account, and if cash is spat out, an account will be debited.

Cash machines are the most successful example of either of these technologies to date. The truly adventurous applications, some of which include food service, have nearly all failed, and, even when operative, they were transmitted only to limited markets or to homes participating in market research for the medium. However, there are new services already in the wings and the corporations involved are very big: AT&T, IBM, Sears, McGraw-Hill, CBS, *The New York Times* and American Express are all vitally interested—and becoming active—in this fast-developing new world of communications.

The capital investment required is huge—Sears, IBM and CBS each pledged $60 million just to get their new services off the ground—but the company that figures out how to make these services work may have the equivalent of the telephone in their hands.

Punch the restaurant

First in the world of interactive services came CBS's entry: Venture One, of Ridgewood, New Jersey. Alas, now defunct, Venture was an early videotex system, programmed to

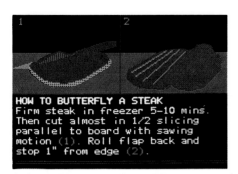

HOW TO BUTTERFLY A STEAK
Firm steak in freezer 5–10 mins.
Then cut almost in 1/2 slicing
parallel to board with sawing
motion (1). Roll flap back and
stop 1" from edge (2).

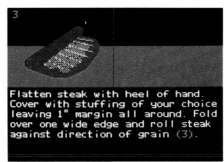

Flatten steak with heel of hand.
Cover with stuffing of your choice
leaving 1" margin all around. Fold
over one wide edge and roll steak
against direction of grain (3).

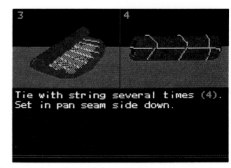

Tie with string several times (4).
Set in pan seam side down.

Animated how-to-cook graphics were a unique feature of Time Teletext's electronic food magazine. Stored in a VAX computer, they

perform specific tasks when asked.

One of the innovations offered by Venture One was a restaurant database. To read restaurant reviews, you first chose a neighborhood by punching a button whose number corresponded to a section on a map. You then chose the type of food you wanted from a list of cuisines available in that location: For example, you might have chosen "4" for Italian food in the center of town.

Once you selected a restaurant, you didn't have to reach for a phone book or copy down a telephone number from the screen. All you had to do was punch another number: Venture One was programmed to dial the restaurant for you automatically, enabling you to make a reservation without leaving your screen.

"Time" for cooks

While restaurant databases like Venture One's have always been a bright blip for electronic services (they bring in advertising the same way restaurant reviews in a magazine do) Time Inc.'s teletext entry, Time Teletext (also now defunct), brought electronic technology to the cook.

Along with good recipes (listed either by category or in a full-menu format) came animated "how-tos" that ranged from shelling shrimp to dicing carrots. These teaching tools could be called up whenever needed, without losing one's place in a recipe.

"Food" was greatly appreciated by its viewers and doubtless paved the way for the food services to come, but it died a common death: The technology was too expensive to deliver to the user.

The above services were the major precursors of the food on the tube: There were others like them, but they were the first and the best, respectively. Is it even worth discussing them? The answer is yes. Individual services, like individual newspapers and individual books, come and go; some of the best are the first to go. But creative, forward-thinking people take note of them and that has far-ranging effects.

Now designers of the avant-garde often put up to three monitors in their kitchens: one for the VCR, one for the TV and one for the computer. Someday, recipes using the

freshest produce in our markets will be waiting for use every morning on our computer screens, with a button to push for home delivery of all ingredients needed. It may be a long wait—or it may be just around the corner. ●

A New Way To Cook

There are about 30 million VCRs in use today—30 percent of all U.S. households are prepared to fast-forward and freeze-frame. Jane Fonda has sold 850,000 videocassettes, and nearly all of us eat more than we exercise. Is it any wonder that cooking videotapes are a growing market?

While many of the cooks featured in the most successful videotapes got their experience and honed their on-screen personalities on TV, good cooking tapes differ greatly from TV cooking shows and guest demos on talk shows.

TV is an entertainment medium, and if the viewer doesn't think you're cute, he or she is going to channel-hop. Videotapes can be more confident of their audience: A person who bought (or rented) a Thanksgiving Dinner tape is not going to watch the news during Baste-The-Bird. As a result, cooking tapes are packed with far more information than most of the TV shows.

Tapes can also take advantage of a VCR's features. You can play back something you missed; you can freeze a frame and get a pencil, if you want; tapes can be indexed both for recipes and for important information steps.

Moreover, the cooks who perform on tape can gain more than by appearing on TV shows. Besides the repeated exposure and the possible sales royalties, videos are a natural marketing tool for their books.

Action

Part of the reason so much hash is being flung around behind camera these days is that the American appetite for new releases

was triggered when unreleased movies proliferated. There is a limit to these, yet we still expect new VCR titles every time we go to the store. Enter the celebrity cook.

Just so you know what happens during a filming: Many of those gleaming kitchens over which the cook presides don't have running water, so pots, pans and measuring cups—all of which may be used 10–20 times a day—are washed in buckets of soapy water off the set. It usually takes at least $200 of food to complete a day's shoot, and one four-minute segment can take up to three hours to tape.

The green stuff

Making a cooking video isn't that cheap, either; it can cost over $100,000. But there *are* lower-budget success stories: *A Guide To Good Cooking*, by Jacques Pépin, came in at under $15,000, but Videocraft had donated the producer's and director's time to bring it in at that price. The *Cook's* magazine tapes cost only $10,000 to produce, but once again the director's time was donated, and so was the editor's: Chris Kimball, the publisher of the magazine, did both himself. "You have to be incredibly organized," Kimball said. "You can shoot a one-hour video in three hours, if you're well prepared; it can take you days if you're not."

Even though offering some of the lowest prices in the business, Kimball is wary about the product. "Stores don't know how to sell videos," he said, "and straight recipe tapes may not be that good a concept. You can turn on your TV for free and watch someone cook; a cookbook will give you many times more recipes for far less in price than any tape. Frankly, I don't see how any of these people [other, high-spending producers] are going to make any money; they're spending so much up-front."

The break-even point on cooking videos is usually about 5,000 copies sold versus 20,000 for cookbooks. This difference is partially due to differences in production: You can make a new copy of a videotape each time you sell one, thus keeping your costs very close to the sales figures. When you publish books, you have to gamble on the entire printing—and sometimes you lose.

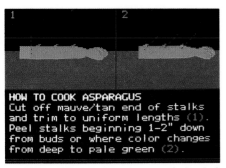 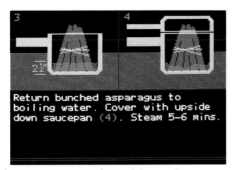

HOW TO COOK ASPARAGUS
Cut off mauve/tan end of stalks and trim to uniform lengths (1). Peel stalks beginning 1-2" down from buds or where color changes from deep to pale green (2).

Return bunched asparagus to boiling water. Cover with upside down saucepan (4). Steam 5-6 mins.

Tie asparagus in bunches of 6-8 spears. Stand in deep pot and pour in water to a level of 2 1/2" (3). Remove asparagus and bring water to a boil with 1T salt.

could be called up whenever needed to help viewers prepare recipes of the week.

A carp or two

Even the best videocassettes don't do everything. Most VCRs are not in the kitchen—despite the fast-forward-looking designers who are now putting them there in showrooms. Although one video reviewer was inspired to set up his ironing board in the living room in order to have a surface on which to bone a chicken along with his video instructor, many people find this somewhat impractical.

Packaging of video cookbooks is not all it might be, either. Many feature a grinning cook, or a sumptuous dish on the box, without mentioning whether or not there is a recipe book included (a *must*), or indicating how many recipes are covered or what level of experience is required.

Tapes can't correct viewer errors, either, and many cooking students are convinced they are "doing it right," and the recipe is wrong; it takes an instructor on the spot to see the problem and help correct it.

Mind you, they also said Sesame Street wouldn't work, but a lot of kids who can now read aren't complaining. Here's hoping the same is true of video cooks! ●

Pizza Slice, Pardner?

Any information service that provides news, weather and sports information can also have food articles; the same lines that deliver the headlines carry the by-lined pieces for featuring recipes, good nutrition, regional food, new food and other topics. But Star-Text, a very successful videotex service in Fort Worth, Texas, gives its 2,500 subscribers something more.

Run by the *Fort Worth Star-Telegram* (which is in turn owned by Capital Cities), StarText has over 100 recipes, divided for ease of access into sections like a cookbook: entrées, desserts, soups and so on.

One-third of these recipes is from the syndicated services, as described above; another third is put in by readers as a sort of special interest bulletin board. The final—and most interesting—third is a free-standing section called *The Duke's Cookbook* which is written in a Texas drawl, and with more novelistic concerns than the average "gently beat two eggs" manual.

A recipe for homemade pizza, for example, features Cap'n Pepperoni, a mother ship of dough and a time warp device which you program to speed Cap'n Pepperoni 40 minutes into the future, at a rate of 450 degrees Fahrenheit. What will Pac Man be eating next? ●

Surrogate Shoppers

Cabletext, a very successful, if limited, form of electronic information service, usually consists of computer-created text constantly run on one channel of your TV. Weather information, sports statistics, stock market quotes, TV listings . . . the data transmitted this way is usually repeated at least once an hour, and can be of interest to a group as small as a neighborhood school district.

Vector Enterprises, of Sacramento, California, whose primary job is consulting to the U.S. Government on food-related issues, has been putting out a very successful cabletext TV show for eight or nine years called *Vector Shopping Guide*.

Here's how it works. When a local TV cable system decides to get the guide (for about $700 a week), Vector finds someone in the area to go to five or six of the largest local supermarkets with a shopping list provided by Vector. The person then buys the whole list at each market (a car is a must). Back home, the price of each item and where bought is entered into Vector's Honeywell computers.

Vector then produces a rolling display for the cable company that shows which supermarket has the best prices, both item-by-item and for the list as a whole. This list is broadcast to about 300,000 viewers nationwide, and makes about $250,000 a year for Vector. How about them apples? ●

Screen of plenty CompuServe of Stamford, Connecticut, a massive computer videotex service with over 250,000 users has moved into the food-shop arena with Comp-u-Mall, a group of over 50 on-line boutiques that includes Gourmet Food Shops and a Wine and Liquor Cabinet. Subscribers can order food and liquor directly from computer (or decoder-equipped TV) and bill it to their CompuServe account or to their pre-approved VISA card. Maybe soon there'll be a slot for what computer-users need more: two aspirin, delivered pronto. ●

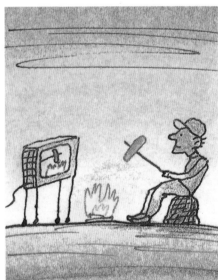

The Top Players In Videocassettes

Paul Bocuse: *Bocuse à la Carte*
Giuliano Bugialli: *Guide to Italian Cooking*
Jane Butel: *A Guide to Tex-Mex Cooking*
Julia Child: *The Way to Cook*
Craig Claiborne: *Craig Claiborne's New York Times Video Cookbook*
Madeleine Kamman: *Madeleine Kamman Cooks*
Master Chefs from Public Broadcasting System television series
Jacques Pepin: *A Guide to Good Cooking*
Stephen Yan: *Wok Before You Run*

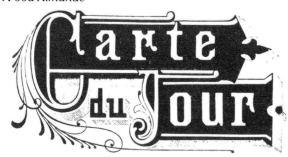

Help With A Byline

For food writers and editors, who operate almost entirely by computer, help has finally arrived. *Recipe Master*, a data management system that runs on an IBM PC and compatible machines, is designed to let food editors:

- enter their own recipes
- keep a record of the source of the recipe and when it was used
- print out recipes
- modify recipes and have nutritional values recalculated
- save recipes in a separate area from running text yet merge the two easily—a tour de force for *Recipe Master*.

Recipe Master is put out by Datatrek of Encinitas, California, and the National Dairy Promotion Board.

I Have It Somewhere

For the "I-have-it-somewhere" cooks, there is now *The Recipe Writer* from At-Your-Service Software of New York City. *The Recipe Writer* has gained a strong following in the food world—both East Coast and West Coast, according to Matthew Starobin of At-Your-Service Software.

The Recipe Writer is one of the best of its type: For example, it will multiply ingredients in practical measures, so multiplying "3 tablespoons of flour" by four gives you ¾ cup of flour, not the oh-so-helpful 12 tablespoons other software packages are prone to provide.

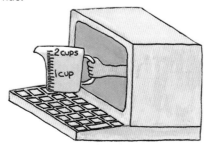

The Recipe Writer will also generate a shopping list from a menu of input recipes, and cross-reference all recipes by up to six categories—food type, cuisine, main ingredient, season . . . whatever you'd like.

If you really can't take the hassle of inputting all those recipes and categories, At-Your-Service is developing other products that Starobin calls "selling the blades, not the razor" in reference to Gillette's "the razor is free" marketing breakthrough. The product Starobin thinks he can get people to depend on like blades for their razor is *Bibliotech*, an index of leading cookbook and recipe magazines. You still have to print it out to use it in the kitchen, but it's one way to look through 30 years of *Gourmet* magazines without tears. ●

High Calorie Input For all those ambitious computer cooks who scaled up their chocolate fudge cake recipe to serve 32 and fed it to four—diet programs abound.

The Original Boston Computer Diet, from Scarborough Systems, in Cambridge, Massachusetts, offers almost everything except willpower: three "diet coaches"—onscreen personalities that range from chirpy to stern-voiced—nutrient tracking, menu generation complete with a shopping list and privacy with your caloric conscience. The program includes 700 somewhat boring foods (no Fettuccine Alfredo here!), lots of charts, a mood indicator and a constant calorie clock to tell you how many have gone down the hatch today. There are whistles for the good guys, and Bronx cheers for the rest of us—and computers never give up. There may be hope!

For those of us who want an old favorite at our widening sides, Bantam has put out a software version of *The Complete Scarsdale Medical Diet*. Nutri-Byte from ISC lets you enter both food intake and exercise output, while MECA's *The Running Program* by Jim Fixx puts its stress on the number of calories consumed by over 25 different kinds of exercise. Carbohydrate, fat, protein, cholesterol and calorie intake are only counted in order to mark how they might affect your fitness level.

Every single one of the above depends on a little bit of real-life help from the user, but still—a new attack on an old problem. ●

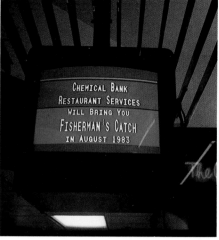

Sea treats on Chemical Bank's video menu

How'd You Get Tunafish? Chemical Bank has video menus at its six New York City dining facilities. Up to five 20- or 25-inch screens display each day's food choices and specials. The food service manager can change the list of items available and the price during the meal and make specials out of leftovers, so to speak. Waiting for the meatloaf to get cheaper?

Tuna Wiggle At Their Fingertips Institutional nutrition, while interesting on an intellectual level and important on a physical level, was for a long time downright exhausting on the desktop level. Paper everywhere: reference books with endless tables, individual charts for each patient, or class, or vegetable. But help has come quickly, in the form of computer programs for institutional feeders which fit the bill pretty well.

The state-of-the-art program for hospitals at the moment is *Nutritionist III*, a $495 update of a now-standard program called *Nutritionist*. *Nutritionist III* graphically presents 58 nutrients and percentages of RDAs (U.S. Recommended Daily Allowances) for foods, recipes, menus and complete diets (including diabetic food exchanges). It also enables nutritionists to keep track of costs and includes a word processor for inputting patient data files.

For schools and other cost-conscious institutions, *Kitchen Help* is another re-worked release (the earlier, perhaps more aptly named, was *Food Cost Explosion*). *Kitchen Help* is unique because its menu system can keep track of non-food items that directly contribute to the cost of the meal: Two napkins per child for Sloppy Joes and extra spoons for soup can put a seemingly inexpensive meal out of reach.

Kitchen Help offers over 1,000 menu items, and its recipes can include up to 8,000 ingredients. It also features recipe recalculation so a recipe can be scaled down for a baseball game or up for an army. ●

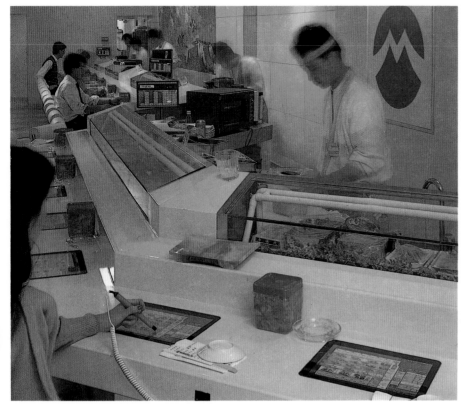

Where else but in LA could you order your lunch with a beam of light?

Sushi By The Board At Sushi-Tron, a restaurant in the financial district of Los Angeles, a customer can peruse an electronic menu of the day's sushi offerings (and their prices) displayed like a placemat at each counter seat. Using a light pen, he or she can then indicate the items wanted while discreetly calling up a running total of the cost of the meal. ●

You Don't Say! There are those who are aggressively moving into electronic distribution, and there are those who are letting nature take its course.

One company is heavily advertising a fast, no-fuss, no-wait food delivery system over electronic services, trying to grab the hungry, time-conscious user.

Another company that until recently portrayed its customers entreating the company (in songs, yet) to move closer so they could enjoy its magnificent features, is now advertising a phone link for greater shopping ease: The customer doesn't even have to visit the store.

Company No. 1? Domino's Pizza. Company No. 2? D'Agostino's. The hot new services?

No. 1: Call for a pizza. No. 2: Tele-D'Ag—place a call to the supermarket and they will deliver. Imagine that.

Fresh Menus Handsome-looking menus can now be printed out by a computer even as the chef decides how to use the day's produce and how each entrée should be priced vis-à-vis its wholesale price. Letter-quality printers can produce menus that are as good-looking as a pre-printed menu. These menu printouts are usually either clipped onto card stock boards with color graphics or photocopied onto expensive paper stock. Customers' first choices may actually be available, and waiters' time is saved for more important tasks than reciting lists of priceless specials at tableside. ●

Give That Cow A Screen Test Ranchers in Texas, Florida and Oklahoma now bid in cattle auctions by video hookup. The cows are taped at home on their Florida range by First American Video (a company 51 percent-owned by Seminole Indians), and ranchers bid after hearing descriptions of the cattle on conference lines. The cows don't have to travel—and First American gets 2 percent of the gross sale.

On Foodies And High-Tech "Food people tend to be nearly the last people to 'get with' high-tech stuff. They're more creative, they're more interested in live produce than they are in machines. Doctors and lawyers have computers already; there aren't going to be any big explosions there soon. But food people are finally catching on to computers; I think we're going to see some really great things."

Matthew Starobin, executive vice president
At-Your-Service Software

THE QUILTED GIRAFFE'S BLACK (BEANS AND TRUFFLES)
Black beans move into the stratosphere.

Serves 4 as a first course

Ingredients:
1 cup dried black turtle beans
6 cloves garlic, peeled
1 medium size onion, finely chopped
1 bay leaf
Salt
6 whole black peppercorns
4 tablespoons unsalted butter
1 fresh black truffle, about 1 1/2 ounces, thinly sliced
Freshly ground black pepper

Method:
1. Wash and pick through the beans. Put them in a bowl with cold water to cover by 2 inches and let them soak overnight.

2. When you are ready to cook the beans, bring 5 cups of water to a boil in a heavy saucepan. Finely chop 4 of the garlic cloves and add them, along with half the chopped onion, the bay leaf, salt to taste, and the peppercorns to the water. Simmer over low heat for 15 minutes.

3. Strain out the solids and return the broth to the saucepan. Drain the soaked beans and add them to the broth.

4. Bring to a boil over high heat, reduce the heat to low and cook the beans, uncovered, for 1 to 2 hours, until they are tender but still holding their shape. Add water as needed during cooking to keep the beans from drying out. At the end of the cooking time, enough liquid should remain to give the beans a thick stew-like consistency.

5. Heat the butter in a 9-inch skillet over moderate heat until it is sizzling. Chop the remaining garlic and add it, along with the remaining onion and the truffle, to the pan. Cook, stirring frequently, for 5 minutes, until the vegetables soften slightly, then add the beans and their liquid. Reduce the heat to low, season to taste with salt and pepper, and cook for 5 minutes.

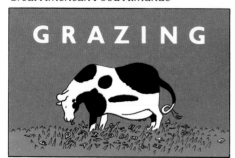

GRAZING

What's The Scoop

Are you puzzled about just what all those fashionable frozen desserts that aren't ice cream *are*? *Changing Times* magazine has sorted them all out for us, as follows:

Semifreddi A lighter version of gelato, an iced fruit mixture to which whipped cream, meringue or pastry cream is added.

Sorbet (In English: sherbet.) A rich blend of fruit and sweetener, sometimes with cream, gelatin or egg white added, but nearly fat-free. It sometimes has more sugar in it than ice cream has.

Frappé Fruit and sweetener forced through a sieve, then frozen hard. It is subsequently eaten after thawing to a mush.

Granité Made from fruits, ice and sweetener. It is a sort of flavored chopped ice, more granular than the others.

Change Partners And Dance With Me

"Breaking bread is a way of making contact....It's part of the dance between the man and the woman, the marvelous meal, the bottle of wine—the civilized way of saying I want to eat with you, I like you."

Art Buchwald, columnist, in the (late) *Cuisine*

At Least They Didn't Unionize Perhaps affected by the warm California sun, a prune grower named Martin Seely decided in 1905 that monkeys would make ideal employees, unlike humans, who seemed to expect cash in return for picking his fruit. He bought 500 monkeys in Panama and transported them to his orchard, where he turned them loose, with instructions to scamper up the trees and pick the fruit. They did so, but as fast as they picked, they also ate—absorbing Seely's potential profits and, incidentally, making a monkey out of him.

Sweet Tooths Vanilla wafers are the favorite cookies down South. Northeasterners and Floridians prefer chocolate-covered marshmallow cookies, while the spice-loving Pennsylvania Dutch are particularly fond of gingersnaps and spice cookies.

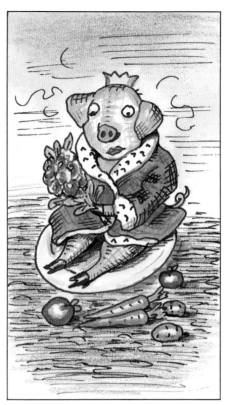

The Diet Trap Advertise a food as "low-cal" and you may be challenged for laboratory proof. And don't use "Spa Cuisine"—that phrase is trademarked by New York's Four Seasons restaurant.

Man Cannot Live By Bread Alone But that doesn't diminish its value. Take the case of a special 15-pound lode of "mother sourdough" that was recently insured for $1 million, secured inside a strong box, given its own airplane seat and transported from San Francisco to San Diego. It was chaperoned by the president of Boudin's Bakery, a man who it is safe to assume got all A's in his How to Get Publicity class at business school. He needed the dough to start a bakery in San Diego.

Or Swordfish/Fish Why do we say tunafish when we don't say salmonfish or haddockfish or solefish?

Did You Know? Prairie oysters are eggs, Bombay duck is fish and Alaskan strawberries are beans.

By The Letter When reporters asked a New York City "traffic spokesman" why it took three Campbell's Soup trucks to clean up when one truck carrying alphabet soup overturned he answered, "One truck took letters A through G, another H through P and the last Q through Z."

New York

Miss Piggy?

Mansura, in Louisiana's bayou country, has been christened (by no less than the governor) La Capitale du Cochon de Lait (The Suckling Pig Capital). Each April, Mansura holds a Cochon de Lait festival, at which rows of suckling pigs, none weighing more than 30 pounds, roast over hickory fires until they are crisp and deep amber on the outside and succulent within. Their enticing aroma fills the air for miles around. A queen is chosen each year and given the hallowed title of Miss Cochon de Lait. (She is not, as one might hope, pudgy and unctuous, but slim and pretty, like all beauty queens.)

How Would You Order The Following If You Spoke Dinerese?

1. Toasted English muffin, coffee with cream and sugar, to go.
2. Beef stew. Coke with no ice.
3. Hamburger with lettuce and tomato, no onions.

Answers:
1. Burn the British, draw one blonde and sweet, walking.
2. Bossie in a bowl. Stretch one, hold the hail.
3. Burn one and drag it through the garden but don't cry on it.

Eat Your Heart Out Fancy Grills: Ice Cream Beats Mesquite 4 to 1

In 1985, the National Restaurant Association asked 2,069 people across the U.S. which types of "specialty restaurants" they had tried in the last three months, or were likely to try. The restaurants which generated the most interest were those offering:

Premium hand-dipped ice cream	57%
Barbecue	57%
Pizza delivery	55%
Pasta	53%
American regional cuisine	53%
Freshly baked cookies	50%

Only 16 percent of those polled were interested in mesquite-grilled foods, and 14 percent in sushi or sashimi.

The Truth At Last!

"Anyone who is passionately interested in food also has to be passionately interested in life."

Alice Waters, food author and restaurant proprietor

COTTAGE INDUSTRIES

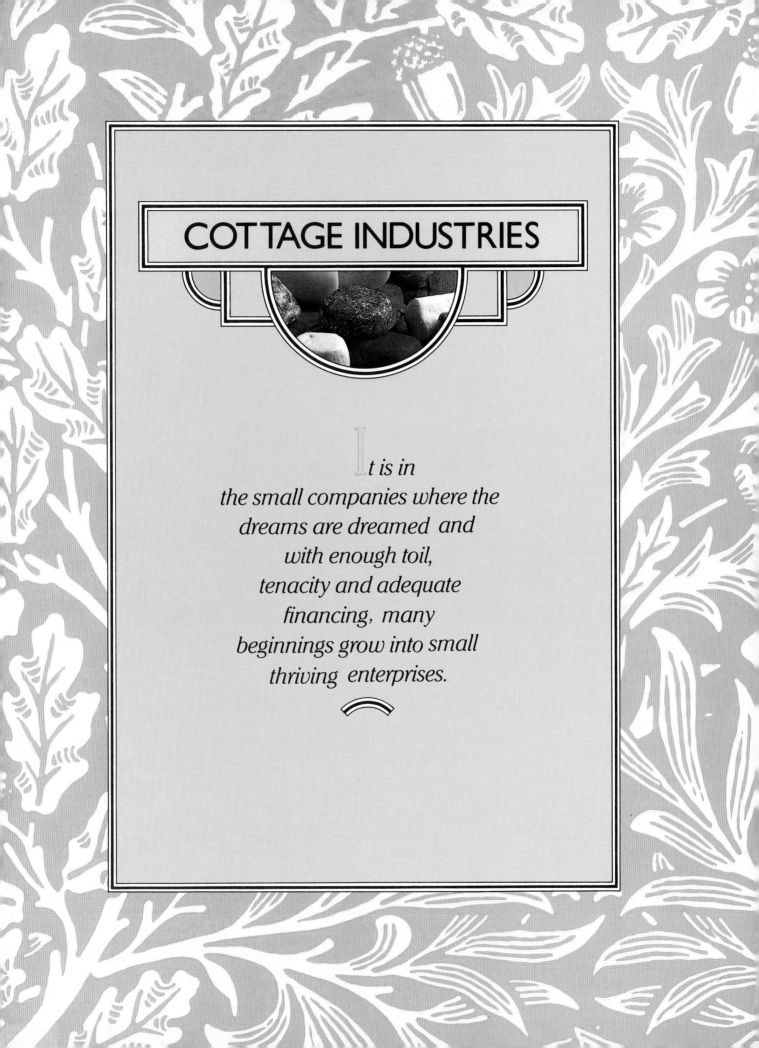

*I*t is in
the small companies where the
dreams are dreamed and
with enough toil,
tenacity and adequate
financing, many
beginnings grow into small
thriving enterprises.

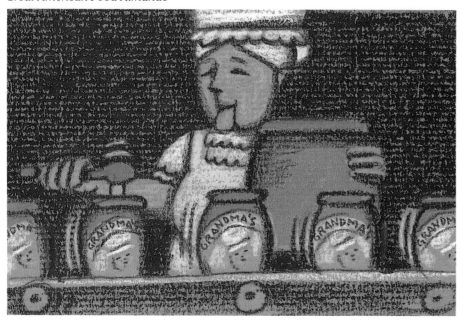

COTTAGE INDUSTRIES

As a general rule, small companies have little chance to expand in an economy that benefits the strongest players. A small company simply doesn't have the resources to compete effectively. It therefore becomes almost a *fait accompli* that a small, successful entrepreneurial company will become absorbed into a division of a larger entity.

Celestial Seasonings is a typical example. Here, a radical health food rebel became a marketing genius whose sales were sufficiently large to begin to offer competition to Lipton, one of the largest tea companies in the country.

So what happened? Celestial Seasonings was bought not, surprisingly, by a tea company, but by Kraft, a forward-looking conglomerate that had the foresight to seize an opportunity.

As for successful small companies that choose to stay relatively small, some, like the one that makes DoveBars, remain both independent and successful, but they tend to be the exception rather than the rule.

More frequently, the pattern is as follows: An entrepreneur has an idea for a product—a sauce or a jar of preserves or whatever. He or she makes it a hobby and gives it to friends, who beg for more. The product is then seen as a way to make a little extra income and the local specialty store is persuaded to put it on the shelf. The product, in the vernacular, flies off the shelf and the store wants more. The pot of gold is glimpsed and opportunity calls.

Off goes the entrepreneur to exhibit at the Fancy Food Trade Show. But no one buys the product. No one even looks at it. Gloom, doom and depression descend, but not for long: The product is terrific—it's the packaging that is at fault. So a designer is hired and uses up a lot of the earlier profit to develop a fancy label for a fancy jar and Neiman-Marcus wants 124 cases—immediately. Now quite extended, and often undercapitalized, the entrepreneur hires more people to fill the jars and spends more money to ship the product in a box rigid enough to prevent the jar from breaking in transit. Sales increase, but now the paper work is overwhelming: the orders and the billing, accounts receivable and accounts payable.

More people are hired to help—and more. But the margin is very thin and there are many times that the payroll can barely be met. Orders continue to come in and the originator of the product who was once making the sauce, filling the jars and delivering them locally begins to spend more and more time away from the kitchen, traveling to promote the product and trying to get more orders. The entrepreneur who started a little business is caught up in all the problems of big business but usually without much depth of experience. Almost always, it means learning on the job—and often learning from mistakes.

All this is not to say that small business is inevitably doomed. That would be far from the truth. Hundreds, and indeed thousands of cottage industries are alive and well, generating ideas for the foods we will be enjoying in the future. The following brief profiles present a few of the shining examples. ●

Magic In The Wrap

Grandmothers! How can there be so many in all the world as there are on jars of jam, or bags and tins of cookies?

Still, the packaging of fine foods seems to scream out for homage to maternal lineage or any other sort of warm, friendly, familiar yet slightly august image. Flowers, log cabins, ships and the occasional long shot of a mill or a winery do nicely as well.

With just a split second—or two—available for visual recognition on the part of the potential buyer, you can't put salad dressing in a soup can or dried beans in a lucite box. Package images may be complex and multileveled (lots of words and squiggles), but they must be instantly recognizable and in keeping with the value of a product. What's all that on the red Italian cookie tin? Who knows, but I just love the crinkly paper inside and, oh yes, the cookies!

Cottage industry, or the look thereof, is hot. And as the need for a good hug grows in today's snappy society, it's going to get downright crucial. That's why paper labels (ostensibly hand-affixed), homey expletives, family stories and pleasant, quixotic histories are never wrong, and often true.

The package is that first hint (or holler) that a magical journey is in store, or a childhood memory is within grasp. What's outside reminds, suggests and seduces. What's inside is the stuff of the good life, adventure and a mini-vacation. The best package enhances self-image (here's a photo of me with my $28.00 bottle of near-extinct Tuscan olive oil) while re-creating the original context (here's me in that lovely little shop in Provence).

Ribbons, seals, ties and extra folds all confirm and assure us that some human being has in fact made this food, especially for us. And when the feeling is right, price is no object. In fact, if it doesn't cost enough, it can't be special enough to bring, this very weekend, to that very fabled *grand-maman*.

It's also helpful if the container itself can remain long after the product has been gleefully consumed. We all look in the fridge to see what isn't there. And when a great empty package becomes part of the household landscape, it's like a constant ad or tiny shop window, crying out for response and repurchase. After all, even if the product inside is underwhelming, at least we end up with a great little someplace to put our pencils. ●

Clark Wolf, specialty food consultant

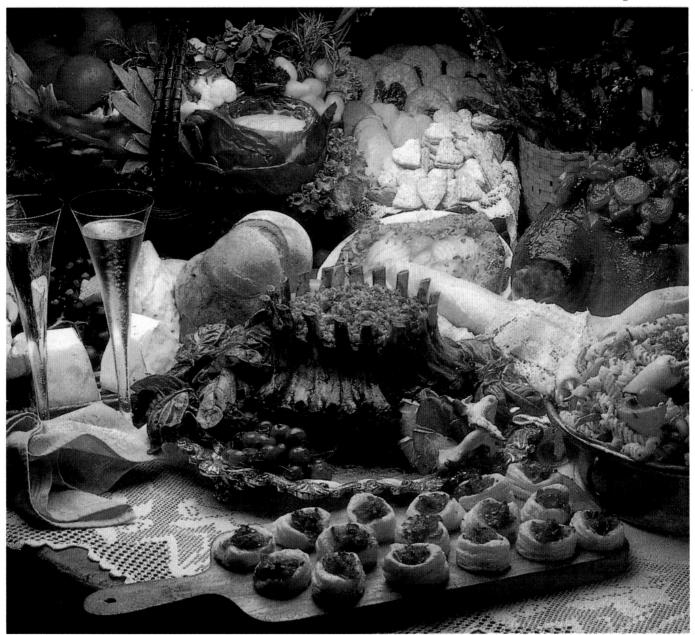

From canapés to dessert, are rack of lamb, peasant loaf, glazed ham and salad. This is Ferrari carry-out.

THE SILVER PALETTE

Julee Rosso and Sheila Lukins went into partnership in 1977 to found and operate a gourmet take-out emporium on Columbus Avenue on the west side of Manhattan—a tiny place, you understand; nothing fancy or uppity. The initial investment for this modest effort was $21,000, and the size of the shop they occupied was 11 feet by 16 feet. They called their establishment The Silver Palate.

Today, Columbus Avenue is the smart part of town where everybody is dying to go to see and to be seen, and one place everybody *must* go is The Silver Palate, where the bon ton all try to cram themselves into that same 11 feet by 16 feet in order to buy

something. This is perfectly acceptable to Julee Rosso and Sheila Lukins, whose business now does something in the neighborhood of $10 million a year. They have a staff of 44 people, a factory set-up near the store, a full-service catering operation and a mail-order business to boot. They produce a line of 122 bottled and packaged delicacies (chutneys, mustards, preserves and vinegars among them) which sell in 1,500 stores in the U.S. and in Europe and Asia. Just lately they added a new line of drink mixes called, quite appropriately for them, Good Times Cheers . . . and their additional plans to take over the entire world are shortly to be

announced to all.

There are those who say that theirs is the perfect partnership, that they are joined at the hip, stuck together for all time. This makes them laugh, because thereby hangs a tale. Early on, they were at a moment quite literally stuck together, on an occasion which neither will ever forget.

Their first commercial order for preserves was from elegant Saks Fifth Avenue, and they worked diligently all through the night before the day of delivery, creating what they were labeling their "Winter Fruit Compote." They stewed up such vast quantities of fruit that the air and their hair and their epidermi became adhesive; after a sticky game of hyper-pattycake, they hailed a taxi and rushed off to Saks with their load of "Compote," feeling just as stuck together as the fruit in their jars.

For the Silver Palate, success and calamity have walked hand in hand from the beginning. On the day they opened their doors, they sold out completely. That's the success part. The calamity part is that Sheila had to turn herself into a cooking dervish to supply demand, rushing from bed to stove at four in the morning, slipping a coat over her nightgown to trundle product to the store. In those times, 20-hour days were common for both; if they had a motto, it might be "Hard Work," and their current prosperity shows the virtue of it. Even now, they sometimes put in the kinds of hours that a Sherpa guide would think twice about.

Their outreach well beyond Columbus Avenue was made manifest in their two eclectic cookbooks: *The Silver Palate Cookbook* and *The Silver Palate Good Times Cookbook*, both published by Workman (1982 and 1985), and both runaway best-sellers.

They also spread their gospel of fresh, clear and distinctive taste by making personal appearances: Julee speaks frequently on the gastronomical circuit, and Sheila takes teaching engagements at major cooking schools. At home, Julee handles advertising, media relations, sales and merchandising. Together, they develop all the recipes and new products and packaging. Sheila supervises the production of fresh and preserved foods and catering. They also publish a newsletter, and have taken on a monthly column in *Parade* Magazine called "Simply Delicious."

All this is a far cry from the fantasy that grew from their first meeting, when Sheila was running a catering business in New York called "The Other Woman Catering"—Motto, "So discreet, so delicious, and I deliver"—and Julee hired her to cater a business breakfast. Each was looking for a hobby, a fun little something to do on the side. Today, of course, there *is* no other side, and 20-hour days are still not uncommon. But it is still fun too, and never more so than when the two women reminisce about the early days, especially about the many triumphs snatched in last, lunatic moments from the jaws of disaster.

Among these tales is one with which any

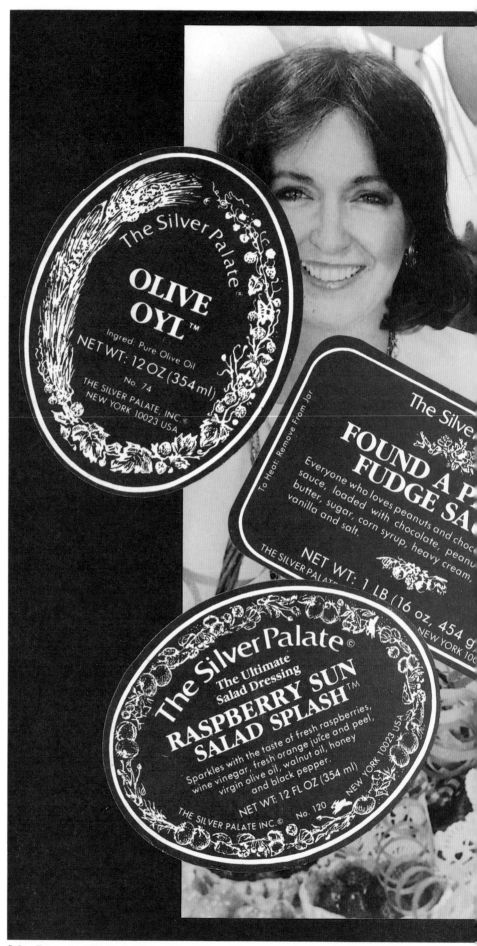

Julee Rosso and Sheila Lukins of The Silver Palate run a class operation. All their stuff tastes

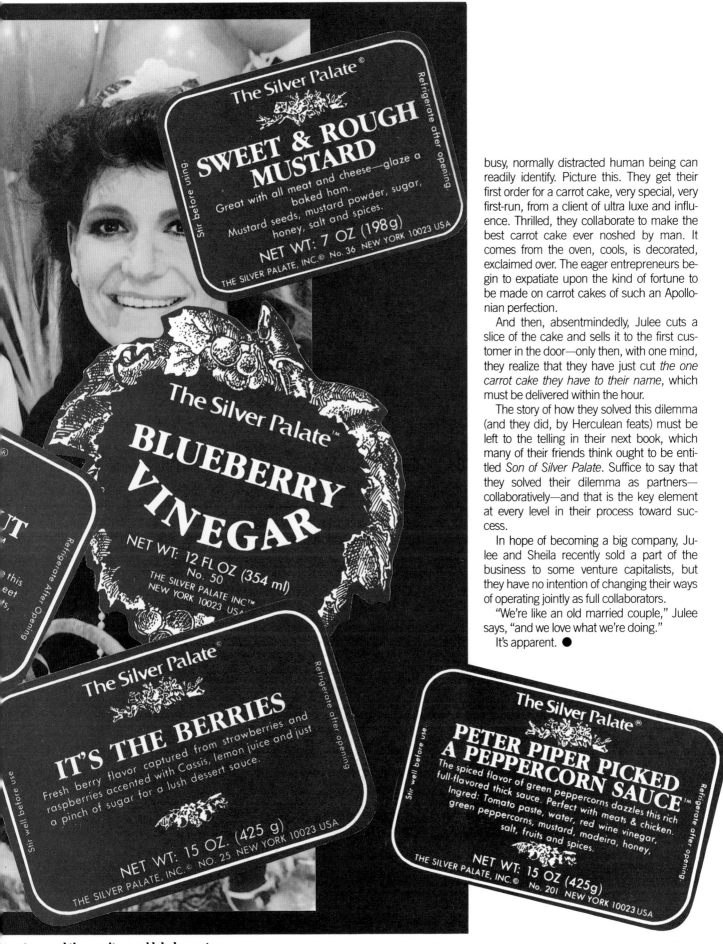

The Silver Palate ©

SWEET & ROUGH MUSTARD

Great with all meat and cheese—glaze a baked ham.

Mustard seeds, mustard powder, sugar, honey, salt and spices.

NET WT: 7 OZ (198g)

THE SILVER PALATE, INC.© No. 36 NEW YORK 10023 USA

Stir before using.

Refrigerate after opening.

The Silver Palate™

BLUEBERRY VINEGAR

NET WT: 12 FL OZ
No. 50 (354 ml)

THE SILVER PALATE INC™
NEW YORK 10023 USA

Refrigerate After Opening

The Silver Palate ©

IT'S THE BERRIES

Fresh berry flavor captured from strawberries and raspberries accented with Cassis, lemon juice and just a pinch of sugar for a lush dessert sauce.

NET WT: 15 OZ. (425 g)

THE SILVER PALATE, INC.© NO. 25 NEW YORK 10023 USA

Stir well before use

Refrigerate after opening

The Silver Palate ®

PETER PIPER PICKED A PEPPERCORN SAUCE™

The spiced flavor of green peppercorns dazzles this rich full-flavored thick sauce. Perfect with meats & chicken.

Ingred: Tomato paste, water, red wine vinegar, green peppercorns, mustard, madeira, honey, salt, fruits and spices.

NET WT: 15 OZ (425g)

THE SILVER PALATE, INC.© No. 201 NEW YORK 10023 USA

Stir well before use

Refrigerate after opening

busy, normally distracted human being can readily identify. Picture this. They get their first order for a carrot cake, very special, very first-run, from a client of ultra luxe and influence. Thrilled, they collaborate to make the best carrot cake ever noshed by man. It comes from the oven, cools, is decorated, exclaimed over. The eager entrepreneurs begin to expatiate upon the kind of fortune to be made on carrot cakes of such an Apollonian perfection.

And then, absentmindedly, Julee cuts a slice of the cake and sells it to the first customer in the door—only then, with one mind, they realize that they have just cut *the one carrot cake they have to their name*, which must be delivered within the hour.

The story of how they solved this dilemma (and they did, by Herculean feats) must be left to the telling in their next book, which many of their friends think ought to be entitled *Son of Silver Palate*. Suffice to say that they solved their dilemma as partners— collaboratively—and that is the key element at every level in their process toward success.

In hope of becoming a big company, Julee and Sheila recently sold a part of the business to some venture capitalists, but they have no intention of changing their ways of operating jointly as full collaborators.

"We're like an old married couple," Julee says, "and we love what we're doing."

It's apparent. ●

great . . . and they write good label copy too.

FRESH COOKIE STORES FEEL BITE

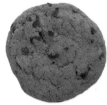

Ever since Wally Amos opened the first Famous Amos cookie store on Hollywood's Sunset Boulevard in 1975, the fresh-baked chocolate chip cookie business has appealed to entrepreneurs.

"The cookie business looked like such an easy business that every doctor or dentist with a brother-in-law out of work opened a cookie store," says Don Sawyer, president of Famous Amos Chocolate Cookie Co. "There was an explosion of amateur cookie store owners." Today, he estimates, there are at least 1,200 cookie stores in the U.S.

But growth is slowing. And the number of independent companies is shrinking as smaller cookie retailers close stores or sell to larger competitors. Even some of the bigger companies are feeling the squeeze. David's Cookies Inc., a market leader with about 170 stores, has lost at least 21 company-owned and franchised outlets, including seven in its New York City home market.

The main reason: The market for munchies on the run is moving on—new confectionary concoctions and other snack foods are competing for consumers' attention. Says Mr. Sawyer of Famous Amos, "The competition for snack dollars is way up."

The stiffer competition illustrates the risk in latching on to a snack-food fad—both for an entrepreneur with a catchy concept and for investors eager to buy franchise rights. In recent years, small businessmen have gambled on outlets specializing in gourmet ice cream, flavored popcorn, tofu-based desserts, crepes, muffins, funnel cakes and other pricey snacks.

"The longevity factor is not there," says Steve Sacks who, as a senior leasing representative at Melvin Simon & Associates, an Indianapolis, Indiana, shopping center developer, has watched food gimmicks rise and fall. Noting one current fad, he says, "Putting M&Ms on ice cream and putting it in a waffle cone is a very clever idea. Would people want to eat it every day? No."

No one is suggesting that the fresh-baked chocolate chip cookie will go the way of the Hula-Hoop. But cookie entrepreneurs agree that expansion will be tougher, particularly for small companies trying to break out of re-

DAVID'S COOKIES

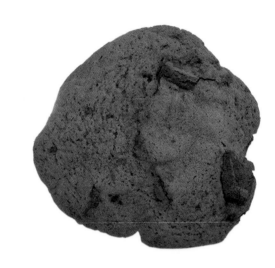
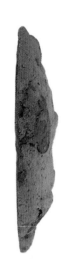

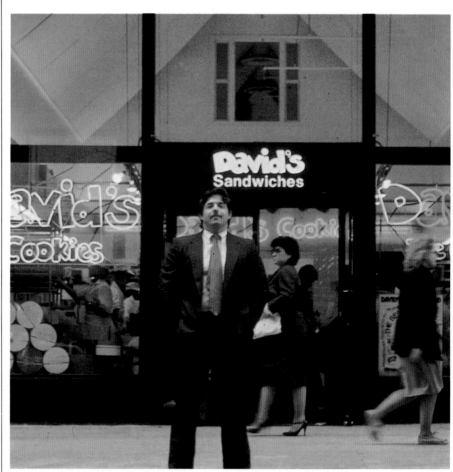

David Liederman, proprietor, David's Cookies: best little cookies in the world

AS SNACK-FOOD MARKETS SHIFT

MRS. FIELDS' COOKIES

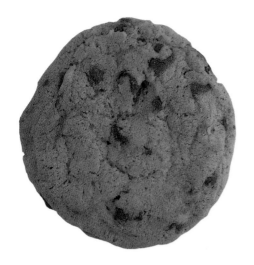
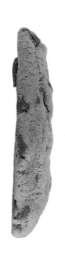

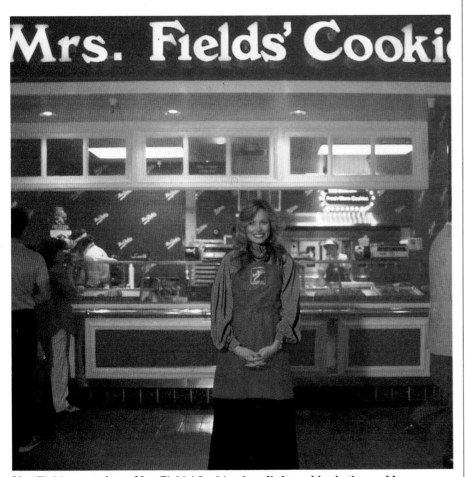

Mrs. Fields, proprietor, Mrs. Fields' Cookies: best little cookies in the world

gional markets. For one thing, the fresh-baked cookie business depends on pedestrian traffic, and the best locations in shopping malls and downtown areas have mostly been taken.

In fact, many mom-and-pop operations are dropping out. Mrs. Fields Inc. alone has gobbled up some two dozen smaller companies that decided to call it quits. Now the company has 250 Mrs. Fields shops, plus about 75 Famous Cookie Co. stores, which it bought in 1984 and plans to reopen under the name Jessica's Cookies.

Other entrepreneurs are determined to stay in the market, but they are finding it tough going. Jackie Kamin, who has launched seven Jackie's Cookie Connection stores on the East Coast since 1979, now is down to only two shops. Though she intends to stay in the business (she has two more stores in the works), Ms. Kamin concedes that the industry "isn't anything like it was. The competition is pretty stiff."

The response of most cookie sellers has been to expand product lines to broaden their appeal. Neal's Cookies in Houston now carries muffins—"yuppie doughnuts," owner Neal Elinoff calls them. Lawrence Rozanki,

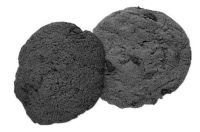

who has eight Larry's Cookies shops in the Washington, D.C., area, is moving away from cookie stores altogether. In the future, he intends to open cafés that sell everything from cookies and croissants to soups and sandwiches.

The trick, though, is to diversify without blurring one's image—a mistake that some say David's Cookies has made. Last year, all but one of the 15 David's franchises in Ohio and Western Pennsylvania closed. Suette Steiner, director of field operations at Dalton Industries Inc. in Cleveland, which owned the franchises, blames the cookies' price. "Being in the Midwest, people preferred to bake the cookies rather than buy them at $6.60 a pound," she says.

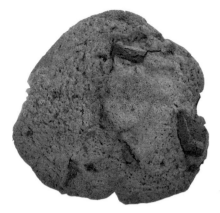

But Cheryl L. Krueger of Cheryl's Cookies Inc. in Columbus, Ohio, who benefited from the closings, says that overdiversification was the problem. David's stores, she notes, now carry ice cream, brownies, muffins, French bread, soft drinks and even mugs and T-shirts. "It looks to me like a lack of focus, and I think it's confusing to the customer," she says.

David Liederman, the owner of David's Cookies, defends the diversification. "The novelty has worn off," he says. "People are not buying the idea of walking into a store just to buy cookies." In fact, he says, he is beginning to rename his stores David's Specialty Foods to reflect their broadened product line.

With even Mr. Liederman hedging his bets, market analysts are looking for the next snack-food fad. Mr. Sacks, the shopping center leasing agent in Indianapolis, says fresh cinnamon rolls have become a hot item in many of his company's malls.

But other items are springing up, too. Sourdough Puff Co. of San Francisco, for example, says it has agreements to open 255 Golden Fresh Puffs franchises in 14 states. The puffs are pieces of fried dough with breakfast, entrée and dessert toppings.

Sourdough's president, Timothy Ryan, is a veteran of the Red Lobster and Magic Pan crepe restaurants and knows something about the fickleness of food fads. "In this business," he says, "if you stand still, somebody gains on you. Food retailing is so dynamic, it changes overnight." ●

Steven P. Galante, staff reporter, *The Wall Street Journal*

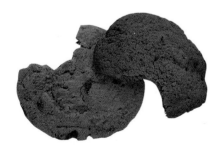

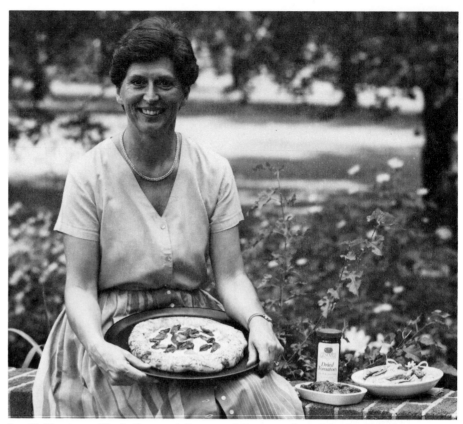

In a Sicilian town, Nicole Genovesi discovered the taste of sunshine in a dried tomato.

Genovesi Food Company
Nicole Genovesi, proprietor

Nicole Genovesi spent the summer of 1958 in Pachino, a little town in Sicily. She and her husband were visiting his relatives and there was not much for a 22-year-old woman to do but observe the people and their ways of living. At that time, her family and neighbors slept on straw mattresses and rearranged the stuffing each morning. They had no stoves, but cooked in the fireplace. And each rooftop had an open porch where the women hung laundry, made tomato paste and set out fresh tomatoes to dry in the hot, steady Mediterranean sun.

At home in Dayton, Ohio, Nicole Genovesi never forgot the intense flavor of those sun-dried tomatoes. The more she thought about them, she recalls, the more she said to herself, "I want some of those." As an experiment, she picked some tomatoes from her backyard vines, salted the halves, dried them for 36 hours in a very slow oven and bottled them in oregano-spiked oil. She did that every summer for years. Friends prized a gift of dried tomatoes from Nicole.

In 1982 she had her first taste of imported Italian sundried tomatoes, and immediately said, "Mine are much better." Friends encouraged her to make a test batch, so the following summer, Nicole Genovesi bought 1,440 pounds of tomatoes and a small dehy-drator. She washed, rinsed, cut, salted, sorted and packed each tomato by hand.

The finished product, first sold in specialty stores in Dayton and Washington, D.C., won raves from *The Washington Post* and orders from around the country. Now during the two-month tomato season she picks up 1,800 pounds of tomatoes straight from the field three times a week. The tomatoes are still handled one by one but Nicole did switch to dried garlic. "I used fresh garlic for the test batch," she says, "but every time I sat down, in the backyard or in front of the TV, I was peeling garlic to be crushed. For a year my hands smelled of garlic." ●

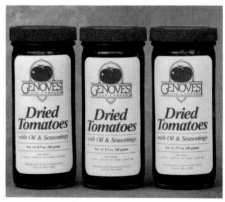

The packaged product, dryly presented

California Chèvre

Laura Chenel, proprietor

The next time you eat goat cheese, think of goats. Think of them the way Laura Chenel does, as intelligent and sensitive animals. Because it was Chenel and her Swiss goats who started the goat cheese industry in this country.

Its seeds were in the anti-war days of the early 70s. On spring evenings, Chenel, her former husband and their graceful white goats would take walks through the apple and plum orchards of their farm in Sonoma County, California. They had moved there to forge a self-sufficient lifestyle. Here, Laura Chenel quickly developed a bond with the goats. "They call you when it's milking time if you're late," she says. "You sit down and start milking and you can lean your head on their nice warm bellies, and they just stand, real calm, and all you hear is milk going into the bucket."

Chenel initially used that milk to make Monterey Jack cheese. It was tasty enough. But in 1977, she had her first piece of chèvre—French goat cheese—and was swept away by the flavor. She had been searching for a project, and producing chèvre became the compelling answer. However, not a single person was making it in the United States; if she wanted to learn, she had to go to France, which she did in 1979. She spent three months with four rural families whose livelihood was making goat cheese.

"I basically went there as an open vessel and placed myself in the hands of the various people with whom I lived and said, 'Fill me up with what you do,'" says Chenel.

Back in California, she made a batch of goat cheese and offered samples to shops which had carried her Monterey Jack. They were wild for it. She bought a farm, set up a fromagerie, and worked at two waitressing jobs to pay the mortgage. When Chenel's health protested the overload, she gave up her goats and the farm, and concentrated on the making of the cheese in a 2,500-square-foot cement fromagerie in Santa Rosa.

Laura Chenel and her six employees make 15 varieties of goat cheese totaling 60,000 pounds a year. The volume is far from staggering. "It's tiny, tiny. When you talk to cow's milk people, it's a joke," she says. "I've never had any kind of goal or five-year plan. I've been doing what I want to do, and the business just sort of lopes along."

Now, however, Chenel is starting to see that there is a growing goat cheese industry in the United States—already 30 companies strong. "America is really changing," she says, and she'd like to help spread the word about chèvre. The time may be ripe for her to increase production and do far better than a comfortable break even. ●

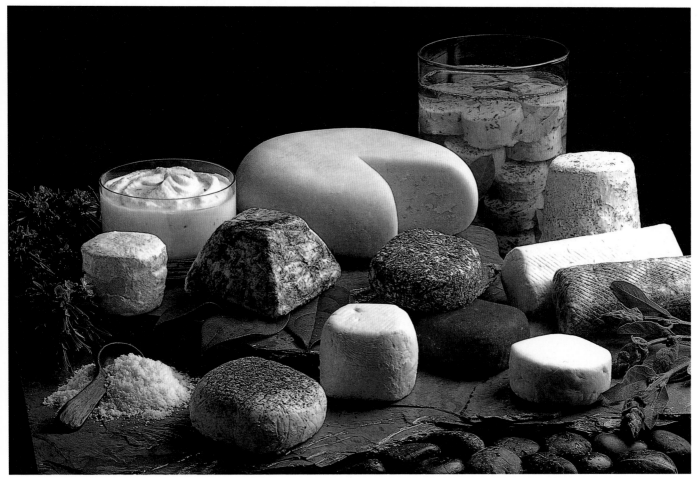

Whatever the shape or form, goat cheese has a bite beyond the common herd, and Laura Chenel made it happen in America.

Bubbies Of San Francisco

Leigh Truex, Proprietor

Leigh Truex was ten years old when she tasted her first kosher dill pickles. She was eating a roast beef sandwich in the kitchen of her aunt and uncle's house in Stockton, California. She sliced and ate one after another until she had eaten six of the big homemade dills. That was enough to make her sick the next day but not sick enough to diminish her passion for the pickles. They were garlicky, briny, tangy hot and spicy, unlike anything that her health-conscious parents in New York City had ever allowed her to eat.

The sassy pickles were made by her aunt's mother, a gourmet kosher cook who became a surrogate grandmother to young Leigh. Years later, after her grandmother died, Leigh Truex experimented with making

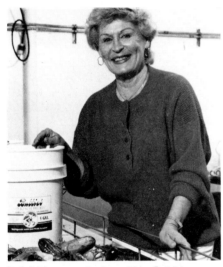

Leigh Truex and a few of her Bubbies

pickles until they emerged with that same tongue-rattling flavor. She switched to small cucumbers for more crunch and cured them in a cloudy, vinegarless brine spiked with hand-peeled garlic cloves, pickling spices, bits of red pepper and fresh dill stalks and flowers.

Leigh Truex gave the pickles to friends and family at holidays, and in 1981, one ended up in the mouth of a business acquaintance of her son. "My God," he said, "what's your mother doing in real estate? *These* should be on the market."

Northern California real estate was flat at the time, anyway. Leigh Truex took a month's sabbatical, rented a plant and put up 350 cases of her assertive dills. She named them Bubbies because the word has double

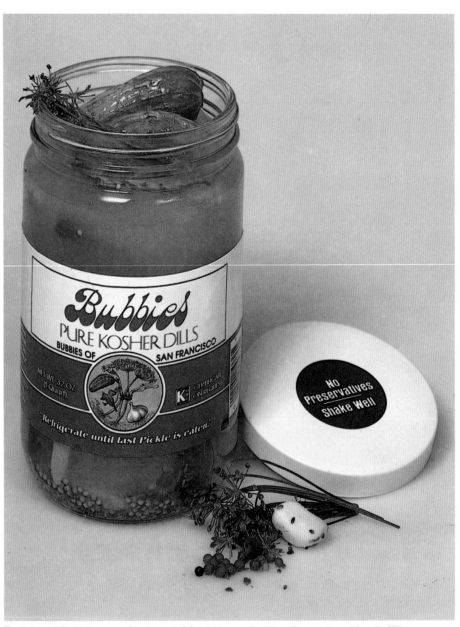

Each jar of Bubbies pure kosher pickles is topped with a flowerette of fresh dill.

meaning: It's a Yiddish term of endearment and nickname for grandmothers. Then she took Bubbies to a San Francisco food show. After a rave review by Jack Shelton, the late Marin County food critic, Bubbies catapulted to become the Bay Area's pickle of choice.

Truex shuttered her San Francisco plant between 1983 and September 1985 while gathering financing for a plant capable of meeting demand. Now curing in Stockton, California, she transforms Mexican and Cali-

fornian cucumbers into snappy dills at a rate of 3,000 cases a month. And in March 1986, she introduced a chunky relish.

Truex doesn't promote novel ways of eating Bubbies. "Just slice 'em long ways," she says, "and eat them with the usual." Her mail tells her that Bubbies have turned otherwise reasonable people into addicts. "It's mind boggling to me that people would take the time to write a letter to a *pickle*," she says. ●

Cheesecakes By J. R.

Janet Rosen, Proprietor

One day in 1980, Janet Rosen phoned the owner of Gene & Georgetti, an Italian restaurant in Chicago and one of the busiest in the city. She asked for an appointment to bring in her cheesecake for him to sample—just as she had done with other local restaurant owners over the previous 18 months.

"No," the man said flatly, "we're not interested. People are too full when they come out of here. And we don't make any money on dessert."

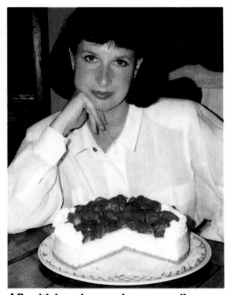

J.R. with her cheesecake nonpareil

Janet Rosen hung up the phone. "This," she said to herself, "is one of the biggest-volume restaurants in Chicago, and the only dessert they serve is spumoni. They *need* my cheesecake."

Besides, she knew he was mistaken about the money. A good slice of cheesecake can command $4 on a menu but costs the restaurant 75¢. That's not a bad profit for merely dirtying a plate. So Rosen grabbed one of her creamy, four-pound cheesecakes, headed for Gene & Georgetti's, asked for the owner and marched up three flights of stairs to his office where she found him doing the payroll. She launched into her pitch. "He didn't look up once," Rosen remembers. "He kept writing checks, just asked a few questions, then said, 'OK, I'll taste it.'"

The sample sold him. And five years later, Gene & Georgetti is still one of her more than 300 accounts in the Chicago area. Back in 1980, when Janet Rosen launched Cheese-

cakes by J.R., many restaurants served frozen cheesecakes hastily thawed or the less-than-expert efforts of their kitchen staffs. The idea of offering fine, locally baked desserts was a novel one which occurred to Rosen while she was studying for her undergraduate and graduate degrees in fine arts.

At that time, Rosen earned money by doing stints in a deli, a family restaurant, a steakhouse and a French Continental restaurant. She was struck by their commonality in one area: No one had desserts nearly as good as the ones that she had eaten around the family dinner table. Her mother was the type who would never think of *buying* a cookie, and everything she baked was rich with butter or chocolate. "I grew up having this around me, thinking it was natural," says Rosen.

By the time she received her M.A. in 1979, Rosen decided to put her ability to conceptualize projects to the test in a new arena: the dessert business. She settled on cheesecake and, after developing the recipe, began baking two days a week. With the help of her mother and sister, her weekly output was 30 cakes. Now 14 employees in a new plant on the northern edge of Chicago produce more than 1,200 cheesecakes weekly. Three-quarters of them are delivered to wholesale accounts in the Midwest. The rest are sold in the bakery's retail shop for $15-$16, and by mail order in the continental United States.

Cheesecake lovers can choose from among 14 different flavors, all developed by Janet Rosen, and each with a different crushed-cookie crust. The chocolate chip cheesecake crust, for instance, is made from light and dark cookie crumbs, walnuts, freshly shaved chocolate and unsalted butter. "My idea of a great cheesecake is everything melding together," she says. "I want the whole picture to say what the flavor is supposed to be"—be it double chocolate chip, cappuccino, raspberry, pineapple-coconut or strawberry.

The majority of Janet Rosen's time is gobbled by the bookkeeping aspects of the business, but she keeps her hand in every pie. "I work and I keep control and when I go out in the bakery, my eyes are all over those cakes. We use the best ingredients, and, in looks, I don't want an air bubble or a brown spot or unevenness," she says firmly. "We don't send an imperfect cake out of here." ●

The Mozzarella Company

Paula Lambert, Proprietor

It wasn't anything so bucolic as a fondness for cows or goats that led Paula Lambert to the cheesemaking business. She wanted fresh mozzarella, the moist kind that oozed milk when cut with a knife, the kind that she'd savored on numerous trips to Italy.

Such mozzarella was not to be found in Dallas. Whenever a new Italian restaurant opened, Paula Lambert called and asked, "Do you have fresh mozzarella?" when told yes, she rushed over to taste it. But it was never the mozzarella like that sold in every corner market in Italy or straight from the cheese factories. It was old and dry and sour.

Lambert had a longtime friend—Suzanne Bartolucci—who married an Italian doctor and moved to the town of Perugia, between Florence and Rome. Lambert went to visit her on a vacation in 1981. One day they were sitting in the garden of the Bartolucci villa, eating fresh mozzarella, when Lambert began bemoaning its absence in the United States. "Why don't *you* make it?" asked Bartolucci.

They struck a deal to be partners; and Lambert—who was fluent in Italian—set out to learn about mozzarella.

Her first stop was a small, family-owned cheese factory at the foot of the hills in Assisi. "It wasn't a place where the milk went into a tube and you never saw it again," she recalls. The family welcomed her to spend time and learn the process. "They just let me put my hands in it and touch the cheese and

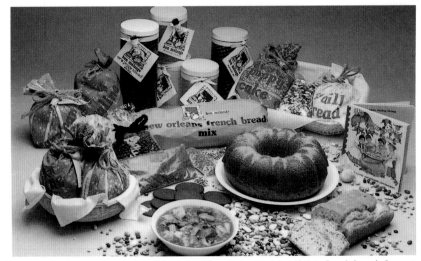

With foods from beans to bundt cakes, Bon Melange highlights Louisiana's bounty.

ask all the questions and make notes and take photographs," says Lambert, who spent a whole month observing and learning. From there she went to visit a renowned professor at a government-run cheesemaking trade school in northern Italy. He, in turn, referred her to a young professor who was excited by the idea of a trip to Texas to help set up a cheese operation.

Back home, Lambert set to work converting an old drugstore in a warehouse district on the edge of downtown Dallas and, in 1982, The Mozzarella Company was born.

The company uses only fresh milk—no frozen curds—in their cheeses and makes them entirely by hand. Patience was the most important lesson Paula Lambert learned from her young Italian consultant. "You've just got to be patient," she says. "The milk is a growing organism and it's different every day. It can come from the same animal and we can make it the same way, but it's different every day. You have to wait. You have to wait for the right moment to go on to the next step."

Lambert made another trip to Italy in 1982 to expand her cheesemaking knowledge and the company now makes 17 varieties. Fresh mozzarella accounts for half of the 6,000 pounds of cheese the company produces each month. "It's really an art and a science. It's all just milk. You vary the temperature and the way you cut it and stir and this and that, and you come up with all these different cheeses," she says with delight. "It really is variations on a theme."

After three years of losing money, The Mozzarella Company moved into the black. Lambert stubbornly refused to raise the prices because, as she put it, "I can't stand inflation. I think everything costs too much." A pound of mozzarella still goes for its original price of $5.50 wholesale and $7.50 retail. ●

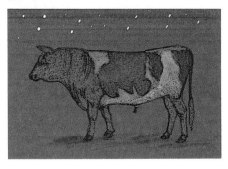

Bon Melange
Malee Hearin, Proprietor

Malee Hearin didn't realize that she was starting a business, but—boom!—that's what happened.

In 1978, when she experimented with a childhood friend's recipe for spicy multibean soup, she thought she was simply tunneling her way out of boredom. Each time her husband relocated with General Electric, Malee Hearin had to give up her own job. When they ended up in Dayton, Ohio, she decided to take a break. She played golf; she played bridge. But faced with a nest newly bare of children, she grew restless without a focus. The soup, at least, was something to *do*.

She bagged a one-pound assortment of 15 kinds of beans, peas, barley, and included a packet of Creole spices and a recipe for adding liquid, meats, onion, garlic and celery. After dubbing it French Market Soup, she took it to a friend who owned a gift shop in Cincinnati. The shop ordered six dozen packets.

Hearin immediately hightailed it to a wholesale bean store, loaded 25 pounds of each of the store's 21 bean varieties into her trunk and started a cottage industry in her basement. She lined up another Cincinnati client and one in Dayton, and for one year, she kept the three shops supplied with bags of French Market Soup. She cooked up pots of soup like mad, she remembers, and served samples at the stores. "I thought I was a howling success," says Malee Hearin dryly, now living with her husband in Mississippi. "I sold $5,000 worth of stuff and thought I was $5,000 richer, which my husband told me wasn't exactly true."

In 1980, her first client urged Hearin to find a sales representative at the Gift Mart in Columbus, Ohio. "I brought one little bag of beans and went into the showrooms and looked for one that carried a nice mix of things," says Malee Hearin. "Then I pulled the bag out of my purse and said, 'Do you want this?' And they said, 'Yeah.'"

It was that easy.

By this time, beans were delivered to Hearin's house by the truckload. Half a dozen women and a couple of high school girls helped with the bagging. "It was fun. It was like a quilting bee," she remembers. And actually, that's the folk history of multibean soups: Women would gather at a friend's house or church, each bringing a bag of beans; there they would mix them, re-bag them and trade recipes.

Malee Hearin grew up in New Orleans, where soups are both plentiful and spicy. "Everything has to be real hot," she says, "because people down here think that if you get hotter on the inside, you'll get cooler on the outside. People eat gumbo all summer long."

When others tried to copy her French Market soup, Hearin defended her trademark and also decided to expand the Bon Melange line. Now the line has grown to include four kinds of bean soup, dill and French bread mixes and a variety of desserts. In 1985, Hearin sold 100,000 products, 42,000 of which were soups retailing for about $5.

Each item is packaged beautifully. Along with the recipes themselves, Malee Hearin believes that the packaging has been critical to the success of Bon Melange. "It looks pretty," she says. "You wanted to bring something to your hostess or a neighbor who's kept the dog, and you didn't want to bring a terribly expensive gift but something *nice*. I think people were tired of giving each other ashtrays." ●

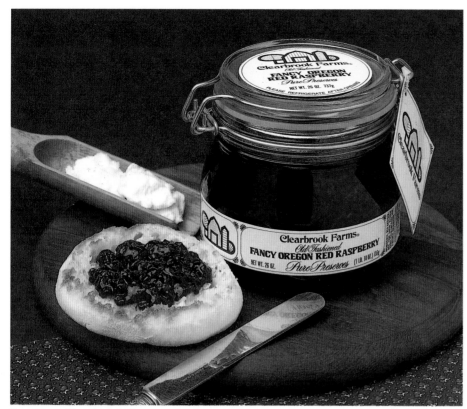

Breakfast, Clearbrook Farms-style: Oregon raspberry jam on a toasted English

Clearbrook Farms

Dan Cohen, Proprietor

Dan Cohen's grandfather once made sweaters in Cincinnati, Ohio, but when textile mills opened in the South, the family could not compete. In scouting around for other work, they heard that the Dolly Madison bakery in Cincinnati needed red raspberry preserves for their coconut-topped jelly rolls. The family needed a living, so in 1924, they opened the Cincinnati Preserving Co.

The new company concentrated on making the jelly roll filling for about 30 years until Dolly Madison switched from preserves to raspberry powder mixed with corn syrup and sugar. In the meantime, the family had also expanded their new business to make preserves for doughnuts, pastries, turnovers and cookies as well as fruity pancake syrups.

Each year at Christmas, this business—like most—sent gifts to their customers: cigars, fruitcakes and the like. Finally, in 1952, they asked themselves, "Why are we running all over town buying fruitcakes when we make fine preserves?" So, without regard to cost, they made six or eight flavors of preserves. They named them Clearbrook Farms Old Fashioned Pure Preserves, filled 16-ounce bottles by hand, labeled them and delivered assortments to clients.

Thank-you letters poured in, raving about the preserves. Word spread, and the following Christmas, they gave assortments to relatives and friends too. The annual tradition continued for nearly another 30 years.

A turning point for the company came in 1979 when Dan Cohen—the next generation—was working on a doctorate in pharmacology and biophysics at the University of Cincinnati School of Medicine. At that time, his father was considering selling the company's preserves to stores. "I—and everyone in the family—thought it was a great idea," recalls Cohen, and he abandoned his doctorate and applied himself to the new venture. He, his uncle and father rounded up red and black raspberries, blackberries and boysenberries from Oregon, tiny wild blueberries from Maine, cherries, strawberries and plums from Michigan, peaches and apricots from California. Cohen adjusted recipes to vacuum kettles, which, because of shorter cooking time and lower temperatures, yield more flavorful preserves than open-air kettles. He made the preserves with cane sugar and the highest grade of fruit and packed them in half-liter French canning jars.

Dan Cohen, who was fastidious with medical research, has a similar passion for perfection with Clearbrook Farms. "I spend my life," he admits with good humor, "being compulsive and concerned about our product. I don't cut corners because it doesn't feel good when I cut corners." ●

Chalif, Inc.

Elizabeth And Nick Thomas, Proprietors

It is Russia, 1906. Sara Chalif receives a message from her husband Louis, who had fled to the United States: "Escape now." Sara sews her jewels into the lining of her coat, also, a recipe for Russian mustard. And Sara crosses the border, soldiers at her heels.

It is Sara's exact recipe that is now sold as Chalif's Hot 'n' Sweet Mustard. In 1981, the Chalifs' great-niece Elizabeth Thomas and her husband Nick took the last $200 of their savings and made a batch of her aunt's mustard. They carried a jar to a cheese shop in Pennsylvania and said to the owner, "Would you like to taste the best mustard in the world?" She told them to come back the following month.

"Can you at least taste it?" Nick pleaded. They didn't even know if it had a chance. The woman dipped her finger into the mustard. "I'll take two cases," she said.

"That was our entire inventory," remembers Elizabeth Thomas, now senior vice-president of Chalif Mustard, Inc. "She paid cash for it, and we ran out and bought more ingredients."

The company is still small but has expanded in sales and products. Whole grain and honey mustards are now also offered as well as five styles of mayonnaise—from Strawberries and Champagne to Dill-Basil-Mint and Stirling Sauce and a tamari-based sauce of peaches and cashews. All the new recipes have been developed by the family and the company expects to do $500,000 worth of business in 1986. "It's a romantic story," Elizabeth Thomas says happily, "vis-à-vis The American Dream." ●

Cottage Industry profiles by Howard Solganik and Janet Filips

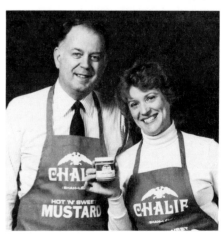

Q: What's hot and sweet and sold all over?

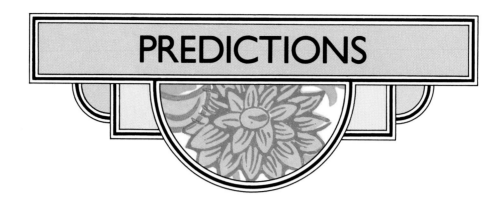

PREDICTIONS

FACING UP TO THE FUTURE

Now, we have come to the end of the Almanac. We have looked to see what is happening in restaurants, in fast-food chains, in homes and in the marketplace. We have examined the mysterious inner workings of food scientists, fragrance makers and genetic engineers. We have peered into the offices of advertisers, the drawing boards of package designers and the ledger books of accountants. We have gasped at the plans of big business and examined the dreams of cottage industries. We have absorbed all this mass of information and we have glimpsed the future.

"And what will the future bring?" you cry.

The future has been decided.

It is a Chicken McNugget!

"No, no," you wail. "This cannot be all there is."

It is. I can prove it.

We can date our recent history from the moment that Herbert Hoover proclaimed to a hungry nation: "Let there be a chicken in every pot."

And there was.

We have found the promised land. Well, not exactly. If there is not a chicken in every pot, there is most certainly one sizzling on every street corner and that is close enough.

The farmers are providing us with more and yet more chickens. The geneticists have already proved that they can engineer chickens without feathers—they can, but the chickens get so neurotic about their nudity that they refuse to eat and will not lay any eggs. So, back to the drawing board with

that idea, but we know it can be done. We have also seen that there are ways—albeit by the judicious use of bleaching agents—to make all-white-meat chickens because that is what researchers say we want.

The chicken is a noble bird. It does nothing but give. Its meat is extruded or stamped out into neat nuggets, its liver is processed into pâté and the giblets are made into gravy. Sadly, they say its eggs will make our hearts break, but happily, its bones, simmered into chicken soup, will make us well again. Even the feathers can be made into a hat. A chicken is no turkey. It is the symbol of plenty in the land of abundance. So what is good for big business, scientists, doctors and politicians—must be good for us too.

Well, it is and it isn't.

It is good for us from a nutritional standpoint. We all know that chicken is better for us than red meat. But take away red meat in the form of a hamburger and you do away with the bun. Alas fear not, less bread for the fast-food chains does not mean less dough. The McNugget is the golden goose feathering its nest beneath the golden arches. And more and more customers flock to the source. A McNugget wrapped like a gift in colorful paper is fun to eat. It is all things to all people. Those who strive to be healthy love it. Those who don't concern themselves with nutritionally-balanced diets, who refuse to fret over such foolishness, like it too—especially when it is deep-fried in beef fat until crispy and crunchy and super-delicious. Cheap too! And fast. We want everything fast

these days. If the evening news reported tonight that Moses handed down ten commandments, we wouldn't have the time or the attention span for them. Dan Rather would just say there was a summit meeting today and the two most important things decided were. . . . Then Johnny Carson would make the news part of his monologue and create funny scenes revolving around McNuggets, and the world would know about them in an instant.

So the fast-food chains are happy, and the healthy people are happy, and the junk-food addicts are enraptured, and the supermarkets overflow with 99 frozen versions of McNuggets and the take-out food places make a hundred variations on the theme. The cooks in the Lean Cuisine kitchens hatch up "lite" renditions. Then low-fat, low-salt versions appear before our wondering eyes. And then they said, "Let there be an upscale version of them," and there will be. There will soon be range-fed chicken nuggets and nifty nuggets with nasturtium blossoms. Nimble fingers will arrange two or three all-natural native Nebraska nuggets on a plate in all the finest restaurants. And these nibbles will nourish the "nattering nabobs," nurture the captains of industry, and feed the fashionable and the feeble. The kids love them and the grazers love them, the MAPAs (Middle-Aged PArents) and the old folk love 'em too. (Though we don't say old folk any more, but rather ROCies, Revered Older Citizens). Everything is becoming miniaturized from our language to our cars, our apart-

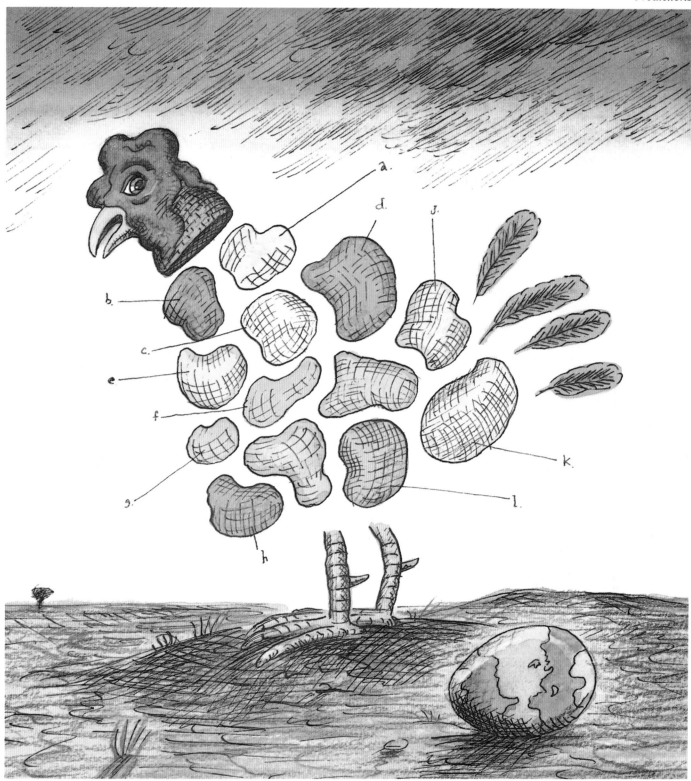

ments and our under-the-counter appliances. . . .

The truth is that we all love McNuggets and there are several reasons why this is so. Some have to do with the 60s, another momentous moment in our sociological history. The 60s, you may have noticed, has stopped being thought of as an era but has shrunk into a single entity—an instant frozen in time. The term 60s is a sort of demographic shorthand—a single word used to describe a generation of babies that grew up without mommies to cut up their food. Nor did they have grandmothers. The grannies were already contemplating taking aerobics classes. So who came along? Why, 'twas Mac and The King of the Burgers and Wendy and Roy Rogers who came galloping to the rescue and DeLited us all with fancy finger food and something to entertain us too. Between mouthfuls, while we are glued to the VCR, we can dunk our morsels of food into a won-derment of ethnic sweet sauces to counter-balance all those calories saved from the calorie-free diet colas.

So, for all these reasons, a McNugget is the perfect food, tooled for the way we live to-day. It satisfies us in every way. But the most fundamental reason for our national affection for the McNugget is that we as a nation have always cherished the idea of being able to sin and repent simultaneously. With a McNugget we can do that triumphantly. ●

U.S. Government Sources On Food

Government Agencies

DEPARTMENT OF AGRICULTURE
Fourteenth Street and Independence Avenue SW
Washington DC 20250
(202) 447-2791

Food and Nutrition Service (FNS)
3131 Park Center Drive
Alexandria VA 22302
(703) 756-3284

DEPARTMENT OF HEALTH AND HUMAN SERVICES
200 Independence Avenue SW
Washington DC 20201
(202) 245-6296

Food and Drug Administration (FDA)
5600 Fishers Lane
Rockville MD 20857
(301) 443-3380

FDA Consumer Affairs Offices

Atlanta GA 30309
(404) 881-7355

Baltimore MD 21201
(301) 962-3731

Boston MA 02109
(617) 223-5857

Brooklyn NY 11232
(718) 965-5043

Buffalo NY 14202
(716) 846-4483

Chicago IL 60607
(312) 353-7126

Cincinnati OH 45202
(513) 684-3501

Cleveland OH 44114
(216) 522-4844

Dallas TX 75201
(214) 767-5433

Denver CO 80202
(303) 844-4915

Detroit MI 48207
(313) 226-6273

East Orange NJ 07018
(201) 645-3265

Houston TX 77009
(713) 229-3550

Indianapolis IN 46204
(317) 269-6500

Kansas City MO 64106
(816) 374-3817

Los Angeles CA 90015
(213) 688-4395

Minneapolis MN 55401
(612) 349-3906

Nashville TN 37217
(615) 251-5208

New Orleans LA 70122
(504) 589-2420

Omaha NE 68102
(402) 221-4675

Orlando FL 32802
(305) 855-0900

Philadelphia PA 19106
(215) 597-0837

San Antonio TX 78204
(512) 229-6737

San Francisco CA 94102
(415) 556-2682

San Juan PR 00905
(809) 753-4443

Seattle WA 98174
(206) 442-5258

St. Louis MO 63102
(314) 425-5021

Center for Food Safety and Applied Nutrition
200 C Street SW

Washington DC 20204
(202) 245-8850

CONSUMER PRODUCT SAFETY COMMISSION
1111 Eighteenth Street NW
Washington DC 20207
(202) 634-7740

ENVIRONMENTAL PROTECTION AGENCY
401 M Street SW
Washington DC 20460
(202) 382-2090

The Office of Pesticides and Toxic Substances
TS788
401 M Street SW
Washington DC 20460
(202) 382-2902

UNITED STATES GOVERNMENT PRINTING OFFICE
Superintendent of Documents
Washington DC 20402
(202) 783-3238

Government Publications

BIBLIOGRAPHIES:
Food, Diet and Nutrition
April 15, 1986
SB-291

Canning, Freezing and Storage of Food
February 13, 1986
SB-005

Cookbooks and Recipes
October 21, 1985
SB-065

Posters, Charts, Picture Sets and Decals
June 28, 1985
SB-057

Consumer Information Catologue
Consumer Information Center
P.O. Box 100
Pueblo CO 81002

SELECTED INDIVIDUAL PUBLICATIONS:
Free booklets listed here are available from the Consumer Information Center. Priced publications may be ordered from the U.S. Government Printing Office.

GENERAL PUBLICATIONS
Breakfast Cereals
S/N 001-000-04283-1 $7

Composition of Foods: Raw, Processed, Prepared. Tables on the composition and nutritive value of foods.
S/N 001-000-00768-8 $7

Dairy and Egg Products
S/N 001-000-03635-1 $7

Fats and Oils
S/N 001-000-03984-9 $7

Fruits and Fruit Juices
S/N 001-000-04287-4 $9

Lamb in Family Meals
S/N 001-000-04098-7 $1

Nut and Seed Products
S/N 001-000-04429-0 $5.50

Pork in Family Meals
S/N 001-000-03640-8 $1

Pork Products
S/N 001-000-04368-4 $7.50

Poultry in Family Meals
S/N 001-000-03895-8 $1.75

Poultry Products
S/N 001-000-04008-1 $9.50

Sausages and Luncheon Meats
S/N 001-000-04183-5 $6

Soups, Sauces and Gravies
S/N 001-000-04114-2 $8

Soybeans in Family Meals
S/N 001-000-03320-4 $3.50

Vegetables and Vegetable Products
S/N 001-000-04427-3 $16

Vegetables in Family Meals
S/N 001-000-04150-9 $1

Vitalize Your Life, Discover Seafood: Your Guide to Nutrition from the Sea
S/N 003-020-00145-9 $1

BUYING GUIDES
Buy Better, Poster
S/N 001-024-00217-8 $2.75

Buying Food: A Guide for Calculating Amounts to Buy and Comparing Costs
S/N 001-000-03811-7 $4.50

Consumer's Guide to Food Labels
600P   Free

Fresh Fruits
S/N 001-00-04406-1 $1.50

Fruits and Vegetables
S/N 001-000-04309-9 $7

How to Eye and Buy Seafood
S/N 003-020-00001-1 $1.50

Meat, Poultry and Dairy Products
S/N 001-000-04308-1 $9

HEALTH AND NUTRITION
Cancer Prevention: Good News, Better News, Best News
560P   Free

A Compendium on Fats
515P   Free

The Confusing World of Health Foods
516P   Free

Diet and the Elderly
517P   Free

Eat Better, Poster
S/N 001-024-00216-0 $2.75

Eating for Better Health
S/N 001-000-04243-2 $3.50

Family Fare: A Guide to Good Nutrition
S/N 001-000-03777-3 $5.50

Food Additives
518P   Free

The Latest Caffeine Scorecard
519P   Free

Nutrition and Your Health: Dietary Guidelines for Americans
520P   Free

The Nutritional Gender Gap at the Dinner Table
521P   Free

Please Pass that Woman Some More Calcium and Iron
522P   Free

Sodium
523P   Free

The Sodium Content of Your Food
114P $2.25

Some Facts and Myths About Vitamins
524P   Free

Sugar
525P   Free

Sweetness Minus Calories Equals Controversy
526P   Free

That Lite Stuff
527P   Free

Vegetarian Diets
528P   Free

What About Nutrients in Fast Foods?
529P   Free

COOKBOOKS AND RECIPES
Cooking for Two
S/N 001-000-03698-0 $5.50

Country Catfish
S/N 003-020-00089-4 $1

Fish and Shellfish Over the Coals
S/N 003-020-00052-5 $1.75

CANNING, FREEZING AND STORAGE OF FOODS
Freezing Combination Main Dishes
S/N 001-000-03559-2 $2.25

Home Canning of Fruits and Vegetables
S/N 001-000-04333-1 $1.50

Home Canning of Meat and Poultry
S/N 001-000-04111-8 $2.25

Domestic Cooking Schools

continued from page 153

La Toque International, Ltd.
(215) 649-0437

To Market, To Market
(215) 925-0948

Rhode Island
Johnson & Wales College, Culinary Arts Division
(401) 456-1192

South Carolina
In Good Taste
(803) 763-5597

Tennessee
Conte-Philips
(615) 352-5837

La Maison Meridien
(901) 722-8892

Texas
The Cooking School
(214) 361-9848

Cooking with Amber, Inc.
(214) 363-3687

The French Apron Inc.
(817) 732-4758

Lepanier, Inc.
(713) 664-9848

The Little House
(512) 573-6684

Maison Bleu Gourmet Shop/Cooking
(512) 226-7116

Peeple's Choice/Cookin' Thyme
(713) 338-2011

The Stockpot Etc. Inc.
(214) 753-6868

Virginia
Dolores Kostelni Cooking School
(703) 261-2304

Giant's School of Cooking
(804) 855-6011

Potluck
(703) 371-2288

Washington
Arcade School: Frederick & Nelson
(206) 382-8307

Bon Vivant School of Cooking
(206) 525-7537

Final Touch Cooking School
(509) 663-6462

Kitchen Kitchen
(206) 451-9507

Magnolia Kitchen Shoppe & Cooking School
(206) 282-2665

Sur La Table
(206) 448-2244

Wisconsin
Cook's Habitat
(414) 274-3166

The Epicure Cooking School
(608) 271-7979

Modern Gourmet of Milwaukee
(414) 351-3679

Directory of Institutional Members
©Copyright International Association of Cooking Professionals 1986

Index

Advertising
  of fast-food chains, 87
  overall, 100
AE1 music, 172
Agribusiness, 155–171
AgrowNautics, 164
Airline food, 52, 190
Air and Travel Food Service, 190
A. J. Canfield Company, 52
Alaskan strawberries, 216
Albertson's, 70, 71
Algin, 178
Alpha Beta, 70
Amaranth, 163
American Cafés, 21
America, 111
American Food & California Wine, 20
American Leadership Group, 76
American Place, An, 22, 23
American School Food Service Organization, 193
American Taste of Japanese Cooking, 200
American Zephyr, 189
Amos, Wally, 222
Amtrak dining cars, 187
Amy, Stan, 65
Anderson, Jean, 18
Andoh, Elizabeth, 152, 200
Antibiotics for livestock, 160
Antoine's, 28
Aquabusiness, 173–181
Aquaculture, 175–176
Aqua Farms, 165
ARA Services, 91
Arby's TV ads, 87
Arcadia restaurant, 16
  lobster club sandwich, 206
Ark Restaurants, 114
Artichoke, 24
  Queen, 24
Artificial sweeteners, 40
Arum, Nancy, 62
Asparagus
  facts and lore, 69–70
  classic, George Lang's, 70
Aspartame, 40
Atemoya, 170
Atlantic Food, Inc., 148
At-Your-Service, 214
Aurora restaurant, 16

Bagel capital of the world, 104
Bagels
  frozen, 104
  increase in sales of, 104
Baldwin, Harley, 71
Balsley, Betsy, 22
Banana, sugar content of, 40
Banana skins, 208
B&B Charcoal Co., 128
Bang! The Explosive Popcorn Recipe Book, 32
Barbecued foods, 127
Barkies, 115
Bartolucci, Suzanne, 227
Bauer, Michael, 106
Baum, Joe, 16, 106, 107, 116, 178
Bay scallops, marinated, the Four Seasons', 131
Beard, James
  and Citymeals on Wheels, 172
  as early cooking instructor, 152

Beard, James, *Cont'd*
  fun food passion of, 33
  on salt, 40
  writing on American food, 200
Beatrice companies, 78, 79, 193, 195
Beef, rare, 208
Bell, Ross, 196
Benet, Jane, 16
Benjamin Company, 203
Berry, Wendell, 157
Better Homes & Gardens
  circulation of, 12
  Consumer Panel Inquiry into Food, 135, 136
Better Than Storebought, 20
Betty Brown's Broadway Dining, 114
Betty Crocker, changing image of, 102
Bildner, J., 58
Biomedical Business International, 196
Biosphere II, 171
Biscuits, ham, Edna Lewis', 145
Black beans and truffles, the Quilted Giraffe's, 215
Blue crab, 177
Bocuse, Paul, 213
Bombay duck, 216
Bon Appétit, 17
Bon Melange, 228
Borst, Bill, 182
Bowl of bossy, 114
Brace of beagles, 114
Bradley, Senator Bill, 34
Braler steer, 161
Braun coffeemaker, 142
Breakfast
  at Bridge Creek, 29
  Coke for, 29
  habits, 28
Breakfast-only restaurants, 28, 29
Brennan, Ella, 19
Brennan, Ralph, 146
Brennan's restaurant, 28
Brickman, Miriam, 184
Bridge Creek restaurant, 29
  peerless corn muffins, 28
Bridgemarket, 71
Brody, Jane, 23, 39, 41, 200
Brody, Laura, 172
Brown, Helen Gurley, 50
Brown, Dr. Robert, 127
Brucken, Robert, 32
Bubbies, 226
Buffalo chicken wings, Janice Okun's, 128
Buffalo roast, 44, 45
Bugialli, Giuliano, 19, 152, 200, 213
Burger King, 84, 85
  growth potential of, 88
  mobile stores, 87
  outlay for ads, 87, 100
Burr, Wesley, 135, 136
Burros, Marian, 19
Butel, Jane, 152, 213

Cabletext, 213
Café des Artistes, 16
Café Beaujolais' sour cream waffles, 189
Caffeine in chocolate, 50
Cagnina, Sam, 112
California Beef Council, 182
California Culinary Academy, 151
California roll sushi, Hallie Donnelly's, 99
Calories, daily consumption of, 76

Campbell Soup Company, 14, 20, 80–83, 195
  and aquaculture, 175
  companies owned by, 80
  day care for workers, 136
  qualities of chicken soups, 198
Campton Place, 21, 28, 108
Candy bars
  consumption of in Salt Lake City, 198
  origin of, 50
Canned goods
  drop in sales of, 59
  storing, 208
Canyon Ranch, 130
Caplan, Frieda, 23
Caraluzzi, Mark, 21
Carambola, 170
Carnation, 195
Carpenter's Drive-In, 26
Carper, Hal, 190
Carrots, daily consumption of, 76
Carver, George Washington, 154
Catered food, 129
Catfish farms, 175
Cattle auctions, by video, 215
Caviar, 178, 198
Caviarteria, 198
CBS's Venture One, 211–212
Celestial Seasonings, 218
Center for Disease Control, 160
Center for Food Safety and Applied Nutrition, 40
Ceriman, 170
Chalif's Hot 'n' Sweet Mustard, 229
Chalmers, Irena: chocolate truffles, 50
Chamberlain, Narcisse, 23
Changing Times, 216
CheckRobot Inc., 62
Cheese
  daily consumption of, 76
  nuclear-explosion tests named for, 148
  see also specific kinds
Cheesecakes by J. R., 227
Chef Paul Prudhomme's Louisiana Kitchen, 200
Chemical Bank's video menus, 214
Chenel, Laura, 16, 225
Cherimoya, 170
Cheryl's Cookies, 224
Chèvre, California, 225
Chez Panisse, 23, 29
Chicago Tribune, 19, 22
Chi-Chi's, 85
Chicken
  and antibiotics, 160
  bleaching of dark meat, 198
  "low-fat", 161
  twenty-four carat gold-plated, Frank Perdue's, 160
Chicken McNugget, 230–231
Chicken soup
  five qualities from Campbell's, 198
  with rice, 197
Child, Julia, 17
  fun food passion of, 32
  on health faddists, 39
  and *Mastering the Art of French Cooking,* 200
  as teacher, 152
  on videocassette, 213
Chili
  Huntley Dent's Texas, 46
  origins of, 44–46

China Rose, 89
Chinese fast food, 89
Chocolate
  annual sales of, 132
  and caffeine, 50
  expensive, 27
  history of, 48–50
  and sex, 50
  truffles, Irena Chalmers', 50
Chocolate chip cookie business, 222–224
Chocolate "fettuccine" alla panna, Martin Johner and Gary Goldberg's, 151
Cholesterol and fat, 24
Christensen, Ivar, 185, 186
Chu, Grace, 200
Chuckwagon cuisine, 44
Church's Fried Chicken, 88
CIA, *see* Culinary Institute of America
City Bites, 21
Citymeals on Wheels, 172
Claiborne, Craig, 18, 178, 213
Clam pie, 148
Classic Indian Cooking, 203
Classic Italian Cookbook, 200
Classic Techniques of Italian Cooking, 19
Clearbrook Farms, 229
Clio awards, 100–101
CM&M Group, 185
Coca-Cola
  and aquaculture, 175
  for breakfast, 29
  design of, 95
Cod liver oil, 41
Coffeemakers, 142
Cohen, Dan, 229
Colbert, Claudette, 132
College food service, 195
Collins Food, 88
Commissary, The, 21
  take-out food from, 147
Complete Scarsdale Medical Diet, 214
CompuServe, 213
Conglomerates, 78
Consumer Reports, 208
Continental Can, 59
Control Data, 164
Convenience food, challenge of, 96–98
Convenience stores, 65
Cookbooks
  authors of, 200
  bestseller list, 207
  color pictures essential to, 203
  covers of, 200–201
  first American, 201
  future of, 201
  mini, 204
  number in American households, 203
  number published in 1985, 200
  proposed title, 201
  sales of, 203
  store devoted to, 202–203
  see also specific titles
Cooke, Phillip S., 18
Cooking schools, 149–153
  domestic, listed, 153, 232
Cooking of South-West France, 200
Cook's magazine, 17
Cooney, Betty, 136
Cornish pasties in Michigan, 24
Corn muffins, Bridge Creek's peerless, 28
Cosby Show, 134, 135
Costello, Jack, 190
Cottage industries, 217–229

Couscous and Other Good Food, 200
Cowboy food, 44–46
Crab, blue, 177
Cracker Jack, 31
Crate and Barrel, 23
Craving Indicator Cards, 76
Creative Gourmets, 146, 184
Croissants, 21, 28
Croissant sandwich, creator of, 21
Crotta, Daniel and Monika, 91
Cruciferous vegetables, 40
Cub Foods, 59
Cucumbers, daily consumption of, 76
Cuisinart, sales of, 142
Cuisines of Mexico, 200
Culinary Institute of America, 16, 150–151
Cunningham, Marion, 22, 29
Czarnecki, Jack, 22, 123
    hominy grits with mushrooms, 123

D'Agostino's, 215
Dairy farming, high-tech in, 158
Dairy Queen TV ads, 87
Dale-Avant, Barbara, 148
Dallas Times-Herald, 106
Dalton Industries, 223
Dart & Kraft, 43
DataTrek, 214
David's Cookies, Inc., 222, 223, 224
Davidson, G. Graham, Jr., 164
Dean, Joel B., 19
Dean & Deluca, 19
Del Monte, 59
DeLuca, Giorgio, 19
Dengler, Ian, 140–141
Denny's TV ads, 87
Dent, Huntley: Texas chili, 46
Dictionary of American Regional
    English, 205
Dienhart, Ligita, 208
Diet
    cookbooks devoted to, 203
    current failings in, 39
    and health, 39–43
    prayer for moderation in, 43
    variety in, 43
    video programs on, 214
Diet chocolate drinks, 52
Diet dinners, sales of, 62
Dill pickles, 226
Dinerese, 216
Diners, modern, 114
Dining Room, The, 107
Dionot, Francois, 18
D'Lites, 84, 85
Dogfish, 176
Domino's Pizza, 90, 215
Donnelly, Hadley: California roll sushi, 99
Donvier Ice Cream Maker, 16, 142, 143
Doolin, Elmer, 35
DoveBar, 10, 21, 218
Dream and the Underworld, The, 208
Dreams and food, 208
Driscoll, Sean, 22, 129
Du-All 8-in-One Food Preparation Appli-
    ance, 128
Dudrick, Dr. Stanley J., 196–197
Duncan Hines Texas-style cake, 148

Eating In, 133–147
Eating out, 105–131

Ecomar Inc., 176
Ed Debevic's, 114
Eel, 179
Egg McMuffin, debut of, 28
Eggroll Express, 89
Eggs
    daily consumption of, 76
    record for peeling hard-cooked, 148
    slices of, 198
Elinoff, Neal, 223
Elmont, Steve, 146, 184
El Paso Chile Company, 96
Embryo transplanting, 158
Engstrom, Daphne and Mats, 178
Entertaining at home, 139
Entertaining with Insects, 132
entrée magazine, 142
Environmental Research Laboratory, 171
Epstein, Jason, 201
Executive dining rooms, 184–186
Exotic fruits and vegetables, 168–170
Expression Unltd., 74, 96

Fairmont hotel, 107
Falcaro, Millie, 95
Family Circle, 12, 17
Family eating habits, 135–136
Famous Amos cookies, 222
Famous Cookie Company, 223
Faneuil Hall Marketplace, 72, 73
Farmers' markets, 67
    computer-operated, 71
Farming
    changes in, 156–157
    chemical fertilizers and pesticides, 157
    dairy, 158
    exotic fruits and vegetables, 168–169
    future in polyculture, 157
    hydroponics, 164–166
Fast and Flavorful, 19
Fast-food restaurants
    as big business, 84, 85
    Chinese, 89
    frequency of robberies in, 87
    pizzerias, 90–91
    takeover prospects for, 88
    TV advertising of, 87
Fat, 24
    and calories, 43
    in chicken and beef, 161
    in diet at North Pole, 43
    reducing intake of, 39–40
Feasts of Food and Wine, 19
Feed, flavored, 104
Fernhame Ned Oceana, 158
Feltman, Arlene, 152
Festivals, food, 181
Field, Carol, 203
Field guide to restaurants, 120–121
Figs, sugar content of, 40
Fine Art of Italian Cooking, 19, 200
Fine Bouche restaurant, 147
Finger food preferences, 154
Firehouse cooking, 122–123
First American Video, 215
Fish
    farming, 175–176
    new facts about, 41
    roe, 178
    trash, 179–180
Fisher, M.F.K., 200
Flakey Jake's, 84

Flavorings, food, 208
Fledermaus, 146
Florida Tomato Exchange, 208
Flowers as flavoring, 182
Foley, Michael, 16, 146
Food and Drug Administration, 20, 40,
    160, 178
Food festivals, 181
Food and Foodways, 203
Food for Friends, 20
Food markets, 53–75
Food poisoning and antibiotics, 160
Food processor, 18, 142
Food service, 183–197
Food on video, 209–215
Foods of Italy, 19
Forbes Magazine dining room, 185, 186
Forgione, Larry, 22, 32, 200
Fort Worth Star-Telegram, 213
Four Seasons, 19, 21, 22, 32, 107, 131,
    171, 216
    marinated bay scallops, 131
Franey, Pierre, 23, 200
Frappe, 216
French Market Soup, 228
Frequent buyers, 62
Fresh mozzarella, 228
Frezier, André, 132
Frito-Lay, 35–36
Fritos, 35
Frog, 21
From the Farmers' Market, 67
Frugal Gourmet, 200
Fruit Smack, 198
Fulton Street Fish Market, 72–73
Fun food, *see* Junk food

Gallup Polls
    finger food preferences, 154
    salad bar preferences, 24
    teenage "fantasy meal," 148
    unloved foods, top ten, 172
Garbage Project, 52
Garbarino, Mario, 178
Garren, Drs. Lloyd and Mary, 43
Gastric Bubble, 43
Gastronome, 18
G.D. Ritzy's, 84
Gene & Georgette's restaurant, 227
General Electric, 164, 165
General Foods, 100, 195
General Mills, 102, 164, 195
Gene-splicing, 162
Genetic engineering, 162
Genovesi, Nicole, 224
Gerard's Haute Cuisine, 98
Glamour, 32
Glaser, Milton, 55
Glie Farms, 166
Glorious American Food, 19
Glorious Food Inc., 22, 129
Goat cheese, California, 225
Goldberg, Gary: chocolate "fettuccine" alla
    panna, 151
Goldberg, Zeus, 146
Golden Door, 130
Golden Fresh Puffs, 224
Goldman, Sylvan N., 60
Goldwater, Senator Barry, 34
Good Cook, The, 21
Gourmet foods, sales of, 65
Graham, Sylvester, 172

Grand Union, 54, 55
Granité, 216
Granola bars, 27
Great Eastern Mussel Farms, 176
Greene, Bert, 23
Greene, Doug, 64
Greene, Gael, 20, 172
Greene on Greens, 23
Grey Poupon Mustard Co., 76
Grilled miniature vegetables, Christopher
    Idone's, 93
Growing Up on the Chocolate Diet, 172
Grunion, 182
Gumbo, 208
Gurney's Inn, 130

Haddix, Carol, 22
Halter, Pieter, 196
Ham biscuits, Edna Lewis', 145
Hands, eating with, 24
Hands Across America, 147
Harborplace, 72
Hardee's TV ads, 87
Hazan, Marcella, 152, 200
Health Food stores, sales in, 64–65
Hearin, Malee, 228
Heflin, Senator Howell, 34
Height and weight tables, 42
Heinz USA, 78
Herbs, hydroponic, 166
Hershey, Milton, 50
Hewitt, Jean, 17
Hickory Industries, 127
Hillman, James, 208
Hilton International, 106, 107
Hodges, Carl, 171
Hoffman-LaRoche, 136
Holly Farms "low-fat" chicken, 161
Holman, William Henry, 57
Hominy grits with mushrooms, Jack
    Czarnecki's, 123
Honchar, George, 52
Hooley, Jack, 59
Horn & Hardart's baked macaroni and
    cheese, 35
Hospital food, 196
    luxury, 154
    Wendy's, 87
Hot chocolate, 48–50
Hot dogs
    in Central Park, 32
    rolls to go with, 208
Hotel dining rooms, 106–107
Hudspeth, John, 29
Hughes, E. Thomas and Meredith, 182
Hussung, M.V. "Buck", 85
Hydroponics, 164–166

IBM, 166
Ice cream
    annual sales of, 182
    consumption of, 182
    popularity by age, 76
Ice cream makers, 142
Idone, Christopher, 19, 200
    grilled miniature vegetables, 93
Il Gelataio, 142
In and Out
    foods, 47–48
    small appliances, 142
Insect-eating, 132

Institute of Ecotechnics, 171
International Association of Cooking
    Professionals, 18, 152
International King's Table, 88
Irradiated food, 99
Italian Baker, The, 203
Itza Pizza, 91
Ivey, Wilbur, 148

Jack in the Box, TV ads, 87
Jackie's Cookie Connection, 223
Jackson, Wes, 157
Jacobs, Don, 195
Jakfruit, 170
Jane Brody's Good Food Book, 23
Jane Brody's Nutrition Book, 23
Jarlsberg, decline of, 74
J. Bildner & Sons, 58
Jean-Louis restaurant, 107
Jerrico, 88, 89
Jessica's Biscuit Cookbook Catalog, 18
Jessica's Cookies, 223
Jette, Jim, 190
Jicama, 170
Joe's Restaurant, 22
Johannen, Gerd, 185
Johner, Martin: chocolate "fettuccine"
    alla panna, 151
Joy of Chocolate, 182
Joy of Cooking, 200
Jukes, Dr. Thomas, 160
Junk food as fun food, 30–37
J. Walter Thompson dining room, 185

Kabler, James H., III, 16
Kafka, Barbara, 20, 76, 172, 201
Kainer, Frank, 128
Kamin, Jackie, 223
Kamman, Madeleine, 213
Kaplan, Steven L., 203
Keillor, Garrison, 121
Kennedy, Diana, 152, 200
Kentucky Fried Chicken, 84, 87
Ketchum Food Center, 17
Ketchup
    and consumer demands, 78
    consumption of in New Orleans, 198
Kimball, Christopher, 17
King, Alan, 190
King Kullen, 54
Kirby, Jane, 32
Kitchen Arts & Letters bookstore, 202
Kitchen Bazaar, 143
Kitchen Help, 214
Kiwi, 168, 170
Kool-Aid, 52, 198
Korean grocers, 64
Koryn, Ted, 21
Kovi, Paul, 19
Kraemer, Carolyn and Jim, 136
Kraft, 18, 22, 218
Krazit, Celia, 196
Kreplach joke, 182
Kroc, Ray, 84, 86
Krueger, Cheryl, 224
Krups coffeemaker, 142

L'Académie de Cuisine, 18, 152
La Camembert restaurant, 147
La Chaine des Rotisseurs, 18

La Champagne Restaurant, 18
La Choy, 193
Lakeville Lettuce, 164
Lalor, William, 114
Lambert, Paula, 227
Lambs, milk-fed, 19
Landers, Ann: meat loaf, 138
Land Institute, 157
Lane, William, 176
Lang, George, 16, 68
    on asparagus, 69–70
    and Citymeals on Wheels, 172
    classic asparagus, 70
    recipe for an American bistro, 113
La Récolte, 208
Larry's Cookies, 223
La Tour, 107
La Varenne Ecole de Cuisine, 16
Laventhol & Horwath, 107
Lawrence Livermore Laboratory, 148
Lay, Herman W., 35
Lay's Potato chips, 35
Lean Cuisine, 10
Legumes and health, 42
Le Menu frozen dinners, 83
Lender's Bagels, 104
Le Peep restaurants, 28
L'Espalier restaurant, 146
Les Trois Petits Cochons, 20
Lettuce
    daily consumption of, 76
    hydroponically grown, 164
Lever Brothers' Sun Light detergent, 24
Lewis, Edna: ham biscuits, 145
Liederman, David, 224
Lister, John, 95
ListerButler, 95
Lite foods, 27
Lobster
    club sandwich, Arcadia's, 206
    daily consumption of, 76
London Chop House, 146
Longan, 170
Long John Silver's Seafood Shoppes,
    87, 89
Longo, Emilio, 123, 124
Los Angeles Times, 20, 22
Losman, Barbara, 190
"Low-cal" in advertising, 216
Lukins, Sheila, 19, 200, 219–221

Macaroni and cheese, Horn and Hard-
    art's, 35
Major League stadium food specialties, 31
Macrobiotic foods, sales of, 65
Madden, Rodney, 186
Mail-order foods, 75
Mako shark, 176
Malnutrition, 196–197
Mamey, 170
Mandel, Abby, 19
Mansura, Louisiana, 216
Maple syrup, 24
Margittai, Tom, 21, 32
Mariani, John, 32
Market of the Commissary, 147
Maroti, Steve, 127
Marriott Corp.
    airline food caterer, 190
    executive food service, 186
    hospital food, 196
Marshall, Lydie, 152

Marshmallows, consumption of in Salt Lake
    City, 198
Mastering the Art of French Cooking, 200
Matsunaga, Senator Spark M., 34
Matthias, Jon, 158
Mattoon, Illinois, 104
Maurice restaurant, 107
Maxim toaster, 142
McCarty, Michael, 154
McCarty-Holman Co., 57
McDonald's
    debut of Egg McMuffin, 28
    designer of flagship restaurant, 21
    first kitchen, 84
    growth potential of, 88
    size of, 86
    as takeover target, 88–89
    TV ads, 87, 100
McGee, Harold, 76
McGovern, R. Gordon, 14, 20, 82, 83
McMahon, Paul, 172
Meals on Wheels, 172
Meat
    antibiotics in, 160
    in diet, 39–40
    in executive dining rooms, 185
    low-fat, 161
Meat loaf, Ann Landers', 138
Melman, Richard, 114
Melvin Simon & Associates, 222
Menus
    on computers, 215
    Nouvelle Hell, 117
    trend food luncheon, 118
Mesquite mystique, 128
Metz, Ferdinand E., 16
Metzger, Juan, 22
Miami Valley Hospital, 87
Microwave ovens
    breakfast prepared in, 28
    sales of, 142
Miles, Michael A., 22
Miller, Jack, 59
Miller, Sanford A., 20, 40
*Mimi Sheraton's Favorite New York Restau-
    rants,* 22
Minyard supermarkets, 60
Miss Cochon de Lait, 216
MissKeet, 128
Monaghan, Tom, 90
Monkeys as fruit pickers, 216
Monkfish, 179
Monroe, Marilyn, 24
Morrison, Pat, 128
Mouli mincer, 143
Moulu, Rona, 185, 186
Mount, Charles Morris, 21
Mount Sinai Hospital, 196
Mozzarella Company, The, 228
Mr. B's restaurant, 146
Mrs. Fields, Inc., 223
Mrs. Winner's Chicken & Biscuits, 85
Mulcrone, Bill, 193
Mussel farming, 175–176
Mussels, 179
Mustard
    Chalif's, 229
    consumption of in past, 76
    specialty, 74

Nabisco package design, 95
Nankin Express, 89

Nathan, Joan, 19
National Academy of Sciences, 21
National Association of College and
    University Food Services, 195
Natural foods, sales of, 64–65
Natural Foods Merchandiser, 64–65
Nature's, 65
Neal's Cookies, 223
Nestlé, Henri, 50
New American Diner, 114
New Doubleday Cookbook, 18
New England boiled dinner, 182
New England Journal of Medicine, 41
Newsletters, 206, 207
New York, 20
    executive dining room, 186
New York Pizza Department, 91
New York Restaurant School, 151
New York Times, 17, 18, 19, 23, 41, 136,
    172, 178
New York Times Heritage Cook Book, 17
Nikkal Industries, 16
Nouvelle Hell menu, 117
Nutri-Byte, 214
Nutrition, 39–40
    of children of working mothers, 42
Nutritionist III, 214

Oak Feed Store, 65
Obesity and dieting, 43
O'Connor, Michael, 59
Ogden, Bradley, 21, 200
O'Grady's potato chips, 36
Okun, Janice: Buffalo chicken wings, 128
Olive oil, virtues of, 52
Olney, Judith, 182
Olney, Richard, 20
O'Malley, Ken and Pat, 135
Omega 3s, 41
Omni/Dunfey, 107
On Food and Cooking, 76
Oranges in segments vs. juice, 208
Ore-Aqua, 176
Original Boston Computer Diet, 214
Oskar, sales of, 142, 143
Out of the Woods, 146
Oysters, 132
    icing of, 177

Package designs
    for fine foods, 218
    then and now, 94–98
Panguad, Gerard, 16
Parkay Margarine, 95
Parker Meridien, 107
Park Hyatt, 107
Parkinson, R. B., 128
Parkland Hospital, 196
Peach fuzz, 148
Peanut trivia, 154
Peanut butter, 154
Peelings, 182
Pell, Senator Claiborne, 34
Pennsylvania Dutch and saffron, 198
Pépin, Jacques, 22, 152, 212, 213
Pepper
    consumption of, 154
    decline of availability of, 76
Pepperidge Farms, 164
Pepper mill in restaurants, 76
Pepsi TV spot, 101

PepsiCo fast-food chains, 89
Perdue, Franklin Parsons, 12, 20, 160
  and "low-fat" chickens, 161
    twenty-four carat gold-plated
      chicken, 160
Perkins, Edwin E., 198
Personality inventory test, 92–93
Peter Kump's New York Cooking School, 152
Philadelphia Inquirer, 21
Philip Morris companies, 78
Photographic food styling, 132
Picnics, 126
Piggly Wiggly, 54
Pillow Puff, 164
Pillsbury, 18
  companies owned by, 78
Pimiento, consumption of, 76
Pincus, Lanie and Max, 146
Pinsel, E. Melvin, 208
Pizza
  in fast-food restaurants, 90–91
  as fun food, 31
  popcorn, 32
Pizza Hut, 84
  comic commercial of, 91
  owned by PepsiCo, 89
  TV ads, 87
Poi, 148
Popcorn
  consumption of, in Dallas, 198
  recipe book, 32
  as snack, 31
  why it pops, 76
Poses, Steve, 21
Potato, healthful effects of, 40
Potato chips
  annual consumption of, 52
  Frito-Lay's, 35–36
  as fun food, 31
  thickness of, 35–36
Potato Jokes, 172
Potato Museum, 182
Potpourri Press, 204
Poverty in America, 147
Power breakfasts, 28
Power Lunching, 208
Pradie, Jean-Pierre, 20
Prairie Home Companion, 121
Prairie oysters, 216
Predictions, 230–231
Preserves, Clearbrook Farms, 229
Pretzels, 32
Prevention, 17
Prince Spaghetti Sauce, 101
Printed Word, 199–207
Printer's Row restaurant, 16, 146
Proops, William, 185
Prudhomme, Paul, 143, 200, 201
Pruess, Joanne, 152
Public Relations associations, 103
Puck, Wolfgang, 200
Pudding Pockets, contents of, 35
Pukel, Sandy, 65
Pummelo, 170
Pyles, Stephan W., 17

Quaker Oats, 18
Quick Wok, 89
Quilted Giraffe, 32, 146
  black beans and truffles, 215
Quincy Market, 72, 73
Quinoa, 162–163

Railroad dining cars, 186–187
  luxury, 189
Rainbow Specialties, 87
Rainbow trout, 175
Raisins as snack, 31
Ralston Purina, 175
Rathje, William, 52
Rattlesnake Club, 17
Rax, 84
Ray, 179
Ready When You Are, 20
Real American Food, 23
Recipe for an American bistro, George
  Lang's, 113
Recipes
  baked macaroni and cheese, Horn &
    Hardart's, 35
  black beans and truffles, the Quilted
    Giraffe's, 215
  Buffalo chicken wings, Janice
    Okun's, 128
  California roll sushi, Hallie Donnelly's, 99
  chicken soup with rice, 197
  chocolate "fettuccine" alla panna, Martin
    Johner and Gary Goldberg's, 151
  chocolate truffles, Irena Chalmers', 50
  classic asparagus, George Lang's, 70
  grilled miniature vegetables, Christopher
    Idone's, 93
  ham biscuits, Edna Lewis', 145
  hominy grits with mushrooms, Jack
    Czarnecki's, 123
  lobster club sandwich, Arcadia's, 206
  marinated bay scallops, the Four Sea-
    sons', 131
  peerless corn muffins, Bridge Creek's, 28
  sour cream waffles, Café Beaujolais', 189
  Texas chili, Huntley Dent's, 46
  twenty-four carat gold-plated chicken,
    Frank Perdue's, 160
Recipes on videotext, 213
Recipe Master, 214
Recipe Writer, 214
Regency hotel, 28
Regional preferences in food, 104
  in sweets, 216
  in three cities, 198
Reichl, Ruth, 20
Renggli, Seppi, 22, 131
Restaurant Business, 198
Restaurant Marketing Associates, 185
Restaurants
  fastest gaining food and beverages
    in, 118
  fast-food, 84–91
  field guide to, 120–121
  "gourmet", 132
  grazing, 110–111
  insurance for, 154
  knowledge of, as status symbol, 24
  in Manhattan, 114
  menus on computers, 215
  modern diners, 114
  music in, 172
  new, 109
  specialty, preferences, 216
  top, in sales, 118
  upscale, take out, 146–147
  see also specific names
Restaurants & Institutions, 65
Retorting, 96
Revsin, Leslie, 17
Rice, William, 19

Richman, Phyllis, 20
Risley, Marie, 152
Ritual meal, 137–138
Ritz Carlton, Chicago, 107
RJR Nabisco companies, 78
Roadfood and Goodfood, 23
Rodale, Robert, 17
  growing of amaranth, 163
Rodale Press, 17
Roe, 178
Rolls, Barbara, 39, 43
Rombauer, Irma, 200
Root beer float, 31
Rosen, Janet, 227
Rosenfeld, Isadore, 18
Rosenzweig, Anne, 16
Rosso, Julee, 21, 200, 219–221
Rouse Company, 72–73
Routh Street Café, 17
Rowenta toaster, 142
Rozanki, Larry, 223
Rubaud, Gerard, 98
Rufe, Fred, 106, 107
Ruffles potato chips, 35
Running Program, 214
Ryan, Timothy, 224

S & W Veri-Green, 59
Saccharin, 40
Sacks, Steve, 222
Saffron consumption by Pennsylvania
  Dutch, 198
SAGA, 195
Sahni, Julie, 203
Salad bar, preferred items, 24
Salmon
  farming, 176
  genetic tinkering with, 180
Salt
  daily production of, 76
  link to hypertension, 39–40
Sanders Associates, 175
San Francisco Chronicle, 16
Sara Lee's frozen bagels, 104
Sawyer, Don, 222
Sax, Richard, 67
Scarborough Systems, 214
Schechter, Alvin, 95
Scheets, Hannah, 176
Schmidt, Jimmy, 17
Schneider, Elizabeth, 20, 170, 203
School cafeteria food, 193
Schowalter, Craig, 89
Schremp, Gerry, 21
Sea claws, 180
Seafood
  farms, 175–176
  and health, 41
  strange, 154
Sea robin, 179
Seaweed, 178
Seeds, hybrid, 162, 163
Seely, Martin, 216
Segal, Gordon, 23
Semifreddi, 216
Seventh Day Adventist's diet, 136
Sex and chocolate, 50
Shake 'n Bake, 101
Shark, 176–177
Shearson Lehman Brothers dining
  room, 185
Shefter, Alan, 143

Sheley, Doug, 85
Sheraton, Mimi, 22, 172
Shoney's, 88
Shooting Stars, 21
Shoplifters, 61
Shopping carts
  facts about, 60–61
  invention of, 60
Showbiz Pizza Place, 84
Shrimp and cholesterol, 24
Silver Palate, 19, 21, 200, 219–221
Simac's Il Gelataio, 142
Simmonds, Amelia, 201
Simpson, Senator Alan K., 34
Sinturel, Alain, 20
Sister's Chicken & Biscuits, 84
Sixteenth Street Bar & Grill, 21
Sizzler TV ads, 87
Skate, 179
Small appliances
  collecting of, 144–145
  sales of, 142–143
Smelts, 179
Smith, Jeff, 200
Sobel, Ilene, 147
Soft-shell crabs, 177
Son-of-a-bitch stew, 45
Sonoma Mission Inn, 130
Sontheimer, Carl G., 18
Sorbet, 216
Soup, annual sales of, 81
Souers, Terry, 190
Sour cream waffles, Cafe Beaujolais', 189
Sourdough Puff Co., 224
South Street Seaport, 72
Spa Cuisine, 216
Spa food, 130–131
Specialty foods
  as big business, 74
  by mail, 75
  mustards, 74
Square Meals, 23
Squid, 179–180
Squire Room, 107
Stadium food specialties, Major League, 31
Star Clipper, 189
Starobin, Matthew, 214
StarText, 213
Steak & Ale, 109
Stefanos, Michael Leo, 21
Steiner, Suette, 223
Stern, Jane and Michael, 23
Stewart, Martha, 22, 32, 200, 201
Stockli, Albert, 178
Stokely's, 59
Stop & Shop supermarkets, 62
Strawberries, Chilean, 132
Strymish, David, 18
Stuart, Julien, 185
Sturgeon, 178
Suckling pig capital, 216
Sugar, harmful effects of, 40
Sunbeam's Oskar, 142
Sun-dried tomatoes, 224
Supermarkets
  changes in, 54–59
  come-ons in, 62
  as place to be seen, 70–71
  shoplifting in, 61
  teen-age shoppers in, 62
  video cassettes in, 62
  see also specific names
Surimi, 180

Sushi
   California roll, Hallie Donnelly's, 99
   by computer, 215
   a negative view of, 116
Sushi-Tron restaurant, 215
Symposium on American Cuisine, 18

Taco Bell, 84, 85, 87, 89
Tait, Elaine, 21
Take out food, upscale, 146–147
Tante Marie's, 152
Teenage "fantasy meal," 148
TeleText, 211
Texas red, 44–46
Thanksgiving
   in food research, 140–141
   as ritual meal, 137
Thomas, Dian, 18
Thomas, Elizabeth and Nick, 229
Tiegreen, Mary, 95
Tilapia, 175
Tilefish, 180
Time Inc., 22, 212
Toaster oven, microwave, 142
Toasters, 142
Tomatoes
   hard, 208
   sun-dried, 224
   vitamin C in, 208
Tomsun Foods International, 22
TOPCO, 57
Top cooking videocassettes, 213
Top restaurants in sales, 118
Total Parenteral Nutrition, 197
Tower, Jeremiah, 23, 200
Trash fish, 179–180
Trillin, Calvin, 168
Tripp, Marian, 18
Truck stops, 118–119
Truex, Leigh, 226
Truffles, chocolate, Irena Chalmers', 50
Tuna, canned, daily consumption of, 76
Tuttle, Bill, 19
Twenty-four-carat gold-plated chicken,
   Frank Perdue's, 160
Twinkies, taster of, 32

Uncle Ben's Rice, 18
Uncommon Fruits and Vegetables, 20,
   170, 203
Union Carbide, 175
Union Square farmers' market, 66
United Nations dining rooms, 185
Universal Marine and Shark Products, 176
Unloved foods, top ten, 172
USA Café, 21
U. S. Government sources on food, 232

Vance Research Service, 203
Vector Enterprises, 213
Venture One, 211–212
Veri-Green process, 59
Video information systems, 211–215
Videotapes, cooking, 212–213
   cost of producing, 212
   top players, 213
Videotext, 211
Vienna Park restaurant, 146
Vietmeyer, Noel, 21, 168
Vining, Wallace, 189

Vivalp microwave toaster oven, 142

Waffles, sour cream, Café Beaujolais', 189
Waitperson
   interview with, 112–113
   new name for, 172
Waldman, Buddy, 28
Waldron, Gary, 165, 166
Waldron, Maggie, 17
Walking and taking off fat, 43
Wall Street Journal, 61, 88, 148, 208
Wang Laboratories' day care, 136
Warner, Senator John, 34
Washington Post, 20, 224
   executive dining room, 185
Watergate Hotel, 107
Waters, Alice, 23, 200, 201
Waxman, Nach, 202–203
Wayman, Doyle, 107
Weight, ideal, 42
Weinstein, Michael, 114
Welmer, Jan, 17
Wendy's, 85
   growth potential of, 88
   hospital lease, 87
   as takeover target, 89
   TV ads, 87
Weyerhauser, 164, 178
Whatley, Booker T., 157
White Castle, 84
Whittaker Corp., 164
Wickersham, Duane, 198
Wick's Sugar Cream Pie, 198
Wilkinson, Steve, 147
Willan, Anne, 16
Williams, Ray and Rozan, 128
Williams, Timothy, 158
Wine, Barry, 32
Wing, Rena, 40
Winners Corp., 85
Wintermyer, Art, 185
Wise, Jonathan Kurland and Susan
   Kierr, 43
Wolfert, Paula, 17, 32, 200
Woman's Day, 12
Wong, Naomi, 136
Woods restaurant take out food, 146
Working mothers and children's nutri-
   tion, 42
World Bank Headquarters dining
   room, 185

Yan, Stephen, 213
Yannuzzi, Elaine, 74
Yaseen, Roger, 18
Yogurt, sales, of, 172
Yum Yum hot dogs, 32
Yuppie Chow, 87

Zagat Survey, 23
Zagat, Tim, 23
Zona Rosa, 112

Text Credits

p.26—"What America Eats" originally entitled "Manduco Ergo Sum" in *The Economist*, January 5, 1985. By permission of The New York Times Syndication Sales Corporation.

p.31—"Major League Stadium Food Specialties," excerpted from the book *Junk Food* by Charles J. Rubin, David Rollert, John Farago, Rick Stark, Jonathan Etra. Copyright © 1980 by Charles J. Rubin, David Rollert, John Farago and Jonathan Etra. Reprinted by permission of Dell Publishing Co., Inc.

p.32—Quotation taken from "The Rapunzel Syndrome," by F. Gonzales-Crussi in the November–December 1985 issue of *The Sciences* published by The New York Academy of Sciences.

p.34—"Fun Food Favorites of Some Solons," from *Junk Food*, Rubin, Rollert, Farago, etc. *Op. Cit.*

p.41—"New Facts About Fish," by Donna Florio appeared in *Commentary*, Vol. 7, No. 7, October/November 1985. Permission granted by Donna Florio.

p.44—"Grease and Gladness," © 1985 by John Thorne. Reprinted by permission of the author, c/o Erica Spellman, William Morris Agency, Inc., New York.

p.46—"Huntley Dent's Texas Chili" is from *The Feast of Santa Fe*, Copyright © 1985 by Huntley Dent. Reprinted by permission of Simon & Schuster, Inc.

p.50—Helen Gurley Brown on chocolate by permission of Helen Gurley Brown.

"Irena Chalmers' Chocolate Truffles," by Irena Chalmers is from *Gifts from the Kitchen*, Potpourri Press, 1979.

p.52—"Food Flies," Copyright 1985 *USA TODAY*. Reprinted with permission.

p.59—"Cashing In On the Wow Factor," excerpted from "Bigger, Shrewder and Cheaper Cub Leads Food Stores into the Future," by Steve Weiner and Betsy Morris, *The Wall Street Journal*, August 26, 1985. Reprinted by permission of *The Wall Street Journal*, © Dow Jones & Company, Inc. 1985. All Rights Reserved.

"Why the Super Warehouse Store?" *The Wall Street Journal, Ibidem.*

p.62—"Cassettes to Keep Kids Safe," *Progressive Grocer* magazine, a Division of Maclean Hunter Media Inc., November 1985.

"Supermarket Expeditions" from Ron Alexander's Metropolitan Diary, *The New York Times*, December 4, 1985. Copyright © 1985 by The New York Times Company. Reprinted by permission.

p.76—"In One Day," from *In One Day* by Tom Parker. Copyright © 1974 by Tom Parker. Reprinted by permission of Houghton Mifflin Company.

p.84—Excerpt from "Fast Food's Changing Landscape," by H. R. Kleinfield, *The New York Times*, April 14, 1985. Copyright © 1985 by The New York Times Company. Reprinted by permission.

p.85—"On The Run Exponentially," Quotations are from "An Affluent Long Island Village Resists Intrusion of Burgers and Fries," Special to *The New York Times* by Clifford D. May, February 26, 1986. Copyright © 1986 by The New York Times Company. Reprinted by permission.

"No Cha-Cha at Chi Chi's." "Buck" Hussung quotation reprinted from the March 22, 1985 issue of *BusinessWeek* by special permission, © 1985 by McGraw-Hill, Inc. All Rights Reserved.

p.86—"McFacts," from "McDonald's Planning 500 New Outlets in '86." Reprinted with permission of *ADWEEK*, February 3, 1986.

p.87—"How Now Dow Chow?" Reprinted with permission of *ADWEEK*.

p.88—"I Can't Believe I Ate the Whole Thing," excerpted from "Heard on the Street: Fast-Food Stocks Could be on Shopping List for Their Earnings Growth," by Dean Rotbart, *The Wall Street Journal*, September 25, 1985. Reprinted by permission of *The Wall Street Journal*, © Dow Jones & Company, Inc. 1985. All Rights Reserved.

p.89—"Chinese Fast Food, Sweet & Sour," adapted from "Assembly-Line Chinese Food," *The New York Times*, January 22, 1985. Copyright © 1985 by The New York Times Company. Reprinted by permission.

p.90—"The Untapped Demand," excerpted from "Domino's Delivers," November 13, 1985. With permission from *Restaurants & Institutions*, a Cahners Publication.

p.91—"One with Anchovies, Hold the .38," *Time*, March 10, 1986. Reprinted by permission of *Time*.

p.92—"Mother Hubbard's Multiflavored Personality Inventory Test," originally entitled "A Food Personality Test," © Ariel Swartley, from *The Boston Phoenix*, October 8, 1985.

p.93—"Christopher Idone's Grilled Miniature Vegetables," from *Christopher Idone's Glorious American Food*, by Christopher Idone. Copyright © 1985 by Christopher Idone. Reprinted by permission of Random House, Inc.

p.99—"Hallie Donnelly's California Roll Sushi," from *Sushi and Sashimi and Soup and Tempura* by Hallie Donnelly. Copyright © 1982 by Hallie Donnelly. Published by Irena Chalmers Cookbooks, Inc.

p.100—Leading National Advertisers and Broadcast Advertisers Reports, Inc.

p.114—"A Bowl of Bossy," by Jane Freiman. Copyright © 1986 by News America Syndicate. Reprinted with the permission of *New York* magazine.

p.118—"High On The Hog," by Russell Baker, *The New York Times*, October 23, 1985. Copyright © 1985 by The New York Times Company. Reprinted by permission.

p.121—Peggy Katalinich's quote of Miss Manners appeared in *Newsday*, March 11, 1985.

p.123—"Jack Czarnecki's Hominy Grits with Mushrooms," from *Joe's Book of Mushroom Cookery* by Jack Czarnecki. Copyright © 1986 Jack Czarnecki. Reprinted by permission of Atheneum Publishers, Inc.

p.127—"Hearts Remain Aflame For Our Beloved Bar-B-Q," originally entitled "Barbecuing lights fire in foodservice," by Julie Franz. Reprinted with permission from the September 19, 1985 issue of *Advertising Age*. Copyright 1985 by Crain Communications, Inc.

p.128—"Mesquite Mystique," excerpted from "Mesquite Mystique Has Bred Fanatics, Like R. J. and Rozan," by John Huey, *The Wall Street Journal*, January 20, 1986. Reprinted by permission of *The Wall Street Journal*, © Dow Jones & Company, Inc. 1986. All Rights Reserved.

p.131—"The Four Seasons' Marinated Bay Scallops," from *The Four Seasons Spa Cuisine* by Seppi Renggli, Paul Kovi and Tom Margittai. Copyright © 1986 by Seppi Renggli, Paul Kovi and Tom Margittai. Reprinted by permission of Simon & Schuster, Inc.

p.132—"In Which Case Look In the Door But Turn Your Steps Elsewhere" reprinted from *The Official Gourmet Handbook* © 1984 by Pasquale Bruno, with permission of Contemporary Books, Inc., Chicago.

p.137—"On The Ritual Meal," from *Comforting Food*, Copyright © 1979 by Judith Olney. Reprinted by permission of Atheneum Publishers, Inc.

p.138—"Ann Landers' Meat Loaf," by Ann Landers, from *The Daily News*, February 26, 1986. Copyright News America Syndicate. Reprinted by permission.

p.139—"Who's Coming to Dinner?" from *Food for Friends*, Copyright © 1984 by Barbara Kafka. Reprinted by permission of Harper & Row, Publishers, Inc.

p.140—"Clues in the Cranberries," originally entitled "Food Sleuth," by Ruth Reichl, *New West*, December 3, 1979.

p.145—"Edna Lewis' Ham Biscuits," from *The Taste of Country Cooking* by Edna Lewis. Copyright © 1976 by Edna Lewis. Reprinted by permission of Alfred A. Knopf, Inc.

p.148—"What's My Line? Egg Peeler," from "Boiled-Egg Peelers Aim for Perfection, and That's no Yolk" by Valita Sellers, *The Wall Street Journal*, July 9, 1985. Reprinted by permission of *The Wall Street Journal*, © Dow Jones & Company, Inc. 1985. All Rights Reserved.

p.151—"Martin Johner and Gary Goldberg's Chocolate 'Fettuccine' Alla Panna," from *Successful Parties Simple and Elegant* by Martin Johner and Gary Goldberg, a Great American Cooking Schools Book. Copyright © 1983 by Martin Johner and Gary Goldberg. Printed and published by Irena Chalmers Cookbooks, Inc.

p.172—*Potato Jokes*, Copyright © 1984 by Paul McMahon. Reprinted by permission of Pocket Books, a division of Simon & Schuster, Inc.

p.181—From *Food Festival* by Alice Geffen and Carole Berglie. Copyright © 1986 by Alice Geffen and Carole Berglie. Reprinted by permission of Pantheon Books, a division of Random House, Inc. Available in paperback @ $9.95 from Pantheon Books.

p.189—"Cafe Beaujolais Sour Cream Waffles with Toasted Pecans and Sauteed Apples," from Cafe Beaujolais by Margaret S. Fox and John Bear. Copyright © 1984. Used with permission of Ten Speed Press, Box 7123, Berkeley, CA 94707.

p.205—"Why You Order Crawfish and I Order Crayfish," by Stanley Dry. Excerpted by permission from *Food & Wine* magazine, March 1986. Copyright © 1986 by The International Review of Food & Wine Associates.

p.206—"The Quilted Giraffe's Black Beans and Truffles," reprinted by permission of Barry Wine.

p.222—"Fresh Cookie Stores Feel Bite as Snack-Food Market Shifts," by Steven P. Galante, February 24, 1986. Reprinted by permission of *The Wall Street Journal*, © Dow Jones & Company, Inc. 1986. All Rights Reserved.

Picture Credits

Illustrations by Juan Suarez-Botas: pp. 28, 40, 42, 46, 59, 76, 92–93, 113, 119, 120–21, 123, 127, 136, 139, 145, 148, 160, 182, 187, 192, 197, 198, 204, 218.

Illustrations by Marc Rosenthal: pp. 24, 52, 62, 63, 100, 104, 132, 138, 141, 146–47, 154, 172, 208, 213, 216, 231.

Illustrations by Nadia Pignatone: pp. 75, 103, 181, 207.

William Morris prints, Courtesy Arthur Sanderson & Sons.

pp. 16–23 Portraits courtesy of food celebrities plus 16 Joe Baum: Dan Wynn 17 Paula Wolfert: William Bayer; Julia Child: James Scherer 18 Jean Anderson: Rudy Muller; Craig Claiborne: Lou Manna Studio; Roger Yaseen: Dan Wynn 19 Marian Burros: Gene Maggio, N.Y. Times Studio; Paul Kovi: © Jill Levine, 1985; Ella Brennan: Frank Lotz Miller Photography, Inc. 20 Elizabeth Schneider: © Kelly/Mooney 21 Charles Morris Mount: Armen Kachaturian; Tom Margittai: © Karsh, Ottawa 22 Juan Metzger: William Lulow Photography; Martha Stewart: George Bennett, 1985 23 Pierre Franey: Bill Aller, N.Y. Times Studio; Tim Zagat: Mary Hilliard; Jane E. Brody: © Thomas Victor 26–27 Los Angeles County Museum of Natural History 27 UPI 28 top: New York Public Library 29 Courtesy Bridge Creek 30 both: H. Armstrong Roberts 31 William Hubbell—Woodfin Camp, Inc. 32 R. Dias—H. Armstrong Roberts 33 Dan Wynn; Cheerios by Matthew Klein 34 *The New Yorker* 35 Courtesy Pillsbury Company 36–37 Matthew Klein 38 Henry Wolf 39 *The New Yorker* 41 American Heritage Publishing Company 43 Susan Gray 44 University of Oklahoma 45 Buffalo Bill Historical Center, Cody, Wyoming 46

American Heritage 47 National Palace Museum, Taiwan 48 Frederick Lewis Agency 48–49 Museum of Modern Art, New York 50 Matthew Klein—Chocolate, Courtesy Krön Chocolatier 51 Courtesy Nahum Waxman 54 all: American Heritage 55 top: Robert Levin, center: Theresa Fasolino 56–57 American Heritage 57 Courtesy McCarty-Holman Company 58 top: Courtesy J. Bildner & Sons, bottom: Ira Wyman 59 top: Courtesy Super Value Stores, Inc. 60–61 J. Anderson—H. Armstrong Roberts 61 left: Courtesy Minyard Food Stores 63 Courtesy National Turkey Federation; sunglasses by Marc Rosenthal 64 Lynne Weinstein 66 Elisabeth Meryman 67 Lynne Weinstein 68 Henry Groskinsky 69 Courtesy Café des Artistes 71 Courtesy Bridgemarket 72–73 all: Courtesy The Rouse Company 74 both: Courtesy Elaine Yanuzzi 79 Courtesy Beatrice Corporation 80–83 all: Courtesy The Campbell Soup Company 84 Lester Sloan—Woodfin Camp, Inc. 85–87 all: John Margolies—ESTO 88 top left: Courtesy McDonald's, right: Courtesy Wendy's 89 top left: Courtesy Burger King, right: Courtesy White Castle 90 Courtesy Domino's Pizza 91 Courtesy New York Pizza Department 94 Fossil Films & Photos 95 top & center left: Lister/Butler, Inc., center right: The Schechter Group, bottom: Falcaro & Tiegreen Graphic Design 96–97 all: Reprinted with Permission of *Food and Drug Packaging*, © 1986, Harcourt, Brace, Javonovich 98 Courtesy Radiation Technology, Inc. 100 Courtesy Clio Awards 101 top left: Courtesy BBDO, top right: Courtesy Ogilvy & Mather, bottom: Courtesy Fallon McElligott 102 Courtesy General Mills 106 Compte de Hamal, Paris 107 Courtesy Omni-Berkshire Place 108 Fred Lyon 109 Bibliothèque Nationale, Paris 110 bottom: Timothy Eagan—Woodfin Camp, Inc. 111 Courtesy Ark Restaurants 112 Lynne Weinstein 114 Lynne Weinstein 115

Frederic Lewis Agency 116 top: Matthew Klein bottom: Courtesy Sapporo USA, Inc. 119 Jeff Lowenthal—Woodfin Camp, Inc. 122 Neal Slavin 124–25 Neal Slavin 126 Louvre, Paris 127 American Heritage 129 Courtesy Glorious Food 130–131 Lilo Raymond 134 top: Phototeque, bottom: Courtesy NBC 137 Matthew Klein from Judith Olney, *Entertaining*, Barrons 140 Janet Fries 142 Courtesy Sunbeam 143 Courtesy Kitchen Bazaar 144 Matthew Klein 150 *Taste Magazine*, Winter 1986 152 Dan Wynn 156–57 M.H. Cronberg, *National Wool Grower* 158 Courtesy Clover Matt West Farms 159 Bill Strode—Woodfin Camp, Inc. 161 Courtesy Perdue 162–63 Rodale Press, Inc. 164–65 Courtesy Lakeville Lettuce 167 Anthony Wolff 168–69 all: David Wasserman 170 New York Public Library 171 Courtesy Space Biospheres Ventures 174 Terrence Moore 175–80 Pacific Kitchens 177 top: Terrence Moore 184 Courtesy CM&M Group, Inc. 186 Roberta Raeburn 186–87 Courtesy Bloomingdale's 188 American Heritage 189 *Daily Press—Times Herald*, Newport News, Virginia 190 Courtesy Marriott Corporation 191 Vincent Lee 193 H. Armstrong Roberts 194–95 Courtesy University of Rochester 196 *The New Yorker* 197 Courtesy Mount Sinai Medical Center, Miami 210 *The New Yorker* 202 Diane Raines Ward 205 New York Public Library 210–11 Bill Rothschild, Vogel-Mulea 212–13 Thom Lepley, Teletext © Time, Inc. 214 Courtesy Chemical Bank Restaurant Services 215 Kathryn K. Russell 219–21 Courtesy The Silver Palate 222–24 Cookies by Matthew Klein 222–23 bottom, both: Nubar Alexanian 224 both: Courtesy Genovesi Food Company 225 Courtesy Laura Chenel 226 Courtesy Bubbies of San Francisco, Inc. 227 Courtesy Cheesecakes by J.R. 228 Courtesy Bon Melange 229 top: Courtesy Clearbrook Farms, bottom: Courtesy Chalif Mustard

We would like to hear from you with suggestions for the next Food Almanac. Please write to Irena Chalmers, Box 988, Denton, NC 27239.